SCLERODERMA

Publication Number 925

AMERICAN LECTURE SERIES ®

A Monograph in

The BANNERSTONE DIVISION *of*
AMERICAN LECTURES IN LIVING CHEMISTRY

Editor

I. NEWTON KUGELMASS, M.D., PH.D., SC.D.
*Consultant to the Department of Health and Hospitals
New York City*

SCLERODERMA

(Progressive Systemic Sclerosis)

By

ALFRED J. BARNETT

M.D., F.R.A.C.P., M.R.C.P.(Lond.)

Specialist Physician

and

Associate Director of Clinical Research Unit

Alfred Hospital

Melbourne, Australia

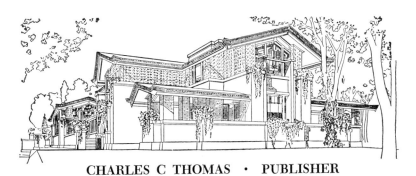

CHARLES C THOMAS · PUBLISHER

Springfield · Illinois · U.S.A.

Published and Distributed Throughout the World by
CHARLES C THOMAS · PUBLISHER
Bannerstone House
301-327 East Lawrence Avenue, Springfield, Illinois, U.S.A.

© 1974, by CHARLES C THOMAS · PUBLISHER
ISBN 0-398-02955-5
Library of Congress Catalog Card Number: 73-12160

*With THOMAS BOOKS careful attention is given to all details of
manufacturing and design. It is the Publisher's desire to present books
that are satisfactory as to their physical qualities and artistic possibilities
and appropriate for their particular use. THOMAS BOOKS will be true
to those laws of quality that assure a good name and good will.*

Printed in the United States of America
K-8

Library of Congress Cataloging in Publication Data

Barnett, Alfred John.
    Scleroderma (progressive systemic sclerosis)

    (American lecture series, publication no. 925.
A monograph in the Bannerstone division of American lectures in living
chemistry)
    1. Scleroderma. I. Title. [DNLM: 1. Scleroderma, Systemic.
WR260 B261s 1974]
RL451.B37   616.5′44   73-12160
ISBN 0-398-02955-5

To my wife Hazel, and sons Mark and Derek,
for their patient forbearance
during the rather long gestation of this book.

FOREWORD

OUR LIVING CHEMISTRY SERIES was conceived by Editor and Publisher to advance the newer knowledge of chemical medicine in the cause of clinical practice. The interdependence of chemistry and medicine is so great that physicians are turning to chemistry, and chemists to medicine in order to understand the underlying basis of life processes in health and disease. Once chemical truths, proofs and convictions become foundations for clinical phenomena, key hybrid investigators will clarify the bewildering panorama of biochemical progress for application in everyday practice, stimulation of experimental research, and extension of postgraduate instruction. Each of our monographs thus unravels the chemical mechanisms and clinical management of many diseases which have remained relatively static in the minds of medical men for three thousand years. Our new Series is charged with the *nisus élan* of chemical wisdom, supreme in choice of international authors, optimal in standards of chemical scholarship, provocative in imagination for experimental research, comprehensive in discussions of scientific medicine, and authoritative in chemical perspective of human disorders.

Dr. Barnett of Melbourne unravels the progressive transformation of hardened skin with increased deposition of collagen into horrifying solidification of body tissues. It is one of the most terrible of all human ills; like Tithonus, the Greek mythological hero, to wither slowly, "beaten down, marred and wasted" until one becomes a mummy, encased in an ever-shrinking, slowly contracting hard skin, is a horrible fate not pictured in any dramatic tragedy of human history. The hardening process appears to be the establishment of more and more cross links between collagen chains with a consequent stiffening of the molecules. Such changes are probably responsible for the degeneration of the elastic tissues, irreversible because the collagen does not turn over. Indeed, there is some relationship between the overall metabolic activity of tissue and the rate of its collagen turnover. The story of scleroderma has been thought to its conclusion when it has taken its most possible turn embodying localized plaque forms, linear forms, diffuse forms, acrosclerosis and CRST syndrome, yet all these forms are capable of self-limitation and spontaneous resolution in the face of nonspecific therapy.

> *To despise the little things of functional disorders*
> *is to fall little by little into organic disease.*

I. NEWTON KUGELMASS
Editor

PREFACE

THIS IS NOT the first monograph on scleroderma. Books on this subject have been written as early as 1895 by Lewen and Heller and as recently as 1967 by Sackner. There have been several large review articles and numerous case reports and studies of particular aspects of this disease.

One may question the purpose of a new monograph at this stage. Scleroderma, although uncommon, is not a rare disease and every physician is likely to encounter such cases and needs a reference more extensive than the sketchy accounts in text-books of medicine. Also scleroderma has interest to clinicians and medical scientists extending beyond the clinical problems of individual patients. It is an outstanding example of a *connective tissue disease* and researches on collagen and connective tissue disorders in scleroderma may also have important bearing on the understanding of other connective tissue diseases such as rheumatoid arthritis, disseminated lupus erythematosus and dermatomyositis. It is frequently associated with auto-immune disturbance and studies on these features may add to our understanding of the importance of auto-immunity in disease generally. For these various reasons there is a place for a modern monograph on scleroderma.

A study of the literature indicates that many of the reports by medical scientists on the pathological, biochemical and immunological studies are published in journals not commonly read by clinicians and also that some scientific investigators are not fully aware of the clinical aspects, particularly the different types of this disease. It is hoped that this book will bridge that information gap and inform the clinician of the extensive investigational studies that have been conducted on the basic aspects of the disease and also give the medical scientist a fuller appreciation of the clinical aspects, particularly its various types.

The present writer's qualification for this task is a long-term interest in this disease and a personal follow-up of cases over a period of up to twenty years. The writing of this book has been a rewarding but, at the same time, humbling experience. There are various larger series (in the case of the Mayo Clinic much larger) and each chapter could probably have been written by someone more knowledgeable in the particular aspect. However it would have been difficult to have enlisted a suitable team and one can only imagine the difficulties of keeping the various sections to an appropriate length with each person engrossed with the importance of his particular viewpoint. It is hoped that, although the present writer cannot claim to be expert in all fields, he has presented a balanced account, understandable by both scientists and clinicians, and with adequate reference to original work for those desirous of further study.

ACKNOWLEDGMENTS

I must acknowledge my debt to numerous fellow-workers in the subject of scleroderma, on whose published work I have drawn extensively and who are mentioned in the text. I am grateful to the authors and editors who have allowed me to quote from their work or reproduce tables and figures.

My thanks are due to Dr. T. E. Lowe (Director of the Baker Medical Research Institute) for encouragement and helpful criticism of the manuscript, to various colleagues for advice on special sections, to Dr. Essex of the Pathology Department of the Alfred Hospital for discussion on the pathological aspects and supply of photomicrographs, to the Departments of Diagnostic Radiology and Photography of the Alfred Hospital for help with the illustrations, to Mrs. Mary Rae and Miss Sherry Dudley for help with the references and Mrs. Elaine Kern for typing the manuscript. The Board of Management of the Alfred Hospital gave generous financial support.

A. J. B.

CONTENTS

SCLERODERMA

Chapter I

INTRODUCTION AND
BRIEF HISTORICAL SURVEY

INTRODUCTION

IN 1895, JONATHAN HUTCHINSON wrote: "The group of affections which have been described under the names *Morphoea, Hide-bound skin, Scleroderma* and *Scleriasis cutis* offer some of the most interesting and at the same time, very difficult problems." Although much has been added to the knowledge of these conditions since that time, they are still of interest and provide many unsolved problems.

Scleroderma is uncommon, but not a rare condition and is of interest and importance out of proportion to its incidence. Its aetiology is unknown, and it does not fit into the commonly accepted classifications of disease (such as congenital, inflammatory, degenerative, neoplastic) and is classed with other disorders (rheumatoid arthritis, disseminated lupus erythematosus, dermatomyositis, polymositis, polyarteritis nodosa) of unknown aetiology in the group *connective tissue disorders*.

Some confusion has existed in the variety of terms with ill-defined meaning such as those quoted above. Other terms used in connection with this or allied disorders include *sclerodactyly, sclerodactylia, diffuse systemic sclerosis*, and *progressive systemic sclerosis*. No attempt will be made at this stage to define these various terms. It is necessary however, to define the meaning of *scleroderma* as used in this monograph. It literally means *hard skin* (*scleros* = hard and *derma* = skin) and is applied to a condition of the skin in which it is harder than normal and has reduced mobility on deeper tissues. By common usage it is also now applied to all features of a disease (or diseases) in which hardness of the skin is a prominent feature, even when discussing manifestations remote from the skin. Thus we may speak of the *scleroderma kidney* or the *kidney in scleroderma* to indicate the condition of the kidney found in the disease scleroderma, although the expression "scleroderma of the kidney" (literally *hard skin of the kidney*) is not acceptable.

The difficulties in classification experienced by Hutchinson have continued until the present. Although this problem will be discussed more fully in a later chapter, it is necessary to briefly define certain terms in common use. *Sclerodactyly* (or *sclerodactylia*) refers to tightness and hardness of the skin of the fingers. *Acrosclerosis* refers to a type of scleroderma in which the skin changes are confined to extremities (fingers, hands, face). *Diffuse scleroderma* refers to the condition where the skin changes are extensive—involving trunk as well as the extremities. *Progressive systemic sclerosis* is used to indicate the involvement of other systems (particularly viscera) in association with skin changes. *Morphoea* is used for the condition characterized by circumscribed hard white patches of skin. *Linear scleroderma* refers to the occurrence of bands of hard skin and *guttate scleroderma* to the presence of small patches of hard white skin (*gutta* = drop).

Particularly in the early phase, the vascular disturbance consists of paroxysmal ischaemic episodes of the digits which become white or blue on exposure to cold. These will be described as *Raynaud's phenomenon* which will be used in a broad descriptive sense in contradistinction to *Raynaud's disease* which is reserved for a (presumed) primary vascular abnormality in which ischaemic episodes also occur.

HISTORICAL SURVEY

Early Descriptions

It is possible that scleroderma was known to the ancient physicians for Hippocrates (460–370 B.C.) described the case of "a certain Athenian whose skin was so indurated that it could not be pinched" and Galen (130–200 A.D.) described an illness characterized by "a sort of obstruction of the pores of the skin with thickening, white spots, pigmentations and absence of sweat glands." However the descriptions are not sufficiently precise for these to be accepted as definite cases of scleroderma as now defined.

Also, it is difficult because of lack of detailed information to be certain of the first description in modern times; different authors being cited by various writers (Zacutus, 1634; Curzio, 1753; Watson, 1754; Thirial, 1845). Rodnan and Benedek (1962) who have made a careful study of the history of scleroderma state that the first convincing description of the disease is found in a monograph written by Carlo Curzio and published in Naples in 1753, translated into English in 1754 under the title "An account of an extraordinary disease of the skin and its cure" and into French in 1755. This described the case of a young woman of seventeen years with generalized hardness of the skin, more severe in the forehead, eyelids and neck, difficulty in opening her mouth and impaired movement of her neck and of her limbs, attributed to the tightness of the skin rather than to any affection of joints or muscles. If it is accepted that this was a case of diffuse scleroderma, the outcome was most remarkable: complete relief from treatment consisting of warm milk, vapor baths and "small doses of quick silver," so that after a period of eleven months, the patient's skin had become "perfectly soft and flexible and capable of being moulded, raised, extended and of performing all its natural functions," a result far beyond that expected from potent modern drugs, including corticosteroids! It should be noted that Curzio's case has been claimed by other authors (Tourraine *et al.* 1937) as the first reported case of a different disease, *scleroedema adultorum*.

There was a strange lack of further observations on this condition for almost a century until 1847 which proved a vintage year for scleroderma with three case reports: Grisolle ("Cas rare de maladie de la peau"), Forget ("Mémoire sur le chorionitis où la sclérosténose cutanée") and Thirial ("De sclérème des adultes"). Gintrac (1847) reviewed eight cases comprising those of the above authors and previous possible cases including that of Curzio and called the disease *Sclérodermie,* the French equivalent of the name by which it is now commonly known. In 1854 Gillette collected reports of twelve cases.

Raynaud in 1862, in his classical thesis on "Local asphyxia and symmetrical gangrene of the extremities" noted hardness of the skin in several patients who were probably suffering from scleroderma.

Late Nineteenth Century Descriptions

Scleroderma excited considerable interest among physicians writing in the last quarter of the nineteenth century. Weber (1878), a Swiss physician, described subcutaneous deposits of calcium in some cases of scleroderma, a feature reported later by Thibierge and Weissenbach in 1910. Jonathan Hutchinson (1893, 1895) recognized the association between Raynaud's phenomenon and scleroderma. He stated that the most characteristic type of *Raynaud's malady* was not associated with induration of the skin, but also described cases of acroteric sclerosis followed by Raynaud's phenomenon and Raynaud's phenomenon followed by *acroteric sclerosis.* He distinguished between the form affecting predominantly the extremities (*acroteric sclerosis*), the diffuse form and localized patches. Lewen and Heller, in a monograph published in 1895, were able to collect 507 cases. Osler (1898) described eight cases and gave a dramatic picture of the severe generalized form: "In its aggravated form, diffuse scleroderma is one of the most terrible of all human ills. Like Tithonus to 'wither slowly,' and like him to be 'beaten down and marred and wasted,' until one is literally a mummy encased in an ever shrinking skin of steel, is a fate not pictured in any tragedy, ancient or modern." The first post mortem report on a patient with scleroderma was made in 1898 by Steven, who noted changes in the vessels of the pons, medulla and cord, and *intersitital nephritis* in the kidneys.

Progress in the Twentieth Century

During the twentieth century, scleroderma has continued to evoke interest. Following extensive clinical studies, the occurrence of visceral disturbance in scleroderma has been generally recognized, scleroderma has been classified into types (although there is still not uniformity in nomenclature) and pathological and physiological studies have been extended.

The pathological lesions in scleroderma were described in detail in 1924 by Matsui who found increased collagen and thickening of walls of small vessels in the skin and similar changes in various viscera. The changes in the digital vessels (sclerosis of the adventitia and media, thickening of intima and narrowing of the lumen) were confirmed by Lewis (1937, 1938).

The physiological aspects of the vascular abnormality was studied by various workers. Brown and O'Leary (1925) observed the nailfold capillaries and found a reduction in the number of loops, the presence of giant loops, and sluggish capillary flow. Brown *et al.* (1930) found that the heat elimination from the hand was low, that the vasomotor index (rise in skin temperature per degrees rise in oral temperature after intravenous injection of foreign protein) was lower than primary Raynaud's disease, indicating a structural occlusive factor, as well as a vasospastic factor. Lewis and Landis (1931) found that there was a diminished volume change of the digital pulse in response to heating and reached the same conclusion.

Classification of the various types of scleroderma continued to present a problem. O'Leary and Nomland (1930) in an extensive clinical study, distinguished between *diffuse* (or generalized) and *circumscribed* (or morphoea) forms and concluded "generalized scleroderma is a cutaneous manifestation of a systemic disease in which changes in the vascular system play a leading part."

Sellei (1931) distinguished between two types of *dermatosclerosis* (scleroderma): *acrosclerosis* and *scleroderma verum* a term applied to various types of scleroderma with purely dermatological features. O'Leary and Waisman (1943) also recognized these two types and defined the differences between them. There thus developed a distinction between scleroderma as a generalized disease and scleroderma as a dermatological disease, although there remained difficulties in nomenclature and some differences of opinion as where to place certain types.

Study of the early reports reveals symptoms in some cases which may have been due to visceral disturbance, but the significance of these does not seem to have been realized and, until the beginning of the twentieth century, scleroderma was regarded as either a dermatological or dermatological *plus* peripheral vascular condition. Ehrman (1903) remarked on the oesophageal lesions in scleroderma, indicating that the disorder was not confined to the skin. Matsui (1924) found vascular lesions in visceral as well as cutaneous blood vessels. Goetz (1945) showed that in patients with scleroderma, lesions might extend down the gastro-intestinal tract to the colon, stressed the importance of the visceral lesions and suggested the name *progressive systemic sclerosis* which has subsequently been widely used. Beerman (1948), in a review article, emphasized the importance of visceral lesions which he recorded in practically every organ. About the mid-century there were numerous reports of involvement of particular viscera in scleroderma: *gastro-intestinal* (Olsen *et al.*, 1945; Skouby and Teilum, 1950; Prowse, 1951; Cullinan, 1953); *cardiac* (Weiss *et al.*, 1943; Hurly *et al.*, 1951; Barritt and O'Brien, 1952; Mustakallio and Sarajas, 1954; Bauer, 1955; Meltzer, 1956); *pulmonary* (Murphy *et al.*, 1941; Getzowa, 1945; Lloyd and Tonkin, 1948; Spain and Thomas, 1950; Church and Ellis, 1950; Dawson, 1955); *renal* (Moore and Sheehan, 1952; Hannigan *et al.*, 1956; Rodnan *et al.*, 1957). The state of knowledge of scleroderma by the 1950's may be briefly summarized as follows.

Numerous clinical studies had been made and it was apparent that two types of diseases were described under this name: a purely dermatological condition and a condition associated with other disturbances such as vascular and joint and visceral lesions. In the latter type, acrosclerotic and diffuse forms were recognized. There does not however seem to have been general agreement as to whether these two forms were different conditions or extreme manifestations of the same underlying disease. There was no knowledge as to the cause of the condition and there was no effective treatment.

Developments since 1950 include elaboration of the previous observations, studies on immune phenomena, more precise pathological studies using modern techniques including electron microscopy, studies on collagen metabolism, and trial of numerous remedies, mainly on an empirical basis. Much of this work still needs evaluation as to its importance and will be referred to in subsequent chapters.

Chapter II

EPIDEMIOLOGY AND ETIOLOGY

GEOGRAPHIC DISTRIBUTION

M OST DESCRIPTIONS OF SCLERODERMA are from European countries as could be expected on the basis that these were the countries with greatest interest in clinical medicine. During the past quarter-century there have been various reports of large series from the United States of America dealing with both European and Negro populations.

The first detailed report of pathological changes in scleroderma was made by Matsui of Japan. Although there have been no reports of large series, the condition is well known in that country as evidenced by the fact that Nakashima *et al.* (1966), when reporting a fatal case of visceral scleroderma were able to find an additional forty such cases reported in the Japanese literature since 1952.

However, the condition appears to be rare in other parts of Asia. Tay and Khoo (1970) in Singapore were able to find only sixteen cases (thirteen Chinese and three Malays) in ten years in a large hospital admitting 10,000 new cases per year. They commented on the rarity of the condition in Asia and over the same period could find reports of only seven Chinese cases from Taiwan and eight Indian cases. However Panja *et al.* in a report from Calcutta in 1960 on the vascular changes in scleroderma based it on fifteen cases (eight of systemic sclerosis and seven morphoea).

Enquiry by letter has elicited the information that the disease is rare in India, only two or three cases being seen per year in a dermatological department in New Delhi seeing approximately 6,500 new patients per year (Rattan Singh, 1972), not particularly rare in Iran (Ala, 1971; Sardadvar, 1971), rare in Taiwan with only seven cases in two large general hospitals in five years (Nong Ting, 1972). Tay and Khoo commented on the differences in symptomatology between Asian and European cases. In the Asian cases, there are fewer facial lesions but more involvement of the feet, and relative absence of ischaemic ulcers. These differences may lead to cases being overlooked.

The disease is also apparently rare in Black Africa. Privat *et al.*, in a case report in 1968 of "generalized scleroderma in an African," stated that this was one of the first such cases. It also appears to be rare in Egypt. El Zawahry (1966) describing a case of systemic sclerosis in an Egyptian regarded it as a rare and interesting condition.

It is not clear in most cases whether the differing incidence in countries depends on geographic or racial factors. However the disease does not appear to be particularly rare among American negroes.

PREVALENCE

Although scleroderma is an uncommon disease, it is not excessively rare and it is to be expected that all large hospitals, at least in Western communities, will have several patients with this disease attending at one time.

As it is not notifiable and does not present a great problem as regards community health, there is no detailed knowledge of its prevalence, which probably varies greatly between communities.

Kierland *et al.* (1969) in a study of epidemiological features of diffuse connective tissue disorders in Rochester Minnesota in the ten year period 1957–1967 found eight cases of *diffuse systemic sclerosis* giving a prevalence (cases per 100,000 at any particular time) of 10.5 and incidence (new cases per year per 100,000) of 1.2.

Masi and d'Angelo (1967) studied the epidemiology of fatal scleroderma in Baltimore (population approximately one million) in the fifteen year period 1948 to 1963. They found reports of fifty-three deaths from scleroderma (including thirty-four residents) indicating a mortality rate between two and four per million per year, considerably less than the incidence rate in Rochester. The reports suggest to us that there is either a different incidence in the two cities or that scleroderma is often not a fatal disease. The observed mortality for negro females exceeded that for white females, but this did not apply in case of males.

Medsger and Masi (1971) conducted an epidemiological survey of all the hospitals in Skelby County, Tennessee for the period of 1947 through 1968 and found eighty-six patients. The annual incidence was 2.7 new patients per million population. The sex incidence was three females to one male. The incidence was the same in whites and negroes. The condition was rare in childhood and no male cases were found under the age of twenty-five years; the peak occurrence was in patients over sixty-five years. No socio-economic or infective factors were identified.

FAMILIAL OCCURRENCE

The occurrence of scleroderma in several members of one family is very rare and is not mentioned in most of the larger series. I have not observed a single instance in a personal series of approximately eighty cases. However, five instances of familial scleroderma are reported:

1. Father and daughter with morphoea (Reese and Bennett, 1953).
2. Two sisters with acrosclerosis (Orabona and Albano, 1958).
3. Two brothers with acrosclerosis (Blanchard and Speed, 1965).
4. One brother with progressive systemic sclerosis, one brother with acro-

sclerosis and one sister and mother with flexion deformity (McAndrev and Barnes, 1965).

5. Two sisters with childhood scleroderma without visceral involvement (Burge *et al.*, 1969).

In spite of hundreds of cases of scleroderma in the literature, reported cases of familial scleroderma are limited to single figures, indicating that in the vast majority of cases, scleroderma is not a familial disease.

POSSIBLE ETIOLOGICAL FACTORS

Chromosomal abnormalities

Housset *et al.* (1969) reported a much greater incidence of chromosomal abnormalities in cells from ten patients with scleroderma compared with control studies. His group has since confirmed these findings in a larger group of seventy patients (Emerit *et al.*, 1971). Abnormalities include chromatid and chromosome type aberrations and increase in hyperploid cells. Marker chromosomes are significantly more frequent in severe cases. However the authors cannot state whether these abnormalities are the cause or the effect of the illness.

Infection

Scleroderma does not show general features such as fever and tachycardia or histological features such as accumulation of inflammatory cells indicative of an infective process. Although infection has been considered as a possible cause by some early writers, no infective organism was demonstrated.

Two types of possible infecting agents considered recently are atypical acid-fast bacilli and viruses. Wuerthele-Caspe *et al.* reported the presence of acid-fast bacilli in nine patients with scleroderma in 1947 and this was confirmed by Delmotte and van der Meiren in 1953. More recently, reports of acid-fast bacilli in tissues from scleroderma patients have been reported by Cantwell and Wilson (1966) in one patient, and by Cantwell *et al.* (1968) in seven patients and by Cantwell and Kelso (1971) in six patients. The significance of these findings is doubtful and they have been criticized on bacteriological grounds (Fite, 1971). Although it would be too much to demand the fulfillment of Koch's postulates, it should at least be required that before an organism is seriously considered as cause of scleroderma, it should be found consistently in scleroderma patients, or in a significantly higher number of patients than control subjects.

Norton (1969) observed inclusion bodies similar to those in myxovirus infection in tissues of certain patients with subacute disseminated lupus erythematosis and scleroderma, studied by electron microscopy, although he could not demonstrate specific myxovirus antibodies in the patients' tissues or serum. He suggested as possibilities that the inclusions were (a) viral or (b) a reactive phenomenon at the site of the active disease. Haas and Yunis (1970) found these inclusion bodies not only in the tissues of patients with subacute disseminated lupus erythematosus, but also in several other unrelated diseases and concluded that they were due to reaction to cellular injury.

Toxic agents

The chronicity of the condition and the absence of evidence of infection lead to the suspicion that a toxic agent may be responsible. (Vascular disease from injection of ergot and renal disease from lead poisoning are analogous examples). The recent widespread use of chemical substances as additives to food, industrial solvents and pesticides would provide many suspects.

Industrial chemicals

Walder (1965) reported that following a claim by two patients with scleroderma that their condition followed working with solvents, he questioned a further five patients and four of these gave a history of use of solvents or industrial chemicals (benzol, toluene, dry cleaning agent, solvents in aircraft factory, miscellaneous chemicals). There does not seem to be any follow-up of this observation.

Starr and Clifford (1971) reported a case of scleroderma in a man who had been a pesticide formulator for many years. They attributed the high level of *Dieldrin* in his blood a year before his death to excessive absorption due to his skin condition, but do not comment on the possibility that the long contact with chemicals might have caused the scleroderma. I have not been able to find a history of excessive contact with industrial chemicals in any of my eighty cases.

Silicosis and mining

There appears to be an increased incidence of scleroderma in subjects in contact with silica dust. In 1914 Bramwell in Scotland reported on nine cases of scleroderma which had occurred in his personal practice. He commented that this was a greater number than would be expected for such a rare condition, and noted that five were stonemasons and one was a copper smith, whose occupations required working with a cold chisel, and who considered the use of this tool in cold weather might be the cause of the condition.

In 1957 Erasmus in South Africa reported on an apparent increased incidence of scleroderma among gold miners in the Witswatersrand. He found sixteen patients with scleroderma among 8,000 case records of underground miners, but only one in 25,000 case records of Pretoria Hospital. In ten patients the onset was acute, usually with pulmonary symptoms, and in six there was concurrent definite or probable pulmonary silicosis. Although he suggested a possible relation to contact with silica dust, he also observed that miners were subject to many other noxious influences, including rapid descent to great depths. One patient had also worked in an asbestos mine.

In 1967 Rodnan *et al.* reported on twenty six consecutive men with scleroderma in the Pittsburg area in America, who had been found to be coal miners or who had been exposed to silicious dusts for a long time. Co-existant silicosis was found radiologically or at necropsy in eleven cases. They conducted an epidemiological study in the area and found the prevalence of scleroderma among hospital discharges to be seventeen per 100,000 for coal miners (all males), six per 100,000 for male non-miners, giving approximately three-fold increased incidence among miners when compared with non-miners.

The association of scleroderma with silicosis has also recently been reported from European countries. (Miguères *et al.*, 1966; Thieme, 1967; Gunther and Schuchardt, 1970.)

The evidence for increased frequency of scleroderma in the groups mentioned (stone-masons, gold miners, coal miners) seems fairly convincing and it is tempting to attribute this to silica dust as the common factor. However Denko (1969) considered that mechanical vibration could be the factor. Support for this view was obtained from the finding that when animals subjected to vibration were fed substances containing ^{35}S, there was a greater incorporation of the ^{35}S into the connective tissue in most organs than occurred in control animals not subjected to vibration. He assumed that this was due to a greater synthesis of connective tissue in the animals subjected to vibration.

Psychological factors

In view of the stated increased incidence of scleroderma in European countries as contrasted with Asian and African societies, it is tempting to look for some factor in the Western way of life, one of which is mental stress associated with a competitive type of existence. In the 1950's there was a tendency to look for a psychosomatic origin of obscure diseases. This was suggested in the case of scleroderma by Mufson (1953), who stated that patients with scleroderma were dependant types of person and their disease tended to relapse when there was a threat to the security of their existence. I have been impressed by apparent psychological disturbances in scleroderma and submitted a group of twelve patients with this disease and a group of patients with other skin lesions to examination by a panel of psychiatrists and a psychologist. All were found to be psychologically abnormal in some respect, but the scleroderma patients not more so than the other patients with skin diseases.

Auto-immunity

As will be discussed more fully later, in common with other connective tissue or *collagen* diseases, scleroderma patients present a fairly high incidence of positive tests for antinuclear factors and other auto-antibodies and this has led to the inclusion of scleroderma and other connective tissue diseases under the heading *Auto-immune diseases* (See chapter VI). This implies that these diseases result from a disturbance of the immune mechanism so that the body forms antibodies to its own tissues and that these are in some way harmful. Difficulties in this concept are (a) that such auto-antibodies are only found in less than half the cases, and one would still have to account for the occurrence of the disease in the patients without the antibodies, (b) the reason for the derangement of the normal immune process would still have to be explained, and (c) one would still have to demonstrate that the auto-antibodies were harmful.

COMMENT

In spite of the work outlined in this chapter, the cause of scleroderma remains unknown and there are indeed few clues to help in the search.

There is no convincing evidence of infection. In spite of the occasional reports of the disease in patients in contact with chemicals, this is not usually the case. In looking for a common toxic agent, one would have to consider one operative before 1900, that is, prior to the development of modern industrial chemicals.

The increased prevalence in certain occupations (stone masons, gold miners, coal miners) causes suspicion of contact with silica in these cases, but this cannot be operative in most cases.

It is not a familial disease. However the increased incidence of chromosomal abnormalities is interesting but this may be an effect rather than a cause. Although psychological disturbance is probably common in scleroderma, it would seem unlikely that it is the prime cause as similar disturbance is found in many peoples without scleroderma.

Although immunological disturbance is common in scleroderma, this does not mean that auto-immunity plays a causative role.

Chapter III

PATHOLOGY

HISTORICAL SURVEY

A̲LTHOUGH SCLERODERMA WAS RECOGNIZED at least as early as the middle of the eighteenth century and there were numerous clinical reports by the end of the nineteenth century, there were no comprehensive pathological studies. At that time, scleroderma was generally regarded as a disorder of the skin and peripheral circulation. However, fibrosis of the lungs had been reported by Dinkler in 1891, in two of the cases collected by Lewen and Heller in 1895 and by Notthafft in 1895.

The first general reports of the pathological changes in scleroderma with particular reference to internal organs were made by Kraus in 1924, who described both cardiac and pulmonary fibrosis and by Matsui in the same year, who gave detailed descriptions based on complete autopsy findings in five cases and examination of the skin in one additional case. Matsui described the histological changes in the skin, comprising atrophy of the epidermis, fibrosis of the dermis, and changes in the blood vessels. The latter included reduction in number of capillaries, sclerosis and hypertrophy of media of small arteries, decreased lumen, and in some cases, presence of thrombi. He stated that the medial hypertrophy was not due to simple fibrosis but also to hypertrophy of the smooth muscle. He also described hypertrophy of smooth muscle of other situations: *arrectores pili* of the skin, gastro-intestinal tract, uterus and ureter. Changes in the small arteries similar to those in the skin were found also in the heart, lungs, esophagus, uterus, thyroid gland and ovaries. Connective tissue changes consisting of excessive growth and thickening of collagen fibres occurred also in skeletal muscle and internal organs—intestinal tract, lungs, kidney, urinary tract and uterus. He gave detailed descriptions of the changes in particular organs. In skeletal muscles there was atrophy and degeneration of fibres (without changes in the nervous system to account for them). The bones of the extremities and particularly of the digits showed resorption of the bone substance and reduction in size of the terminal phalanges. The lungs showed severe interstitial fibrosis, and intimal thickening and medial hypertrophy of the small arteries. Pleural effusion or pleuritis might be present. Although tuberculosis was often associated with diffuse scleroderma, pulmonary findings described above had been observed in the absence of tuberculosis. In the alimentary tract, there was fibrosis of the submucosa, slight hypertrophy of the muscularis

14

mucosae, and hypertrophy or atrophy and fibrosis of the muscle coat. In the kidneys he found marked connective tissue proliferation, but no marked vascular changes. He discussed the primacy of the arterial changes and connective tissue changes and concluded that both were equally important and not causally related.

Heine (1926) in his detailed report of the necropsy findings in one case described changes in the arteries of the skin (consisting of proliferation of the intima resulting in narrowing of the lumen and fibrosis and hyalination of the media) and fibrosis in various organs. The changes in the arteries in the finger were confirmed in 1938 by Lewis who found sclerosis of adventitia and media, conspicuous thickening of the intima by connective and elastic tissue and obliteration of the lumen in places. Pathological changes in the skin and alimentary canal were described in 1931 by Rake who commented on dilatation of the lower part of the esophagus and of the intestine in the absence of muscular hypertrophy indicating that the dilatation was not due to obstruction.

The first report of the florid changes in the kidney (now sometimes designated *true scleroderma kidney*) was made in 1938 by Masugi and Yä-Shu who reported on one case in whom they found patchy changes in small arteries consisting of fibrinoid necrosis, thickening of the intima by connective tissue hyperplasia and narrowing of the lumen. An illustration in their paper shows fibrinoid in an afferent glomerular arteriole and in neighbouring capillary loops.

Linenthal and Talkov (1941) reported on the fibrotic changes in the lungs in a patient in whom involvement had been diagnosed previously by radiography.

Weiss *et al.* (1943) reported on nine patients with scleroderma and heart failure in two of whom autopsies were obtained. The hearts contained scars of unusual type in that they were not associated with vascular occlusion and myocardial fibres were present in the centre of the scars. The connective tissue contained numerous fibroblasts and large numbers of capillaries (contrasting with the affected skin in these cases which was characterized by scarcity of fibroblasts and of capillaries). Other pathological changes observed in these cases were focal areas of fibrosis and vascular changes (thickening of walls and diminished lumina of vessels) in the lungs, and areas of atrophy and cellular infiltration in muscles.

In 1945 Goetz gave a detailed clinical and pathological account of a patient whose illness had commenced with the acrosclerotic type of scleroderma and who later developed severe dysphagia and various systemic symptoms (asthenia, wasting, dyspnoea, cyanosis, loss of weight, pigmentation, loss of axillary and pubic hair, amenorrhoea), and died following myotomy of the lower end of her esophagus. In addition to the characteristic changes in the skin, there were pathological changes in various organs. In skeletal muscle, there was atrophy, homogenization and loss of striation of cells, proliferation and degenerative changes in nuclei in perimysium and accumulation of lymphocytes and other cells. In the heart, there were areas of replacement of muscle cells by fibrous tissue and other areas showing increase of vascular connective tissue between muscle cells and degenerative changes in the cells. In the oesophagus there was hypertrophy of the muscle coat near the cardia and inflammatory changes and scarcity of ganglion cells in the myenteric plexus. In the lungs, there were areas with thickened alveolar septa and gland-like outgrowths of alveolar epithelium. The kidneys showed changes similar to those of an arteriosclerotic kidney. The changes in the small arteries of the skin and in those of the viscera were similar, consisting of necrosis and fibrosis of media, hyperplasia of the intima and presence of thrombus in some vessels. He emphasized that these changes affecting a variety of organs indicated a generalized disease and suggested that it should be called *progressive systemic sclerosis.*

Changes in the renal arteries similar to those described by Masugi and Yä-Shu were found by other writers in individual cases (reviewed by Moore and Sheehan, 1952). Some of the patients, but not all, had been hypertensive. Moore and Sheehan (1952) gave detailed histological findings in three patients with scleroderma who had died from rapidly advancing renal failure. Macroscopically the kidneys had an uneven nodular surface with pale or dark-red elevations. Microscopically the most marked changes were in the small arteries and arterioles. The proximal parts of the intralobular arteries showed concentric thickening with *mucoid* material. The more distal part of the intralobular arteries and the afferent glomerular arterioles showed patchy segmental fibrinoid necrosis sometimes extending to loops of the glomerular tufts. The renal parenchyma showed relative or complete ischaemia (infarcts). The authors considered that the renal lesions of scleroderma could be distinguished from those of hypertension. However, Fisher and Rodnan (1958) following a detailed comparative study concluded that the renal changes in scleroderma with renal failure were indistinguishable on morphology and staining reactions from those of malignant hypertension.

A very detailed study of the lung changes in two patients with scleroderma was published in 1945 by Getzowa who described two types of lesions which she called *cystic pulmonary sclerosis* and *compact pulmonary sclerosis.* In the former the cystic lesions occurred in the subpleural region except at the apices and hilar regions and were associated with diffuse fibrosis of alveolar walls. The histological findings suggested that the cysts resulted from ischaemia of the alveolar walls leading to hyaline change and later avascular necrosis. There were also other cysts lined by bronchiolar epithelium. *Compact pulmonary sclerosis* consisted of diffuse alveolar fibrosis with the thickening of inter-alveolar septa without dissolution of the walls. The association of intact bronchi and bronchioles and surrounding fibrosis produced an adenoma-like appearance.

The histological features of the skin in the various types of scleroderma were described in detail by O'Leary *et al.* (1957) on the basis of a study of over two hundred cases. They stated that the fundamental changes were oedema, *homogenization* (loss of detail of fibrillar appearance), fibrosis and vascular changes. These varied with the stage of the disease, oedema being more prominent in the early stage. There were differences (usually of degree) between the different forms of scleroderma—diffuse systemic, acrosclerotic and circumscribed (morphoea). The dermis was usually thick in the diffuse systemic form, thin in the acrosclerotic form and variable in the circumscribed forms. There was a relative increase in elastic tissue in the upper part of the dermis in the acrosclerotic form but not in the other forms.

Since 1950 there have since been various reports of pathological findings based on a relatively large number of cases. Leinwand *et al.* (1954) in a general article on scleroderma based on a study of over 150 cases, included typical pathological descriptions, although the number of post mortem studies was not given. They found changes in individual organs generally similar to those previously described. They divided lesions in blood vessels into three types: (a) acute and subacute arteritis, (b) intimal proliferation leading to obstruction or marked reduction of the lumen and (c) *arteriosclerotic* lesions in the kidney. They considered the pathological changes in general could be summarized under three headings: (a) changes in collagen, (b) changes in arteries and (c) immediate and remote results of these lesions: fibrosis, parenchymatous degeneration, infarction.

Piper and Helwig (1955) described the visceral manifestations (clinical and pathological) in thirty one cases of generalized scleroderma from the files of the American Armed Forces Institute of Pathology, and listed the frequency of involvement of various systems as shown in Table I.

TABLE I *

FREQUENCY OF INVOLVEMENT OF VARIOUS
ORGANS IN A SERIES OF THIRTY-ONE
SCLERODERMA PATIENTS

| | Number Involved | |
Site	*Clinical*	*Pathological*
Joints	30 (97%)	—
Gastro-intestinal tract	30 (97%)	20 (64%)
Heart	30 (97%)	28 (90%)
Kidneys	30 (97%)	23 (70%)
Lungs	29 (93%)	28 (90%)

* From Piper and Helwig: *Archiv Dermatol, 72:*535–546, 1955. Copyright 19—, American Medical Association.

The remarkably high incidence of systemic lesions suggests that the series was a selected one of severe cases. The findings in skin, esophagus, heart, lungs and muscle were similar to those described previously. Additional features not included by earlier workers were sclerosis of submucosa of stomach (thirteen of seventeen cases), obliteration of the pericardial sac (five cases) fibrosis of anterior lobe of pituitary (three cases), atrophy of seminiferous tubules of testis, foci of ischaemic necrosis of cerebral cortex in three and increased gliosis in two of the seventeen brains studied, portal necrosis of the liver in one case, and focal necrosis in three cases.

In his monograph, Sackner (1967) described pathological features based on autopsy experience of some thirty cases. He confirmed changes previously described and emphasized the following features: The main abnormality in the esophagus is atrophy of both smooth and striated muscle, fibrous tissue being minimal. Muscle degeneration is also a prominent feature in small and large bowel. Renal lesions in scleroderma are of two types: (a) in patients dying from rapidly progressive renal failure, the lesions are morphologically, histochemically and immunochemically indistinguishable from those in malignant nephrosclerosis and in these cases necrotizing arteritis may also be found in muscle; (b) in patients dying from non-renal causes, there is a high incidence of vascular sclerosis with mild to moderate glomerular damage and minimal tubular changes.

Although, as indicated by the above survey, the presence and general nature of visceral involvement in scleroderma is well established, there has been some doubt as to the frequency of disturbances of various systems. Some reports are written by people interested in a particular system, e.g. cardiac, pulmonary, gastrointestinal, and stress the involvement of that particular system. Also many of the deaths from scleroderma occur in middle-aged or elderly people when degenerative changes are common and it is possible that these changes may be attributed wrongly to scleroderma. In order to determine the incidence and type of involvement of the various systems in scleroderma, D'Angelo *et al.* (1969) carried out an important study in which they analysed the post mortem reports on fifty-eight autopsy cases of scleroderma in the city of Baltimore and fifty-eight matched control cases which were provided by the next autopsy case in the same hospital of the same race, sex and age decade. In certain cases the control figures were corrected by subtracting lesions due to a specific illness (e.g. cardiac valve lesions in patients known to have suffered from rheumatic fever, pericarditis due to tuberculosis, pleural disease due to specific causes). They found that the organs principally involved in systemic sclerosis were as follows: skin (98 percent), esophagus (74 percent), lungs (59 percent), kidney (49 percent), small intestine (46 percent), pericardium (41 percent), muscles (41 percent), large intestine (39 percent), pleura (29 percent), myocardium (26 percent). The figures in brackets are the excess prevalence in the scleroderma patients over that in the controls. Other organs showing less frequent involvement in scleroderma were adrenal glands, lymph glands, thyroid gland and peripheral arteries.

A comparison was made between the scleroderma patients and controls as to the type of involvement in each organ. Thus in the case of the *gastro-intestinal tract* there was a significant increase of muscle atrophy and/or fibrosis of the oesophagus (74 percent in scleroderma cases versus 0 percent in controls), esophagitis (40 percent versus 19 percent), muscle atrophy and/or fibrosis of the small intestine (48 percent versus 2 percent), and muscle atrophy and/or fibrosis of the large intestine (39 percent versus 0 percent). Peptic ulcer and carcinoma were no more frequent in the scleroderma patients and diverticulosis only slightly more frequent (16 percent versus 10 percent). In the *kidneys* the most frequent lesions were fibrinoid necrosis in afferent arterioles of glomeruli (35 percent versus 0 percent), hyperplasia of interlobular arteries (33 percent versus 4 percent), thickening of basement membrane or wire-looping 32 percent versus 7 percent). Unexpectedly there was an increased frequency of renal artery stenosis (14 percent versus 5 percent). Arteriosclerosis and pyelonephritis were *not* more frequent. In the *lungs* the features showing increased frequency were interstitial fibrosis (70 percent versus 21 percent), arteriolar thickening (29 percent versus 2 percent), pneumonitis (57 percent versus 33 percent), emphysema (45 percent versus 29 percent). Bronchiectasis, oedema or congestion, infarction and atelectasis were not more frequent. *Pericarditis* was more common in the scleroderma patients: fibrinous (35 percent versus 5 percent), fibrous 24 percent versus 7 percent), or adhesive (28 percent versus 9 percent). Pericardial effusions, however, were not more common. *Fibrous pleuritis* (29 percent versus 12 percent) and pleural adhesions (66 percent versus 48 percent) were more common in the scleroderma patients, but not fibrinous pleuritis. There was no increase in the incidence of peritonitis or peritoneal adhesions. In the *heart* the incidence of myocardial fibrosis (81 percent versus 55 percent) and arteriolar sclerosis (17 percent versus 2 percent) was higher in the scleroderma patients but the frequency of coronary arteriosclerosis similar to that in the controls. Minor lesions of the mitral and aortic valves were equally common in the scleroderma patients and in controls. The pathological changes in *muscle* found in the scleroderma patients were atrophy (41 percent versus 0 percent), round cell infiltration (8 percent versus 0 percent). Lesions of *other organs* showing an increased incidence in scleroderma were atrophy of the adrenal glands (26 percent versus 4 percent), fibrosis of lymph nodes (12 percent versus 0 percent), fibrosis of thyroid gland 24 percent versus 7 percent, non-inflammatory intimal proliferation of arteries (24 percent versus 0 percent). Organs without any increased incidence of lesions in

TABLE II*

PATHOLOGICAL FINDINGS IN FIFTEEN CASES IN CURRENT SERIES

Case	Age	Sex	Type*	Brief Clinical Notes	Skin			Eso-phagus			Heart					Lungs				Arteriosclerotic Changes	Kidneys			Other
					Apparent Increase in Collagen	Atrophy of Appendages	Vessel Changes	Submucosal Fibrosis	Muscle Replacement	Vessel Changes	Pericardial Effusion	Pericarditis	Fibrosis	Vessel Changes	Coronary Atheroma	Pleural Effusion	Pleurisy	Fibrosis	Vessel Changes		Intimal Thickening of Interlobular Arteries	Fibrinoid	Cortical Infarcts	
1 HH	60	M	3	Duration 1½ years. Died in renal failure.	+		+				+	+				+		+	++	+	+	+		
2 IW	57	F	2	Duration 12 years. Died in renal failure.	++													+		+	+	+	+	
3 LB	78	F	1	Duration 28 years. Died from cerebral haemorrhage.	N.E.			+	+				+		+				+	+	+			
4 AH	63	F	2	Duration 10 years. Died in cardiac failure.	+	+	+	+	+						+				+	+				Lymphocyte collections in oesophageal wall.
5 DB	52	F	2	Duration 33 years. Long history of gastrointestinal involvement. Died following resection of colon.	+		±	+	+	+		+			±	+		+	+	+				Fibrinoid in dermis & renal arterioles. Honeycomb lung. Alveolar carcinoma. Adrenal infarct.
6 GR	47	M	3	Duration 4 years. Severe joint involvement. Sudden death shortly after stopping steroid medication.	++	+	+						+	+					±	+				Adrenal cortical atrophy.
7 RR	54	F	3	Duration 11 years. Multi-system involvement particularly heart and lungs. Died suddenly when under treatment for C.C.F.	+	+	++	+	+				±		+			++		+				Skin thin. Collections of lymphocytes in myocardium.
8 LW	35	M	3	Duration 3 years. Recurrent arrhythmias. Died suddenly.	++	+	++	±					+		+			++	+					Collections of lymphocytes in oesophageal wall and myocardium. Metaplasia of alveolar endothelium.

TABLE II (Continued)

Case	Age	Sex	Type*	Brief Clinical Notes	Skin			Esophagus			Heart					Lungs				Kidneys				Other
					Apparent Increase in Collagen	Atrophy of Appendages	Vessel Changes	Submucosal Fibrosis	Muscle Replacement	Vessel Changes	Pericardial Effusion	Pericarditis	Fibrosis	Vessel Changes	Coronary Atheroma	Pleural effusion	Pleurisy	Fibrosis	Vessel Changes	Arteriosclerotic Changes	Intimal Thickening Interlobular Arteries	Fibrinoid	Cortical Infarcts	
9	RL	58	M	1	Duration 4½ years. Malabsorption and stasis. Died in renal failure.	++	N.E.	N.E.	N.E.	N.E.	N.E.										+				
10	ED	76	F	2	Acrosclerotic type. Duration over 30 years. Marked calcinosis. Hypertensive. Died from cerebral haemorrhage.	++								+		+					+	+			
11	LB	44	F	2	Duration 5 years. Diabetes mellitus. Admitted with congestive cardiac failure and renal impairment. Steadily progressive renal failure and death in 10 days.	++		+						+		±			+		+	+	+	+	Haemorrhagic entero-colitis. Fibrinoid necrosis of intestinal blood vessels. Cortical infarcts in kidney. Loss of renal tubules.
12	EB	46	F	3	Duration 6 months. Severe multisystem involvement. Died in renal failure.	++		+	+	+							+			±		+		+	Acute ulceration with haemorrhage of lower end of stomach. Small cortical infarcts in kidney.
13	RS	53	F	3	Duration 1 year. Admitted with bronchopneumonia and renal failure. Died within three days.	++			+	+			+	+					±		+				Acute myositis. Accumulation of lymphocytes and polymorphs in heart muscle. Patchy necrosis and vasculitis of thymus.
14	LV	45	F	3	Duration 2½ years. Died in renal failure.	++	+											+				+	+		Cystic changes in lungs. Infarction of glomeruli.
15	WW	66	M	2	Marked systemic involvement. Duration 6 years. Rapid progression in 6 months prior to death. Died in renal failure.	++	+	±	+					±					+	+	+	+		±	Plasma cell collection in oesophagus. Myocarditis. Honeycomb lungs.

* See Chapter Seven. ++ marked changes, + moderately severe changes, ± mild changes, N.E. = not examined.

scleroderma were liver, spleen, pancreas and brain. Cancer was conspicuously rare (2 percent).

SUMMARY OF CHANGES IN PARTICULAR ORGANS

The following is a summary of the main pathological changes in progressive systemic sclerosis based on a study of the descriptions discussed above and illustrated from fifteen of our own cases in which post mortem examinations were made (Table II). Special points will also be referred to later in the chapters concerned with the particular types of systemic involvement.

Skin

The thickness of affected skin may be normal, reduced or increased. The epidermis is thin and the rete pegs shorter than normal. The main change is in the dermis, which is acellular and relatively avascular. The

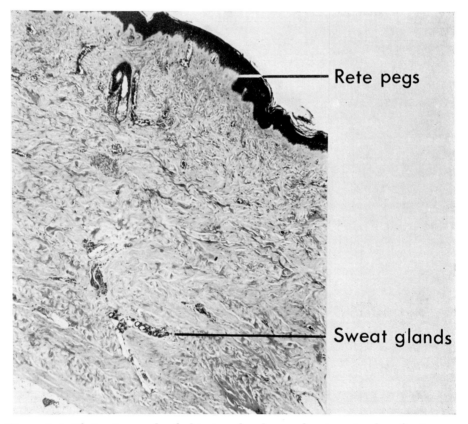

Figure 3–1. Photomicrograph of skin in scleroderma showing atrophy of rete pegs, and dense avascular collagenous tissue extending deep to sweat glands. H. and E. stain. Magnification: Approximately x 100.

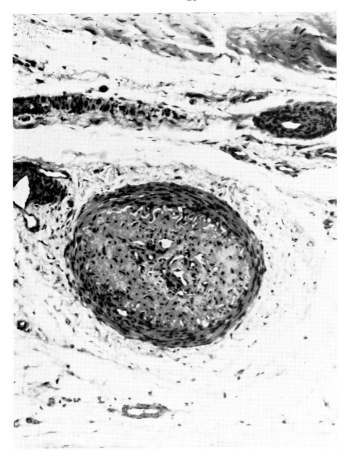

Figure 3–2. Photomicrograph of a small artery from the deeper part of the dermis in scleroderma, showing occlusion by old organized thrombus and partial recanalization. H. and E. stain. Magnification: Approximately x 260.

collagen is altered in appearance in that the fibres appear broader and structural detail is blurred (*homogenization*). This altered collagenous tissue extends deep to the sweat glands. The skin appendages (sweat glands, sebaceous glands) are reduced in number. Arterioles and small arteries show fibrosis of the media and hypertrophy of the intima, with narrowing of the lumen and obliteration by thrombus in some cases. Calcification of the deep layer of skin may occur, particularly in patients with subcutaneous nodules. (See Figs. 3–1 and 3–2.)

Muscle

Skeletal muscle is commonly involved and shows features of myositis. The muscle cells show degenerative changes, including loss of the normal bands, with the exception of the Z band, and degenerative changes in the nuclei. The interstitial tissue is increased and cellular. There may be ac-

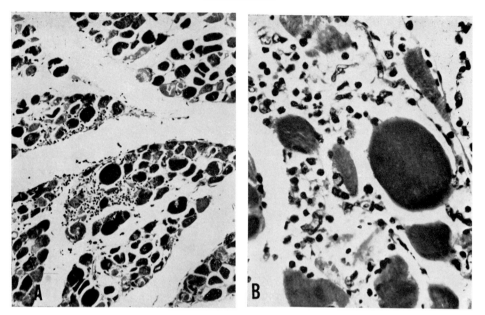

Figure 3–3. Photomicrographs of voluntary muscle from a patient with scleroderma, showing myositis. There is separation of the muscle bundles and fibres by edema fluid, accumulation of inflammatory cells and atrophy and fragmentation of muscle cells. H. and E. stain. Magnification A. Approximately x 215; B. Approximately x 860.

cumulation of lymphocytes either singly or in small collections. (See Fig. 3–3).

Gastro-intestinal Tract

Esophagus

The most prominent change is atrophy and degeneration of the muscle coat, involving mainly the smooth muscle of the lower two-thirds but also affecting the striated muscle in the upper third. Fibrosis is a less marked feature (see Fig. 3–4). There may be secondary features of esophagitis, ulcer or stricture in cases with reflux esophagitis.

Stomach

The stomach does not usually show characteristic features although fibrosis of the muscular coats has been described.

Small Bowel

The small bowel may show dilatation of the duodenal loop or other segments and histologically this may be associated with muscular atrophy and fibrosis.

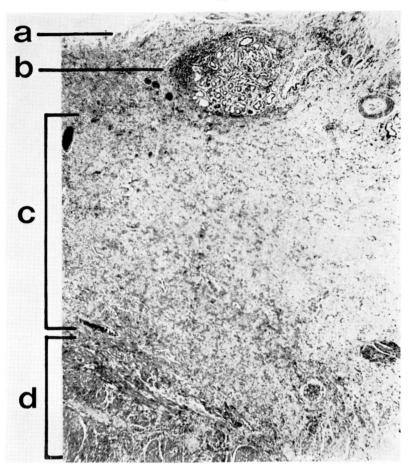

Figure 3–4. Photomicrograph of esophageal wall from a patient with scleroderma showing: (a) ulcerated mucosa, (b) residual mucus-producing glands, (c) dense fibrosis of submucosa, (d) muscle coat infiltrated with fibrous tissue. H. and E. stain. Magnification: Approximately x 50.

Heart

The characteristic change is patchy fibrosis in the myocardium and in subepicardial and subpericardial regions. The fibrous tissue in the myocardium is often of a loose type with numerous nuclei and contains isolated intact muscle cells (Fig. 3–5). Sometimes there is a type of myocarditis with degeneration of muscle cells and infiltration with lymphocytes. (Fig. 3–6) The arterioles may show intimal proliferation, but the coronary arteries are not particularly affected. Pericarditis is common, being fibrinous or fibrous with or without adhesion.

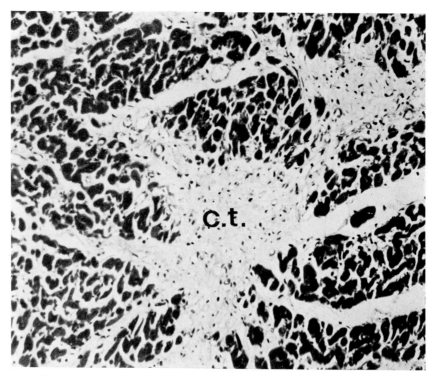

Figure 3–5. Photomicrograph of myocardium from a patient with scleroderma showing fibrosis. The connective tissue (c.t.) is relatively cellular and vascular. H. and E. stain. Magnification: Approximately x 260.

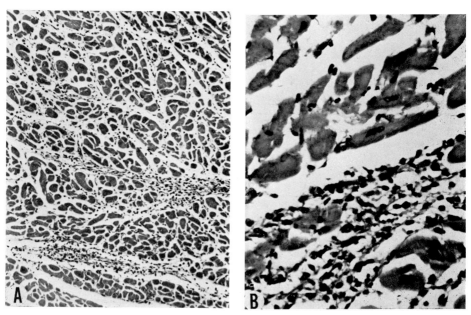

Figure 3–6. Photomicrographs of myocardium from a patient with scleroderma showing myocarditis. The muscle cells are fragmented, separated by edema fluid and there is infiltration by inflammatory cells. H. and E. stain. Magnification: A. Approximately x 230; B. Approximately x 700.

Lungs

The main feature is interstitial fibrosis with thickening of the alveolar septa. In severe cases, there is marked reduction in alveolar spaces at the expense of their greatly thickened walls (compact sclerosis) or cyst formation (cystic sclerosis). Other changes include columnar metaplasia of

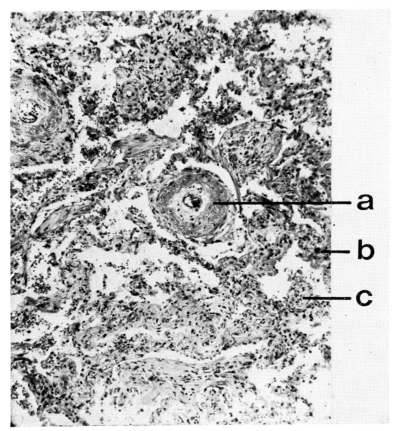

Figure 3–7. Photomicrograph of lung from a patient with scleroderma showing: (a) arteries with thick walls and decreased lumen due to proliferation of mucoid connective tissue in the intima; (b) interstitial fibrosis; (c) organizing exudate in small air spaces. H. and E. stain. Magnification: Approximately x 300.

alveolar lining cells, and localized emphysematous changes. There is frequently thickening of arteriolar walls with reduction of lumen (see Fig. 3–7). Fibrous pleuritis and pleural adhesions are common.

Kidneys

In patients dying of renal failure, there are striking changes in the kidneys. These resemble those of malignant hypertension and comprise cortical infarcts, fibrinoid necrosis in afferent glomerular arterioles and in glomerular capillaries, and thickening of the wall, particularly intimal, of interlobular arteries with reduction of their lumen (Fig. 3–8). Thickening of basement membrane of glomerular capillaries producing a wire loop appearance similar to that in systemic lupus erythematosus may be seen. In some of these cases (of acute renal failure) deposits of immune globulin may be demonstrated in the arteriolar walls and in glomeruli (see Chapter VI).

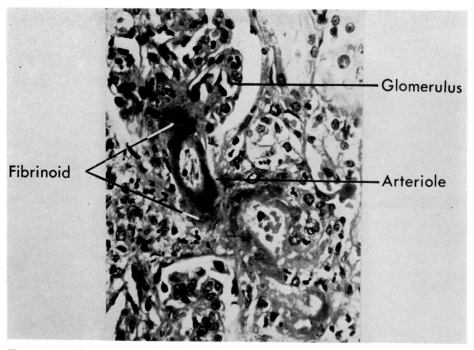

Figure 3–8. Photomicrograph of kidney from a patient with scleroderma showing fibrinoid necrosis of an afferent arteriole and of adjacent glomerular capillaries. H. and E. stain. Magnification: Approximately x 800.

In patients not dying from renal failure, changes are not striking, but there may be an increase in the interstitial connective tissue.

Other Organs

Fibrosis of lymph glands is not uncommon and fibrosis and intimal proliferation of arteries may occur in the thyroid gland. Atrophy of the adrenal glands may be found in patients who have been treated with adrenal steroids. The liver, spleen, pancreas and brain are not commonly involved (although lesions of practically every organ have been described in specific instances).

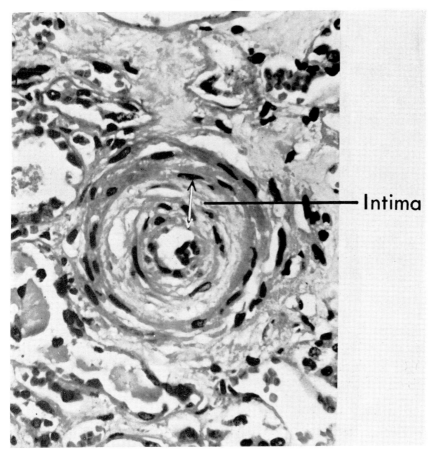

Intima

Figure 3–9. Photomicrograph of a small renal artery from a patient with scleroderma showing marked thickening of the intima by proliferation of mucoid connective tissue and corresponding narrowing of the lumen. H. and E. stain. Magnification: Approximately x 240.

RECENT WORK ON FINE STRUCTURE

Blood vessels

The vascular changes in scleroderma have continued to be the subject of intensive study, being considered by some to be the basic pathological disturbance. The small vessels have also been studied in the living state by the technique of capillaroscopy (See Chapter V).

Recently the observations on the microvasculature have been extended by the technique of electron microscopy. Norton *et al.* (1968) studied the capillary bed in twelve patients with scleroderma of the acrosclerotic type, and in various other diseases including systemic lupus erythematosus. They found that the changes in scleroderma and systemic lupus erythematosus were qualitatively similar but more marked in scleroderma and comprised reduction in number of capillaries, presence of dilated capillaries, endothelial swelling, reduplication of capillary basement membrane and increase in the number of intra-vascular leucocytes.

Muscle

Muscular involvement occurs in approximately half the cases (Rodnan and Medsger 1966) and includes fibrosis of perimysium and endomysium, cellular infiltrates (mainly lymphocytes), and degenerative changes in muscle cells. The changes in the muscle cells on electron microscopy have been described in detail by Michaelowski and Kudejko (1966) who reported lysis, granular degeneration, fragmentation, disintegration, disappearance of bands except Z band in myofibrils and damage of intracellular components: nucleus, sarcolemma, sarcoplasm, and sarcomere. They also observed changes in capillaries similar to those described above. Similar changes on light and electron microscopy have since been reported by Thompson *et al.* (1969).

Skin and Subcutaneous Tissue

Fleischmajer *et al.* (1971) have recently reported on the fine structure of skin and subcutaneous tissue in biopsy specimens through affected skin down to the level of muscle fascia. The changes in the epidermis and dermis on light microscopy were similar to those previously described.

They also found that there was marked replacement of fat in the subcutaneous tissue by abnormal connective tissue which appeared homogeneous with medium power magnification but with high power was seen to consist of fine wavy fibres. With electron microscopy, the collagen fibres of the dermis appeared normal in diameter (mature fibrils) and were surrounded by clear ground substance, whereas in the subcutaneous tissue they were thin (immature fibrils), were arranged in random fashion in an electron opaque ground substance. They suggested that the abnormality of collagen formation in scleroderma resided not in the dermis but in the subcutaneous tissue.

The disturbance in blood vessels and connective tissue are of fundamental importance and will be discussed in detail later (Chapters IV and V).

Chapter IV

CONNECTIVE TISSUE DISTURBANCE

THE APPARENT INCREASE and altered appearance of the collagen in scleroderma has caused it to be classified among *collagen diseases*. However, since collagen does not exist in isolation but is part of a complex of substances in connective tissue and it is possible that there may be associated, or even primary, disturbances in these other components, the term *connective tissue disease* is now preferred.

In order to evaluate recent work on possible disturbances of connective tissue in scleroderma, it is necessary to appreciate the normal distribution and composition of this tissue and it may be helpful to include a brief outline of this subject with emphasis on modern concepts.

GENERAL DESCRIPTION OF CONNECTIVE TISSUE

Histological Features *

Connective tissue is widely distributed in the body, forming the main constituent of the dermis and subcutaneous tissue, the supporting framework of viscera and accompanying blood vessels throughout their distribution. The prototype is the loose or *ordinary* connective tissue forming the frame-work of organs or accompanying vessels. It is modified in various situations to meet special requirements.

Connective tissue consists of two main components: cells and intercellular substance. The morphology and function of the various types of cells (fibroblasts, macrophages, lymphoid cells, plasma cells, mast cells, eosinophil cells, pigment cells) is described in standard histology textbooks. The fibroblasts are those mainly concerned in the manufacture of the non-cellular constituents of connective tissue such as collagen, elastin, mucopolysaccharides.

The intercellular material is composed of fibres and of the apparently structureless *ground substance*. The fibres are of two main types, collagen and elastic, with a third type, reticular, in some tissues. The different types of fibres are recognized by their morphology and by their staining properties. Collagen fibres, as seen by light microscopy (L.M.) are wavy, usually in bundles, are one to twelve μm thick and composed of fibrils 0.3

---

* The following account is based on standard text books such as Bloom and Fawcett (1968): *A Textbook of Histology*.

to 0.5 μm thick. They stain faintly pink with haemotoxylin and eosin stain, but are better shown with special stains such as Van Giesen's picro-fuchsin, which stains them red. With electron microscopy, the fibrils are found to be composed of still smaller structures (micro-fibrils *) about eighty nm in diameter. Elastic fibres are scarce in loose connective tissue. They are of similar diameter to collagen fibres, but more refractile. They are homogenous (not fibrillar) in structure, both in light microscopy and electron microscopy. They also stain pink with haematoxylin and eosin, but are selectively stained dark brown with resorcin-fuchsin. Reticular fibres are fewer than ordinary collagen fibres. They form a network between the basement membrane of epithelial cells and around blood vessels, muscle fibres, fat cells, in the deeper connective tissue and produce a supporting stroma in lymphoid tissue. They do not stain well with ordinary stains, but are stained black by silver stains such as modified Bialchowski and also by periodic acid—Schiff (P.A.S.) stain. Under electron microscopy their structure is similar to that of collagen fibrils and they show the same periodicity.

Ground substance is the term given to the clear, apparently structureless material filling in between the cells and fibres described above. It does not take ordinary stains, but stains metachromatically (purple) with toluidine blue. It is a complex mixture of proteins, including collagen in molecular dispersion, protein-mucopolysaccharides, other glycoproteins and plasma proteins, carbohydrates, lipids and water. The water which is partly bound to the macromolecules and partly free to exchange with capillaries, constitutes *tissue fluid*. The main mucopolysaccharides are hyaluronic acid and sulphated compounds. The basement membranes underlying epithelium and surrounding capillaries can be considered a special type of ground substance.

Among the *specialized* types of connective tissue are included dense connective tissue (of the dermis and submucosa), regular connective tissue (tendons and fibrous membranes), elastic tissue (*ligamentum flavum* and vocal cords), reticular tissue (of lymphoid tissue), adipose tissue, pigment tissue (in eye), and laminae surrounding epithelial elements of various organs. If scleroderma is a disorder of connective tissue one would expect disturbance to occur in the various sites where this tissue is situated.

Biochemical Features †

At any given moment the various components of the intercellular substances are in the processes of formation and breakdown so that precursors and breakdown products are also present. The connective tissue is best

---

* Electron microscopists usually refer to *micro-fibrils* as *fibrils*.

† This description is based on standard texts, particularly the chapter by Bornstein: *Duncan's Diseases of Metabolism*. Sixth edition, 1969. Detailed references may be obtained therein.

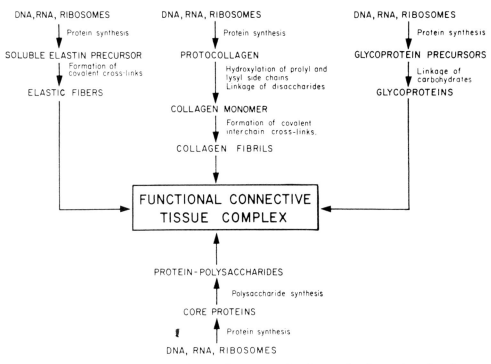

Figure 4–1. The contribution of several macro-molecules to the formation of a functional connective tissue complex. Reproduced with permission from Bornstein, P.: Duncan's *Diseases of Metabolism*, 6th ed. Philadelphia, Saunders, 1969.

regarded as a functional complex of the various components as summarized in the following scheme (Fig. 4–1).

The four main components of the intercellular substance (collagen fibrils, elastic fibres, protein-mucopolysaccharide complexes and glycoproteins) will be discussed briefly.

I. *Collagen*

1. *Distribution and Function:* Collagen is widely distributed through practically all tissues of multicellular organisms. One of its prime functions appears to be supportive, binding parenchymatous elements together and giving the appropriate rigidity and other physical properties. In subcutaneous tissue, the fibres are sparse and loosely arranged; in dense connective tissue the fibres are closely packed and parallel to give the appropriate tensile strength; in the cornea, the fibres are regularly spaced resulting in optical transparency; in bone, collagen fibres are so arranged that they form a basic framework for the regular arrangement of crystals of calcium salts. A collagen-like protein is found in the glomerular basement membrane of blood vessels. Collagens from different tissues show different properties, but this is believed to be due to specific macro-molec-

ular organization of the protein rather than to differences in chemical composition.

2. *Structure of Collagen Molecule and Fibril:* The human collagen molecule is believed to consist of three polypeptide chains (two γ chains and one β chain) each with a molecular weight of approximately 95,000 (collagen monomer). Each chain consists of a left-handed *minor helix* composed of approximately one thousand amino acid residues. The three minor helices are twisted around a common central axis to form a right-handed major helix (collagen molecule; molecular weight approximately 280,000). Collagen molecules aggregate in a specific way: by intermolecular interactions involving amino acid side chains to form fibrils. Observed under the electron microscope, fibrils vary in diameter and demonstrate a characteristic banding pattern with a periodicity of sixty-four to seventy nm. It is suggested that this is due to a *quarter-stagger array* of individual molecules, resulting in *overlap zones* and pale zones (Fig. 4–2).

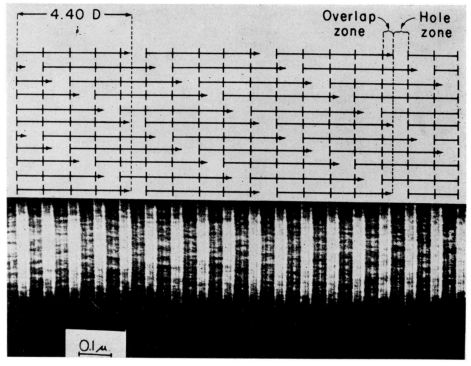

Figure 4–2. Negative contrast electron micrograph of a native collagen fibril stained with sodium phosphotungstate, pH 7.0. The light zones correspond to regions of greater molecular density. The staggered arrangement of the collagen molecules results in the appearance of electron dense zones (overlap zones) and electron sparse zones (hole zones). Reproduced with permission from Bornstein, P.: in Duncan's *Diseases of Metabolism,* 6th ed., 1969. Adapted from Hodge *et al.* in *Structure and Function of Connective Tissue.* London, Butterworths.

3. *Amino Acid Composition and Sequence:* Collagen consists of twenty different amino acids of which glycine comprises one-third and the sum of proline and hydroxyproline one quarter. Tyrosine and tryptophan are sparse and cysteine and cystine absent. The amino acid sequence has not been determined in full, but one-third of the molecule is an orderly arrangement of "triplets" of amino acids in which glycine is present as every third amino acid (position 1), proline occupies position 2 and hydroxyproline (or occasionally another amino acid) occupies position 3.

4. *Metabolism:* (a) Biosynthesis: Collagen is synthesized by fibroblasts through the intervention of collagen messenger R.N.A. The details are still incompletely understood, but an important point is that during the assembly of individual amino acids, proline takes the place eventually to be occupied by hydroxyproline. The protein at this stage is referred to as *proto-collagen.** The appropriate proline groups are then hydroxylated by the enzyme protocollagen proline hydroxylase to produce collagen. Ascorbic acid is required for the activity of this enzyme.

(b) Degradation: A fraction of the collagen can be dissolved in cold neutral salt or weakly acid solution, presumably by breaking inter-molecular bands. In most normal adults only a few percent of the total collagen can be dissolved in this way, but in young growing animals or in tissues undergoing rapid remodelling, a greater proportion of collagen can be dissolved. This is believed to indicate a more rapid turnover in these cases, with a larger fraction of recently synthesized, and therefore incompletely cross-linked, collagen. Collagen is relatively insusceptible to the action of common mammalian enzymes. However to avoid continued accumulation, synthesis must be balanced by breakdown and, in fact, collagenolytic activity has been found in skin and other tissues.

(c) Turnover, urinary hydroxyproline: Provided that ingested gelatin is excluded, the urinary excretion of hydroxyproline as peptides would be expected to serve as an index of collagen breakdown. Recently it has been suggested that collagen fragments can be resorted and re-utilized without breakdown to peptides and amino acids. This would limit the use of urinary hydroxproline as an index of collagen catabolism.

II. *Elastin*

1. *Distribution and Function:* Elastin is less widely distributed than collagen. Elastic fibres are prominent in ligaments, skin and tunica media of arteries. The main function is apparently to produce elastic recoil so that the tissue returns to its previous shape after deformation.

---

* Some workers now believe that protocollagen is an artefact produced in the presence of inhibitors.

2. *Structure of Elastin Molecules and Fibres:* Very little is known of the molecular configuration. Elastic fibres consist of intercommunicating fibrils loosely twisted together to form cords.

3. *Amino Acid Composition:* There is a very high content of apolar amino acid residues (glycine, alanine and valine comprise 80 percent), and a corresponding low content of charged amino acid residues. Glycine comprises one third of the amino acid residues but hydroxyproline contributes only one to two percent in contrast to nine percent in collagen. Amino acid sequence data and other chemical studies are limited. Desmosine, isodesmosine and related compounds formed by interaction of amino acid residues play an important part in the secondary structure of the molecule.

4. *Metabolism:* Elastin is synthesized by fibroblasts as a soluble precursor, but is rapidly polymerized extracellularly. There is evidence that it is also synthesized by smooth muscle. It is relatively inert metabolically. Turnover is required for remodelling during development, but a specific elastase has not been shown in mammalian tissues except the pancreas.

III. *Mucopolysaccharides*

1. *Distribution and Function:* Mucopolysaccharides * constitute the major component of the ground substance of connective tissues, where they are linked to protein to form protein-polysaccharide † complexes. The types of mucopolysaccharides differ in various tissues. They influence the metabolism of cells by affecting molecular transport particularly of water and electrolytes. They are related to the fibrillar elements in determination of the physical properties of the tissue. The resiliency of cartilage can be attributed to the ability of protein-polysaccharides (stabilized by collagen fibres) to trap water and exclude large molecules. Hyaluronic acid is an important lubricant of joints and possibly of tissue planes. Protein-polysaccharides apparently protect cartilage from calcification and may play a similar role in other tissues. Certain mucopolysaccharides have specific important biological properties such as the anti-coagulant and anti-lipaemic functions of heparin.

2. *Chemical composition:* All mucopolysaccharides are composed of long chains of alternating hexosamine and uronic acid groups (sometimes sulphated or acylated). The composition of the different mucopolysac-

---

* † In recent biochemical literature mucopolysaccharides are termed *glycosaminoglycans*, and protein-polysaccharide complexes are termed *proteoglycans*. The old terms have been retained here as they are probably more familiar to most medical readers.

TABLE III *

COMPOSITION AND DISTRIBUTION OF FIVE
COMMON MUCOPOLYSACCHARIDES

Name	*Hexosamine*	*Uronic Acid*	*Predominant Distribution*
Hyaluronic acid	N-Acetylglucosamine	D-glucuronic acid	Vitreous humour Synovial fluid Umbilical cord Skin
Chondroitin 4-sulphate	N-Acetylgalactosamine -4-sulphate	D-glucuronic acid	Cartilage Bone Aorta
Chondroitin 6-sulphate	N-Acetylgalactosamine -6-sulphate	D-glucuronic acid	Cartilage Heart valves Aorta
Dermatan sulphate	N-Acetylgalactosamine -4-sulphate	L-iduronic acid	Skin Heart valves Lung Tendon
Keratan sulphate †	Galactose N-Acetylglucosamine -sulphate	None	Cornea Cartilage Nucleus pulposus

† Keratan sulphate is unusual in that galactose in substituted in place of a uronic acid.
* Adapted from Bornstein, P.; Disorders of connective tissue, in *Duncan's Diseases of Metabolism*, 6th edition. Bondy, Saunders, Philadelphia, p. 677.

charides varies according to the type of glucosamine and of uronic acid. Five common types found in skin are shown in Table III.

Because of the heterogeneity of the complex, the precise nature of the protein component in ground substance is not fully known. However the amino acid composition is different from that of collagen or elastin. It has been suggested that multiple polysaccharide chains possibly of different nature extend outwards from a central protein core.

3. *Metabolism:* A. Biosynthesis: Synthesis depends on the activity of the fibroblasts or, in cartilage and bone, by chondrocytes or osteoblasts. The intermediate stages and enzymatic steps in the production of hexosamines and uronic acids from sugars are now reasonably well known. The metabolic turnover of protein-mucopolysaccharides is more rapid than that of fibrous proteins. The rate of synthesis of various mucopolysaccharides is influenced by hormones. The sex hormones, insulin, corticosteroids and thyroid hormone have all been shown to have some effect.

B. Degradation: The degradation of mucopolysaccharides and protein-polysaccharide complexes is better understood than that of the fibrous proteins. Testis and a number of other mammalian tissues contain lysosomal enzymes capable of degrading hyaluronic acid and chrondroitin sulphate. Proteases capable of degrading the protein moiety of the complexes have been found in cartilage and other tissues.

C. Urinary excretion: Urinary excretion of mucopolysaccharides in a normal adult varies from five to twenty mg. per twenty-four hours. Approximately ninety percent of this is chrondroitin sulphate plus chondroitin but there is also a measurable amount of other mucopolysaccharides.

IV. *Glycoproteins*

According to a recent review (Spiro, 1970) "glycoproteins can be simply defined as proteins which have carbohydrate covalently attached to their peptide portion." They are widely distributed in the body: plasma fibrinogen, globulins, hormones, enzymes, mucins, connective tissue proteins, extracellular and cellular membranes. The carbohydrate units range from mono-saccharides or disaccharides to complex units. In most glycoproteins there are many amino acids per carbohydrate unit. If the hexuronic acids are included in the list of sugar elements, the mucopolysaccharide-proteins would be included in the glycoproteins. However, the marked differences in the structure of the carbohydrate units of the protein-polysaccharides from those of other glycoproteins justify their consideration as a special group (as has been done above). Collagen which is also included among the glycoproteins in the review cited has already been discussed. In addition to these special glycoproteins, other glycoproteins are present in connective tissue. These include aorto-glycoproteins, acid glycoproteins of bone, traces of the numerous glycoproteins occurring in the plasma as immunoglobulins and hormones, tissue enzymes, and components of cell membranes. Further discussion of these numerous and complex proteins is beyond the scope of this work.

CONNECTIVE TISSUE DISTURBANCE IN SCLERODERMA

Collagen Disturbance

One of the most characteristic features, clinically, of scleroderma is stiffness of the skin and one of the most characteristic features on histological examination is an alteration in appearance and an apparent increase in amount of collagen (See Chapter III). Hence it has seemed reasonable to various workers that some clue to its pathogenesis might be obtained from study of collagen, which might be altered in quality or in amount, and, in either case, may have an altered metabolic turnover. The observations concerning these possibilities will be reviewed.

The Quality of the Collagen

PHYSICAL PROPERTIES: Rasmussen *et al.* (1964) excised strips of skin parallel to the skin creases in normal subjects, patients with scleroderma and with keloids and scars and studied the isotonic and isometric contraction in a water bath at various temperatures. They found that in the scleroderma patients all the parameters studied were normal. These comprised temperature at which rapid shrinkage begins, total amount of isometric contraction, rate of change of tension with temperature and maximum tension developed per millimetre thickness. By contrast, in scars and keloids all these values were decreased, this being a characteristic of young collagen.

Recently, Neal (1973) has made an important study of the abnormal skin compliance in scleroderma. Strips of skin from a patient with scleroderma showed a greatly decreased compliance (measured by increase in length with increase in tension) when compared with specimens from control subjects. Microscopic examination of the skin under polarized light showed the fiber structure in the scleroderma patient to be comparable to that in control subjects, but there was wide separation of fibrils, which tended to obscure fiber boundaries and contribute to the "illusion" of homogenization.

The main differences were shown in horizontal sections, where collagen fibers were shown to be arranged in interlacing plates. In normal skin this was only well seen when the skin was fixed in the stretched state, whereas in scleroderma it was equally obvious in the stretched and unstretched state. When fresh specimens from controls were examined microscopically during stretching, the fibers and plates were seen to slip over each other, but this did not occur in scleroderma. Since the fibers were not apparently structurally abnormal, it would seem that this inability to slip under tension resulted from increased interfiber bonding, probably due to a qualitative abnormality of the ground substance.

ELECTRON MICROSCOPY AND X-RAY DIFFRACTION FINDINGS: Fisher and Rodnan (1960) stated that the electron microscopic appearance of collagen fibrils from scleroderma patients was normal. Braun-Falco and Rupec (1964) also found that fine structure of the fibrils was normal, but there was abnormality of fibril diameter so that as well as fibrils with a normal maximum thickness of eighty nm to ninety nm, there were also groups of finer fibrils with maximum diameter of fifty nm to eighty nm. Fleischmajer (1964a) found the X-ray diffraction picture of collagen fibres in the affected skin of patients with scleroderma was the same as in the apparently normal skin of the same patients. More recently Fleischmajer *et al.* (1971) found the main abnormality in scleroderma in the subcutaneous tissue where the fibrils were more numerous and finer than normal. Hayes and Rodnan (1971) counted fibrils of different diameters in homogenates of skin from scleroderma patients, normal subjects and in human embryo skin. In the scleroderma patients there was a higher proportion of finer fibrils giving a profile similar to that in embryos (Fig. 4–3). Also they observed a large number of thin fibrils (twenty nm to forty nm in diameter) with incomplete cross banding pattern (Fig. 4–4) and also embryonic *beaded filaments* (Fig. 4–5).

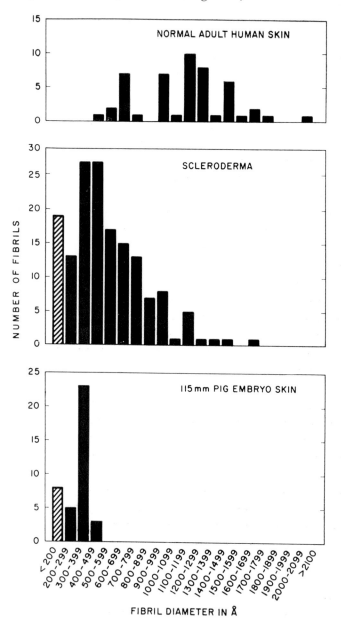

Figure 4–3. Profiles of populations of pooled collagen fibrils from (A) normal adults, (B) scleroderma patients and (C) human embryos. Reproduced with permission from Hayes and Rodnan, 1971, *Amer J Path*, 63:433–440.

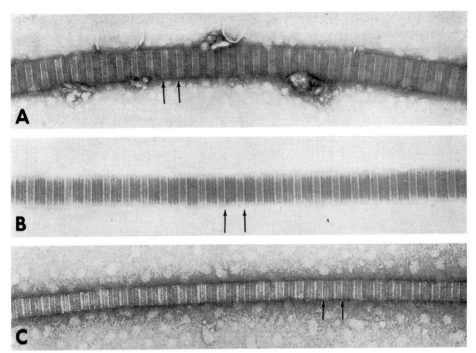

(1) Mature collagen fibrils: A. Control: 38 year old male. B. 20 year old female with scleroderma. C. 55 year old female with scleroderma. All fibrils reveal normal 640Å (64 nm) periodic cross-banding pattern (arrows) with normal intraperiod cross striations (x 76,250).

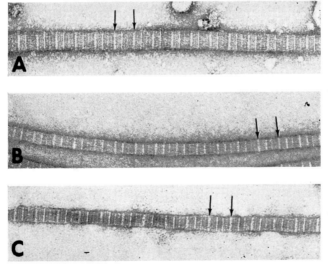

(2) Thin collagen fibrils, 200–500Å (20–50 nm) in diameter: A. 10 week human foetus. B. 150 mm. foetal pig. C. 20 year old female with scleroderma. These fibrils are not observed in adult control tissues. Although 640Å (64 nm) periodic striation pattern is established (arrows), intraperiod cross banding is incomplete. Reproduced with permission from Hayes and Rodnan, 1971, *Amer J. Path*, 63:433–440.

Figure 4–4. Collagen fibrils from skin biopsies revealed by negative staining of un-fixed dermal homogenates.

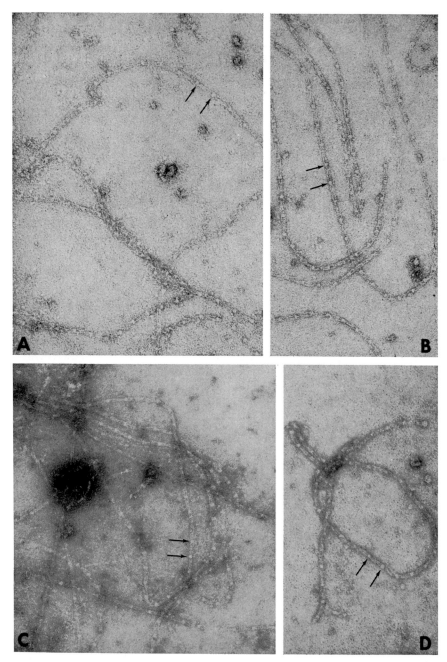

Figure 4–5. Beaded filaments revealed by negative staining of unfixed dermal homogenates. A. 10 week human foetus. B. 115 mm. foetal pig. C. 50 year old female
with scleroderma. D. 29 year old female with scleroderma. Note double strands,
30–40Å (3–4 nm) in diameter joined at 640Å (64 nm) intervals (arrows) by single
spherical beads 120–140Å (12–14 nm) in diameter. These structures are not seen in
homogenates of adult control tissues (x 76,250). Reproduced with permission from
Hayes and Rodnan, 1971, *Amer J Path,* 63:433–440.

CHEMICAL QUALITIES: Fleischmajer (1964a) found the water content and the amino acid composition of affected skin in scleroderma patients to be the same as in the unaffected skin of the same patients. Neldner *et al.* (1966) also found the amino acid content of dermis from scleroderma to be normal. Although these studies were done on dermis and not on collagen, one would expect any abnormality in composition of the collagen, which is the main constituent, to show up in the amino acid analysis of the skin.

Much attention has been paid by some workers to solubility studies. When compared with normal subjects the proportion of soluble collagen in the skin from scleroderma patients varies according to the solvent used. Various workers (Korting *et al.*, 1964; Laitinen *et al.*, 1966; Uitto *et al.*, 1967; Uitto *et al.*, 1971) have reported an increased proportion of collagen soluble in weak salt solution in scleroderma patients compared to that in normal subjects. However Harris *et al.* (1966) reported a reduced proportion of collagen soluble in dilute acetic acid in scleroderma compared with control subjects. Following penicillamine treatment there was an increase in the acid-soluble collagen believed by the authors to be due to disruption of intermolecular bands. The significance of these observations, which have usually been made on small numbers of subjects, is not clear. One interpretation of the increased proportion of collagen soluble in weak salt solutions is that it is young collagen, based on the finding that there is a higher proportion of such soluble collagen in young than in old persons. The decreased amount of collagen soluble in weak acetic acid has not been explained. Protein solubility is usually minimal at the iso-electric point. It could be that the iso-electric point of collagen in scleroderma is closer to the pH of dilute acetic acid than normal collagen.

The Quantity of the Collagen

There is lack of uniformity among workers in the method of expressing the collagen content of the skin — per unit of wet weight, volume, dry weight or surface area.

The weight of collagen per unit wet weight will depend on the hydration of the tissue. In established disease, the water content is apparently normal (Fleischmajer, 1963; Harris and Sjoerdsma, 1966a). Unless there is a marked change in density (which has not been demonstrated) weight per unit volume will have the same significance as weight per unit wet weight. The ratio of weight of collagen to dry weight will indicate the ratio of the content of collagen to the content of total solids (collagen plus ground substance), and will be altered by a disproportionate change of these two components. It is apparent that these values depend on the proportion of collagen and non-collagen and do not give a measure of the actual collagen content of the skin. A determination of collagen content per unit area would seem to be the appropriate measurement for this purpose. But there are difficulties. One would have to ensure that the core of tissue went to the bottom of the dermis. Also caution would be necessary in extrapolation from the content of a small biopsy area to that of the whole limb. Because of reduction of the coarse and fine skin wrinkles in scleroderma patients, the ratio of skin surface to volume would tend to be decreased.

Most of the studies have expressed the collagen content in terms of weight of hydroxyproline per unit of dry weight (mg. per one hundred gm. or µg per mg.). These have shown either slight (probably not significant) decrease (Fleischmajer, 1964a, Harris and Sjoerdsma, 1966b) or no change (Laitinen *et al.*, 1966; Laitinen *et al.*, 1969; Uitto *et al.*, 1967; Uitto, Helin *et al.*, 1970).

Black *et al.* (1970) measured the thickness of the skin of the radial aspect of the forearms in thirteen women with systemic sclerosis. They then took biopsies with a punch of five mm diameter from these regions in twelve of these patients and determined the hydroxyproline content. Skin specimens were subdivided into those from areas *affected* and *not clinically affected* by systemic sclerosis. It was possible to determine the thickness of the skin (mm), collagen per unit surface area (µg per sq. mm) collagen percent of fat-free dry weight, and collagen per unit volume (µg. per c.mm). Compared with values in normal controls, the skin in the affected regions was thin, and the collagen per unit area reduced, but the collagen per unit weight normal. In the non-affected regions, the skin was slightly thinner than normal, but the other values did not differ significantly from normal. Their findings in systemic sclerosis are in contrast with those of Shuster *et al.* (1967) in morphoea, where there is an increased content per unit area (mg. per sq. mm.). in some of the active plaques.

The finding by Black *et al.* of decreased thickness of the skin and decreased collagen content per unit area in scleroderma is contrary to the general impression of increased skin thickness and collagen content in this disease. It should be noted that in the study of Hayes and Rodnan (1971) that in each of five cases where the weight of a seven mm. diameter plug from the dorsum of the forearm from a scleroderma patient was compared with that of a plug from a similar site in a non-affected relative, the skin plug from the scleroderma patient was heavier, indicating (unless there was a change in density) that it was thicker. It would seem that further studies are necessary to decide the simple matter of skin thickness in scleroderma.

Metabolism

TISSUE METABOLISM: Tissue metabolism of collagen has been investigated along two lines: (a) by measuring the rate of synthesis of collagen as indicated by the rate of incorporation of radio-actively labelled proline and (b) by measurement of the activity of the enzyme protocollagen proline hydroxylase, which is concerned in the final stage of collagen synthesis. Uitto *et al.* (1967) found that when ^{14}C-proline was incubated with skin in a Krebs-Ringer bicarbonate medium for ten hours the mean specific activity of the ^{14}C-hydroxyproline produced was more than three times as great in skin from scleroderma patients than from healthy subjects. Laitinen *et al.* (1969) similarly reported increased incorporation ^{14}C-proline into scleroderma skin and (in one case) that the same degree of incorporation occurred into the soluble and insoluble fractions. However Keiser and Sjoerdsma (1969) found increased incorporation of ^{14}C-proline into the skin in only three of thirteen patients with scleroderma. The highest incorporation occurred in patients with very active disease; it was greater in the affected forearm skin than in the apparently unaffected buttock skin of the same patient.

The activity of the enzyme protocollagen proline hydroxylase has been assayed in punch biopsies of human skin by a method involving determination of the amount of ^{14}C-hydroxyproline produced from ^{14}C-labelled protocollagen substrate. Uitto and his co-workers (Uitto *et al.*, 1969; Uitto, Hannuksela and Rasmussen, 1970) found increased activity in certain cases of scleroderma. Keiser *et al.* (1971) found a marked increase (about four-fold) of the activity of this enzyme in the forearm skin of twenty patients with scleroderma when compared with similar skin from control subjects, but also an increase (two-fold) in the clinically unaffected (presacral) skin when compared with skin from the same area from control subjects. Stein *et al.* (1970) found that although the serum protocollagen proline hydroxylase activity was increased in liver disease, it was not significantly raised in scleroderma.

The characteristics of connective tissue metabolism in scleroderma have been studied in a tissue culture preparation (Leroy, 1971). A striking increase in soluble collagen (as indicated by the media hydroxyproline) was observed in eight of nine scleroderma cultures when they were compared with identically handled controls matched for age and sex of the donor and the anatomic site of the donor skin. "Glycoprotein" content as estimated by hexosamine and sialic acid was also significantly increased in the scleroderma cultures.

BLOOD LEVELS OF COLLAGEN-LIKE PROTEIN: Keiser *et al.* (1963) found a collagen-like protein in human plasma. However, Sjoerdsma *et al.* (1965)

found that the level of this protein is normal or low in scleroderma. Holzmann *et al.* (1967) reported that the content of collagen-like protein (CLP) in the serum of scleroderma patients was normal or low but increased during treatment with gestagens.

URINARY HYDROXYPROLINE: Urinary total hydroxyproline excretion, while the patient is taking a gelatin free diet, has been used as an index of collagen catabolism. Under these conditions, the hydroxyproline absorbed from the gut is minimal and appears in the blood as free hydroxyproline, which is almost completely reabsorbed from the renal tubules. On the other hand, hydroxyproline from tissue sources appears in the blood mainly as peptides, which are reabsorbed from the renal tubules in much smaller amounts and as much as twenty percent is excreted in the urine (Sjoerdsma *et al.*, 1965). Ziff *et al.* (1956) found no significant difference in the urinary excretion of total hydroxyproline in a group of eight patients with collagen diseases (including three with scleroderma) compared with a group of eight normal adults. Rodnan and Cammorata (1963) found increased excretion of total hydroxyproline in only three of sixteen patients with progressive systemic sclerosis, two of whom had rapidly progressive disease. Keiser and Le Roy (1965) found increased excretion in only one of seven patients with scleroderma. Smith *et al.* (1965) found that among nineteen patients with scleroderma (including seven of the morphoea type) excretion was increased in only three patients, one of whom had systemic sclerosis in an active stage and also a leg ulcer. Uitto *et al.* (1967) found the urinary total hydroxyproline was raised in five of fourteen cases.

Comments

It will be seen that in spite of earlier studies to the contrary, recent electron microscopy studies indicate a morphological difference in collagen from patients with scleroderma, consisting of an increased proportion of fine fibrils and the presence of extremely fine beaded fibrils characteristic of embryonic tissue. These findings are consistent with the chemical findings of an increased proportion of collagen soluble in weak salt solution, both being capable of interpretation as an increased amount of young collagen.

In spite of expectations to the contrary, most studies have shown the collagen content (per unit dry weight, or per unit volume) does not differ significantly from normal. One group have found that the skin of scleroderma patients, at least in the forearms, is thin and that, although the collagen content expressed as a proportion of the dry weight or content per unit volume is normal, the amount of collagen to unit of area is reduced. Since the total surface area (of a limb or body) is certainly not increased, but probably decreased due to lack of folds and wrinkles, this leads to the rather astounding conclusion that the collagen content of the whole skin in scleroderma is reduced. This cannot be extrapolated to the whole body as recent work suggests an increase (on basis of histological and electron microscopic examination) of the collagen in subcutaneous tissue. However the findings of other workers suggest that the skin thickness may be increased and further work is required to decide the question.

Studies on collagen metabolism have given rather inconsistent results. Recent studies are in agreement in the increased activity of the enzyme protocollagen proline hydroxylase involved in the final stage of synthesis of collagen. Although increased synthesis of collagen has been demonstrated, one study has shown this in only a minority of cases, with active disease. Similarly, increased urinary excretion of hydroxyproline regarded as an index of collagen breakdown has only been demonstrated in a minority of cases, usually with active disease.

Ground Substance Disturbance

As outlined in the introductory part of this chapter, the major part of the ground substance is composed of protein-mucopolysaccharide complexes and, in parallel with the studies on collagen disturbance, studies have been carried out on ground substance, particularly mucopolysaccharides. The summary of reports from the literature will be presented in a manner similar to those concerning collagen.

Qualitative Change

Stoughton and Wells (1950) using the McManus stain for mucopolysaccharides could detect no abnormality in the skin specimens from nine cases of localized and generalized scleroderma. Laskin *et al.* (1961) measured intra-dermal electrical potential and its time course following injection of hyaluronidase. They reported an abnormally low negative potential in scleroderma and very slow recovery of the decreased potential following injection of hyaluronidase and believed that this was evidence for abnormal ground substance.

In a histological and electron microscopic study, Fleischmajer *et al.* (1971) found that the changes in scleroderma occurred mainly in the subcutaneous tissue, and affected not only collagen fibres, but also ground substance, both of which were increased at the expense of fat cells. Areas in this region frequently stained "positively" with P.A.S. and Alcian blue stains. On electron microscopy the ground substance showed "an increase in electron opacity".

Quantitative Change

Boas and Foley (1954) stated that "hexosamines" were increased in the corium and subcutaneous tissue in scleroderma. Fleischmajer and Krol

(1967) found increased hexosamines in the total dermis in five of seven scleroderma patients and increase in collagen bound hexosamines in all of six cases studied.

Metabolism

TISSUE METABOLISM: Animal studies have shown that ^{35}S is incorporated into the mucopolysaccharide, chondroitin-sulphate. Denko and Stoughton (1958) used the incorporation of ^{35}S into skin as an index of mucopolysaccharide metabolism. They found that in progressive systemic sclerosis, there was greater incorporation into *affected* skin than normal skin. This contrasted with morphoea, where the greatest incorporation was in non-affected skin.

Kreysil *et al.* (1973) studied the biosynthesis of mucopolysaccharides and collagen in skin slices from sixteen healthy subjects and ten patients with progressive scleroderma, using auto-radiographic histochemical and radiobiological methods. They found that the mucopolysaccharides (glycosaminoglycans) and collagen synthesis was markedly higher in the skin of the patients than in that of the controls. In all cases (controls and patients) synthesis was highest in the corium, intermediate in the prickle cell layer, and least in the basal cell layer.

BLOOD LEVELS: Winkelmann and McGuckin (1965) found elevated levels of total serum protein-bound hexoses in scleroderma and that these correlated with prognosis. Balabanov and Samsonova (1965) found elevations of serum mucoproteins in all of eighteen patients studied.

URINARY EXCRETION: The method of determination and expression of results varies between workers, the results being expressed as mucopolysaccharides, hexosamines or glucuronic acid.

Thompson *et al.* (1966) found that the mean value of *non-dialyzable urinary mucopolysaccharide* in nineteen patients with scleroderma did not differ significantly from normal subjects, but there was a tendency to increased excretion in patients with active progressive disease. Ohlenschaeger and Friman (1968) found a normal urinary excretion of acid mucopolysaccharides in generalized scleroderma. However Holzmann *et al.* (1968a) found urinary mucopolysaccharide levels raised in six of eight patients. Wessler (1967) found a definite increase in excretion of *acid glycosaminoglycan* expressed as mg. uronic acid per gm. creatinine in one case of diffuse scleroderma. In a recent study, Hardy *et al.* (1971) found the urinary levels (expressed in the same terms) were raised above the control normal range on one or more occasions in thirty-four of forty patients with scleroderma and that the patients showing the highest levels were the most severely affected.

Glycoproteins in Scleroderma

As explained in the preliminary discussion, glycoproteins form such a varied and complex group that study of glycoproteins in general would not be expected to yield useful information. Fleischmajer (1946b) reported increased serum α_2 glycoproteins in scleroderma, but Holzmann *et al.* (1968a) reported normal values.

Comment

In spite of the lack of staining abnormalities, there would seem to be consistent evidence of disturbance in ground substance, particularly muco-polysaccharides, in scleroderma. This evidence includes reports of abnormal reactivity (in terms of resting electric potential and response to hyaluronidase injection), increased content, increased turnover, increased blood levels and, in the majority of reports, increased urinary excretion. Unfortunately, in many instances the findings on a particular aspect are limited to single or very few reports and further work to confirm these findings is required. As in the case of collagen, the main site of the abnormality may not be in the skin but deeper in the subcutaneous tissue.

Although the more obvious findings in light and electron microscopy are in the collagen, it is possible that the primary disturbance may be in the mucopolysaccharides of the ground substance. These may influence fibril formation (Öbrink, 1973), may contribute to their appearance and through their bonding action may be largely responsible for the altered physical characteristics of the tissue.

Chapter V

VASCULAR DISTURBANCE

As MENTIONED in the historical introduction, the association of vascular disturbance and scleroderma was recognized early. Some of the patients with ischaemic digits described by Raynaud had sclerodermatous changes and Hutchinson stressed the relationship of Raynaud's phenomenon to scleroderma. The vascular disturbances associated with scleroderma have continued to evoke interest, and studies have been made on the clinical aspects, vasomotor responses and pathological features. The microcirculation has been investigated both in patients using the technique of capillaroscopy and in histological sections.

References to certain aspects of the vascular disturbance will be found in various chapters of this book (Historical, Pathological, Systemic Involvement), but since it is possible that circulatory changes may have fundamental importance, it is considered worthwhile to group the various relevant observations together in one chapter.

Clinical Manifestations

Vascular disturbance is one of the most important clinical features in progressive systemic sclerosis. Raynaud's phenomenon is a common early symptom. The ischaemic attacks may precede the development of skin changes, both may occur concurrently or, rarely, the skin changes may occur first. In the later stages, Raynaud's phenomenon may be replaced by more persistent cyanosis and coldness of the extremities. Other features such as ulceration, gangrene, atrophy of bone, metastatic calcification may be related to circulatory disturbances. These various aspects will be discussed more fully later when dealing with the clinical aspects of systemic involvement.

Another prominent vascular feature is the presence of telangiectases. These are particularly numerous in the Thibierge-Weissenbach syndrome of scleroderma associated with calcinosis. Recently this association has been emphasized in the description of the *C.R.S.T. syndrome* (calcinosis, Raynaud's phenomenon, scleroderma, telangiectasia). However telangiectasia is also common in long-standing scleroderma without calcinosis.

Vascular disturbance plays a prominent part in some of the visceral manifestations of scleroderma as in the acute renal failure and hypertension which is sometimes the terminal event and in right heart failure due to pulmonary hypertension. However, disturbance of the visceral circulation has been demonstrated in the absence of these florid manifestations. Urai *et al.* (1958) found reduction in renal flow (as indicated by para-amino hippuric acid clearance) in patients with scleroderma without renal failure and pulmonary hypertension is frequent, even in the absence of heart failure (Sackner *et al.*, 1964).

Pathological and Arteriographic Studies

The findings by Matsui of thickening of walls and narrowing of the lumen of small arteries and arterioles in skin and viscera and the confirma-

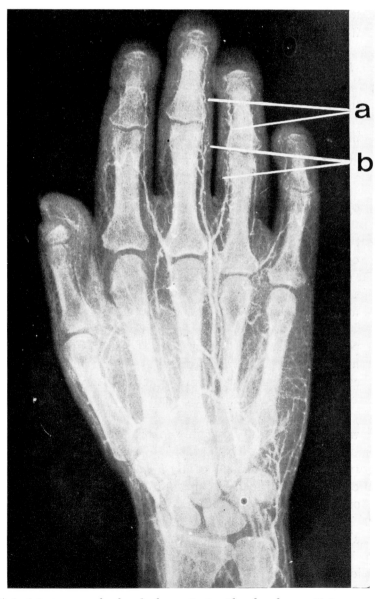

Figure 5–1. Arteriogram of a hand of a patient with scleroderma. Note narrow digital arteries (a) which show blocks in some regions (b).

tion of these findings by Lewis in the case of arteries in the fingers have already been described in the section of the pathology. Similar arterial changes were later described in viscera. The narrowing of the arterial lumen demonstrated pathologically has been confirmed during life by arteriographic studies of the peripheral vessels (Vogler and Gollman, 1953; Barnett, 1959; Schober and Klüken, 1966) (Fig. 5–1). Changes have also been shown in renal arteries (Rodnan, 1966).

Functional Studies

Early workers were interested in the vascular responses to heat and cold in patients with scleroderma and related conditions. Brown *et al.* (1930) found that heat elimination from the hand was low and that the *vasomotor index* (rise in skin temperature per degree rise in oral temperature during artificial pyrexia) was low. He argued that this indicated a structural occlusive element as well as spasm. Lewis and Landis (1931) recorded the volume change in the index finger associated with the digital pulse at different temperatures and found that there was a greatly diminished response of this pulse volume change in scleroderma, and believed that this was evidence for a structural change. Prinzmetal (1936) found that circulatory changes similar to those in scleroderma could be produced by the application of an elastic band and believed that tightness of the skin was important in producing the vascular insufficiency.

Barnett (1959) studied the reactions of the peripheral vessels in scleroderma by observing the effect of immersion of the hands in cold water, by an arterial occlusion reactive hyperaemia test and by measuring the heat elimination from the hand by calorimetry (Table IV). Exposure to cold produced an abnormal degree of pallor or cyanosis in all cases. The time taken for flushing of the finger tips in response to an arterial occlusion reactive hyperaemia test was longer than normal. Calorimetry usually showed a low resting heat elimination and always an impaired response to indirect heating. The results were interpreted as indicating structural arterial narrowing or occlusions, which were demonstrated in some of the patients by arteriography.

The low peripheral blood flow and subnormal response to heat has also been demonstrated by plethysmographic studies (Jablońska and Kisiel, 1957; Kózménska, 1968). More recently isotope methods have been used to measure tissue blood flow. Coffmann (1970) using a Na ^{131}I washout method, found a reduced forehead and fingertip blood flow, but a normal forearm skin and subcutaneous tissue blood flow, even though the forearm was clinically affected. This indicated that the reduction in blood flow and the sclerosis did not run parallel. LeRoy *et al.* (1971) using a ^{133}Xe method, found a low Xe clearance when the finger was cooled, but a normal clearance on warming, although the skin temperature remained lower in

TABLE IV*

VASCULAR RESPONSES OF HANDS IN PATIENTS WITH SCLERODERMA

Case	Type	Effect of Immersion in Cold Water (15° C.)	Response to Reactive Hyperaemia Test†	Heat Elimination (Cal./100ml./min.)	
				Resting‡	From Reflex§ Hyperaemia
1	1	Cyanosis	Normal	11.2	16.3
2	1	"	"	7.6	28.6
3	1	"	"	22	37
4	1	No change		8 / 1	80 (early stage)a / 2 (later stage)b
5	1	Cyanosis	Delay in some digits	10	15
6	1	"	"	15	40
7	1	"	"	2.3	2.7
8	1	"	Delay	9.5	14.8
9	1	"	—	2.9	4.6
10	1	Slight cyanosis	Delay in one digit	11.8	32.2
11	1	Cyanosis with patches of pallor	Delay in some digits	4.1	5.1
12	1	Cyanosis	Delay in one digit	28.9	26.5
13	1	"	Normal	7.1	7.4
14	2	Cyanosis and pallor	Delay	14.9	25.3
15	2	Pallor of some digits	Delay in some digits	6	6
16	2	Cyanosis and pallor	Delay	4	10
17	2	Slight cyanosis	Normal (early stage)c / Slight delay (later stage)d	6 / —	22 / —
18	2	Cyanosis	Normal	5.4	7.2
19	2	"	Slight delay	8.7	10.1
20	2	"	Delay	6.3	18.7
21	3	—	Delay	22	18
22	3	Cyanosis	Slight delay in some digits	4.5	5.6
23	3	"	Normal	21.7	21.7
24	3	"	"	5.8	36.4
25	3			24.5	22.8
26	3			6.5	28.5

† Reactive hyperaemia test: Hands immersed in water at 35°C. for 10 minutes, application of arterial occlusion cuff during immersion for a further 10 minutes, followed by rapid deflation of cuff.

‡ Resting heat elimination: Examination room at 23°C., initial calorimeter temperature 27°C.

§ Reflex hyperaemia test: Immersion of other arm and forearm in water at 44°C. for 20 minutes.

(a) On presentation. (b) After an interval of 2 years. (c) On presentation. (d) After an interval of 3 years.

* Modified from Barnett, A. J.: Alfred Hospital Clinical Reports, 9:33–74, 1959.

the scleroderma patients than in control subjects. These findings are difficult to explain and seem inconsistent with the evidence of other workers
of structural arterial narrowing.

In general, the pathological and arteriographic studies indicate that
there are structural changes of small arteries in scleroderma. However the
part played by the other factors mentioned is conjectural. Tightness of
skin is probably not very important in causing ischaemia as Raynaud's
phenomenon and gangrene of fingertips are often prominent in the early
stages when sclerosis of the skin is minimal. Whether a functional abnormality is also present in the early stages is not proven. Although ischaemic
episodes may result from excessive responsiveness to cold or sympathetic
nervous stimulation, these can also be due to a normal response of the
structurally narrowed small vessels.

Capillaroscopy

In this technique, the skin of the nailfold is cleared by the application
of oil and the vessels are observed in the living state directly by microscopy. Early observations were made in 1925 by Brown and O'Leary who
described nailfold capillaries in normal people, the changes in *diffuse primary scleroderma* and *Raynaud's phenomenon associated with scleroderma
changes*. In normal subjects there was a regular palisade arrangement of
the capillary loops. In *diffuse primary scleroderma* the number of loops
was reduced, giant loops were present and capillary blood flow was slow.
In *Raynaud's phenomenon associated with scleroderma changes* the loops
were less reduced in number, giant loops were less frequent and sluggish
flow (*stasis*) was more marked. They believed this indicated a difference
between these two conditions, although it seems that the changes were
largely a matter of degree. Ross (1966) discussed nailfold capillaroscopy
as an aid in the diagnosis of collagen diseases based on a study of ten
cases. He found that in subacute lupus erythematosus there was disorderly
arrangement of loops beyond the most distal row, in dermatomyositis the
dilated capillaries were not abnormal in form but increased in number
and in systemic sclerosis the capillaries varied in shape and size but were
generally dilated, with slow blood flow and associated haemorrhages.

Buchanan and Humpston (1968) reported a study of the nailfold capillaries in these conditions based on a larger number of subjects (systemic
lupus erythematosis: twenty-nine, scleroderma: fourteen, dermatomyositis:
seven). They found that in normal subjects the diameters of the capillary
loops formed a unimodal curve, but in the connective tissue diseases there
was a bimodal curve with a normal group and a dilated group. At the tips
of the dilated capillaries there were often appearances of successive
haemorrhages. Loop size and presence of haemorrhages did not appear to
provide a basis for separation of the three diseases.

Recently a detailed account of the abnormalities found on capillaro-scopic examination in scleroderma and other rheumatic diseases has been written by Redisch *et al.* (1970) (based on a study of progressive systemic sclerosis: twenty-five cases, *localized* scleroderma: six cases; rheumatoid arthritis: thirty-one cases; systemic lupus erythematosis: thirty-four cases; psoriatic arthritis: nine cases; dermatomyositis: three cases). They divided the changes into rheological and morphological (related to shape, size and number of capillaries). The prominent rheological features in progressive systemic sclerosis were sluggish flow, dusky colour of the blood, cellular aggregation, widening of all three limbs of capillary loops and paucity of capillaries. There was overlap between the various conditions studied in respect to frequency and severity of the abnormalities. The best criterion for separation of systemic sclerosis from the other conditions was the combination of diminished number of loops and presence of enlarged loops which was found in all the cases of systemic sclerosis but only six percent of the cases of rheumatoid arthritis and psoriatic arthritis.

Electron Microscopy

Recent studies of the micro-vasculature by electron microscopy have confirmed the dearth of capillaries and presence of dilated capillaries, and have also shown basement membrane changes and endothelial swelling. Norton *et al.* (1966) found a characteristic laminated appearance of capillaries in muscle from all of eight patients with scleroderma but without clinical muscle involvement or histological changes as demonstrated by light microscopy. These changes were found only infrequently in patients with rheumatoid arthritis or in normal subjects.

Serotonin as a Possible Agent in the Vascular Changes

Serotonin has been suggested as a possible causative agent of the vascular changes in scleroderma. It can produce some of the circulatory changes found in scleroderma: contraction of skin vessels (Winkelmann, 1971), pulmonary hypertension (Page, 1958), decreased renal blood flow (Page and McCubbin, 1953). Also injection of serotonin into normal skin causes fibrosis (Fleischmajer and Hyman, 1961; Scherbel, 1961; Mac-Donald *et al.*, 1958).

Carcinoid tumours have been found in patients with scleroderma (Zarafonetis *et al.*, 1958; Hallen, 1964; Hay, 1964; Asboe-Hansen, 1959), but these would constitute only a minute fraction of all the patients with this disease.

If increased levels of serotonin were indeed a factor, one would expect Raynaud's phenomenon and scleroderma to be common accompaniments of the carcinoid syndrome but this is not so. Conversely the characteristic symptoms of serotoninaemia (violaceous flushing of face and chest and intestinal hurry) are not found in scleroderma. Also if serotonin were responsible for the changes in scleroderma, one would expect either evidence of an increased serum concentration due to increased production or decreased breakdown or an increased sensitivity of the vessels to serotonin. Tuffanelli (1963) found the serum level of this substance to be normal in scleroderma, but Birk (1966) reported a slight increase.

The evidence is against excessive serum serotonin levels as a factor in the vascular changes in scleroderma. The question of possible abnormal vascular responsiveness to normal serotonin levels, and perhaps other vasoactive substances, needs further investigation. The possibility of participation of serotonin or the catecholamines in the vascular disturbances in scleroderma has prompted the study of metabolic pathways involving these substances in patients with this disease (See Chapter XIII).

SUMMARY

From the above survey, it is apparent that from whatever aspect it is studied (clinical, pathological, physiological), there is evidence of abnormality of blood vessels in scleroderma. This involves vessels of various sizes from small arteries to capillaries. The disturbance is widespread being found in skin, muscles and viscera. A strong case can therefore be made out for regarding scleroderma as a vascular disease. Recently the vascular disorder in scleroderma has been reviewed in detail by Norton and Nardo (1970) who sum up by enumerating the following well documented points:

1. "The frequency of vascular abnormalities is inversely proportional to the size of the blood vessels studied."
2. "Vascular abnormalities can be clearly demonstrated in the absence of sclerosis."
3. "The systemic nature of progressive systemic sclerosis is reflected by the distribution of vascular abnormalities as well as by the systemic distribution of sclerosis."
4. "The classic findings of progressive systemic sclerosis (sclerosis and parenchymal atrophy) are well known sequels of vascular dysfunction."

They conclude that "sufficient evidence exists to implicate the vascular system as a primary target organ in the disease."

While agreeing that vascular features play a very important part in the pathology and clinical features of scleroderma we would not accept (nor do Norton and Nardo) that they are the only "primary target organ." We have been impressed (as was Matsui many years ago) by the lack of parallelism between the connective tissue changes and the vascular changes and adopt a *dualistic* approach that both the vascular and connective tissue changes are targets some as yet unknown noxious agent.

Chapter VI

IMMUNOLOGICAL DISTURBANCE

IN RECENT YEARS there have been numerous papers describing immunological features of scleroderma and some authors have classified scleroderma and other connective tissue diseases among the auto-immune diseases. Before describing the immunological features of scleroderma and discussing their significance, the background will be provided by a short outline of (a) the development of the concept of the connective tissue diseases as a clinical group and (b) the concept of auto-immunity.

CONNECTIVE TISSUE DISEASES AS A
GROUP AND RELATED IMMUNOLOGICAL DISTURBANCE

Classically, diseases have been classified according to their aetiological basis or the organ involved. Diseases such as rheumatic fever, systemic lupus erythematosus and diffuse scleroderma do not fit into such classifications as their aetiology is unknown and they affect various organs. Klemperer *et al.* (1942) suggested that these diseases could be grouped together as *diffuse collagen diseases.* He considered that connective tissue (composed of cells, fibres and ground substance) formed a *system,* present in various organs (in a similar fashion to the haemopoietic system occurring in various parts of the body). Rheumatic fever, systemic lupus erythematosus and scleroderma were diseases of this system, thus explaining the multiple-organ involvement. In rheumatic fever, the characteristic lesion was the Aschoff nodule, in systemic lupus erythematosus it was fibrinoid necrosis and in diffuse scleroderma connective tissue proliferation. They emphasized that because the diseases affected the same system, this did not mean that they were the same, or even related, in other aspects (in the same way as diseases of the haemopoietic system may not be related apart from the fact that they affect a common system).

About the same time Arnold Rich was making observations on the pathological changes associated with experimental serum sickness and compared these changes to those in human serum sickness, drug sensitivity and certain diseases—periarteritis nodosa, rheumatic fever, disseminated lupus erythematosus, rheumatoid arthritis (Rich, 1947). Some of these had been included by Klemperer *et al.* in the group *diffuse collagen disease.* He showed that there was much overlap of clinical and pathological features in the conditions listed and that focal collagen degeneration, necrosis and inflammation of arteries occurred in all. He suggested that *anaphylactic hypersensitivity* might be the common de-nominator. Modern writers would use the term *immunity,* which at that time still retained its original connotation of protection from harmful influences. The concept of connective tissue diseases was thus broadened and they were linked with that of *immunity,* an association which has influenced much thinking on these conditions since.

AUTO-IMMUNITY AND ITS RELATION TO THE CONNECTIVE TISSUE DISEASES

In the early period of the study of immunology, it was considered that an animal was incapable of producing antibodies to its own tissues. This idea was epitomised in the term *horror auto-toxicus* coined by Ehrlich and Morgenroth in 1901.

In the mid 1950's certain observations indicated that there were ex-ceptions to the general rule that the body could not form antibodies to its own tissues. First, it was shown that certain haemolytic anemias were due to antibodies in the serum which could be demonstrated by Coomb's antiglobulin test to have adhered to the surface of red cells. A second example was the demonstration that in the serum of patients with Hashimoto's thyroiditis there were antibodies which reacted with thyro-globulin. A third example was the finding that the factor in the serum of patients with subacute lupus erythematosus responsible for the *L.E. test* was an immunoglobulin. This test depends on the phagocytosis of nuclear material by granulocytes, and it is now believed that this occurs following interaction between the nuclear material and an antibody (antinuclear factor, A.N.F.) in the serum. Later this antinuclear factor was demonstrated by other means, including the immunofluorescence method, and auto-antibodies have since been demonstrated in a variety of diseases.

Of particular interest in the present context are the connective tissue diseases. It had already been postulated that these had a *hypersensitivity* (= immune) basis. Auto-antibodies were consistently found in one type, systemic lupus erythematosus. It was therefore reasonable to search for these antibodies in other connective tissue diseases, and, as will be shown presently, these have been found, although not with the same consistency as with systemic lupus erythematosus.

In the case of a particular type of haemolytic anaemia (now called auto-immune haemolytic anaemia) and Hashimoto's thyroiditis, the anti-bodies were directed against the cells showing pathological change and it seemed reasonable to suppose they were harmful (although this was not clear in other instances, including the connective tissue diseases). A new term was therefore introduced into medical literature, *auto-immune dis-ease,* to include those diseases mentioned above and others in which auto-immune phenomena are demonstrable. The concept of auto-immunity as a cause of disease has been expounded by Mackay and Burnet in their now classical book *Auto-immune Diseases, Pathogenesis, Chemistry and Therapy.*

How it comes about that the body produces antibodies to its own tissues (*self*) is not clear, and has been the subject of much discussion among immunologists. Broadly the abnormality may lie in two spheres: the stimulus or the response.

According to the abnormal stimulus hypothesis, the antigenic stimulus from normal tissues might be enhanced so that it becomes exceptionally strong or antigens from infecting organisms may cross-react with tissue antigens, or the tissue antigens may be modified by various agents (infecting organisms, drugs, physical injury). Various examples of the presence of auto-antibodies in diseases of known aetiology could be explained on this basis. Thus in the experimental production of antibodies by the injection of homologous or heterologous tissue, resort is often made to the effect of Freund's adjuvant which forms a chronic granuloma and presumably enhances the stimulus. The presence of auto-antibodies in chronic inflammatory diseases, particularly syphilis and leprosy, may be due to enhancement of the antigenic stimulus of normal tissues by granulomas. Streptococci isolated from a patient with acute rheumatic fever have been shown to have antigens that cross-react with antigens in the human heart. Certain drugs, particularly hydralazine, produce a syndrome similar to systemic lupus erythematosus including the occurrence of the *L.E. phenomenon.* This may be explained on the basis that the drugs modify the patient's nuclear material to make it antigenic.

The second hypothesis involves the response. According to Burnet's clonal hypothesis, clones (or cell lines) able to react against *self* antigens, are constantly eliminated (*forbidden clones*). If surveillance breaks down and these forbidden clones proliferate, auto-antibodies are able to develop and auto-immune disease develops. The details and merits of these hypotheses are beyond the scope of this monograph.

SOME MODERN IMMUNOLOGICAL CONCEPTS AND TERMS

The science of immunology is rapidly developing and the ideas becoming increasingly more complex. Immune responses are believed to be mediated by special cells or immunocytes (lymphoid cells or plasma cells) which are initially produced in foetal liver and bone marrow, are located during early life in the thymus or bone marrow and eventually reside in lymphoid tissue or circulate in the blood. These cells are functionally differentiated into two classes: (1) those derived from thymus (*T cells*) are responsible for cell mediated immunity and reside in *thymus* dependent areas of the spleen and lymph nodes; (2) those derived from the bone marrow (*B cells*) are responsible for humoral antibody production and reside mainly in the corticomedullary junction and medullary cones of the lymph nodes and the red pulp of the spleen.

In cell mediated immunity sensitized lymphocytes proliferate in the lymph glands, migrate to the tissues containing the antigen, react with the antigen to produce a soluble substance which stimulates macrophages and initiates the inflammatory reaction. Cell mediated immunity is involved in various delayed sensitivity reactions, homograft rejection and probably in various auto-immune states.

In humoral antibody production, contact of the appropriate immunocytes with the antigen in some way stimulates them to produce antibodies which circulate in the plasma. These are globulins (the immunoglobulins) and are divided into five main classes designated IgG, IgM, IgA, IgD and IgE with differing structure and involvement in different types of immune reactions. Humoral antibodies are involved in antibacterial, antitoxic and anaphylactic reactions, serum sickness and in auto-immune states.

IMMUNOLOGICAL DISTURBANCE IN SCLERODERMA

The immunological disturbances in scleroderma may be grouped as follows: those related to antibody formation (auto-antibodies, other serological changes, abnormal levels of immunoglobulins), those related to cellular immunity, genetic aspects related to immunity, and association with other diseases with immunological disturbance. Experimental observations made in animals which are possibly related to scleroderma will be mentioned.

A. Features related to antibody formation

Auto-antibodies in serum

A constant feature in systemic lupus erythematosus is the *L.E. cell* described by Hargraves *et al.* (1948). *L.E. cell* formation has since been shown to be dependent on the presence of antinuclear antibodies.

Since, as outlined above, scleroderma had already been linked (by Klemperer *et al.* in 1942) with systemic lupus erythematosus as a connective tissue disease, and it had been suggested (by Rich, 1947) that at least in some connective tissue diseases, hypersensitivity (immunity) played an important role, it was natural to look for the effects of auto-antibodies resulting in *L.E. cells* in other connective tissue diseases including scleroderma. Rowell (1962) found *L.E. cells* in three of sixteen patients with scleroderma (although two of these had some features suggestive of clinical systemic lupus erythematosus in addition to scleroderma) and was able to find four other case reports.

Friou *et al.* (1958) used a more sensitive test (fluorescent antibody test) for demonstration of antinuclear antibodies in systemic lupus erythematosus, and this test has since been used to detect the presence of these antibodies in other connective tissue disturbances. He obtained a positive test in twenty seven of twenty eight patients with systemic lupus erythematosus, in a small production of patients with rheumatoid arthritis and patients with allergic drug reactions, and in one patient with scleroderma. Bardowil (1958) found these antibodies in two of three patients with scleroderma, and various other workers have since demonstrated a variable incidence of auto-antibodies in this disease.

The test has been modified and refined by various workers and it is now believed that there are at least four patterns of nuclear staining, each depending on a different antibody reacting with a different nuclear antigen as listed in Table V.

TABLE V

PATTERNS OF FLUORESCENT NUCLEAR ANTIBODY STAINING

Staining Pattern	*Nuclear Antigen*	*Reference*
Homogeneous (diffuse)	Desoxyribonucleoprotein	Beck (1961, 1969)
Nucleolar	Ribonucleic acid (R.N.A.)	Beck (1961, 1969)
Speckled	Saline-soluble extract	Beck (1962)
Shaggy	Desoxyribonucleic acid (D.N.A.)	Casals *et al.* (1963)

Ritchie (1968) has shown that the homogeneous staining depends on two antinuclear antibodies (nodular and reticular) acting in conjunction. Burnham *et al.* (1969) using the tumour imprint technique have described a fifth nuclear staining pattern, *thready*. The relative incidence of the various types of nuclear staining pattern varies with different diseases. The *speckled* pattern is the most common one in scleroderma. Some of the observations on antinuclear antibodies in scleroderma are listed in Table VI.

Ritchie (1970) found both antinuclear antibodies and antinucleolar antibodies in scleroderma. Although the antinuclear antibody (A.N.A.) was more common than antinucleolar antibody (A.N.$_o$.A.), with incidence 87 percent and 54 percent respectively, the A.N$_o$.A. was more specific. The incidence of positive tests in scleroderma found by different observers varies, no doubt to some extent on the technique and criteria for accepting as positive. Using a sensitive technique Ritchie (1967) found weakly positive tests (titre of less than $\frac{1}{16}$) for antinuclear antibody in a high proportion of normal subjects and patients with non-rheumatic disease, but none had a titre above this level which was taken as the dividing line for a significant positive test. McGiven *et al.* (1968) found that in all of their

TABLE VI

LIST OF REPORTED OBSERVATIONS OF FLUORESCENT
ANTIBODY REACTIONS IN SCLERODERMA

Author(s)	Year	Test tissue	Incidence	Main type of fluorescence
Bardowil *et al.*	1958	Various (human & rabbit)	4 of 6	Not specified
Alexander *et al.*	1960	Leucocytes from healthy donor	2 of 3	Not specified
Hall *et al.*	1960	Normal human skin	7 of 10	Not specified
Beck *et al.*	1963	Rat liver	25 of 32 (78%)	Homogeneous
Rowell & Beck	1967	Rat liver	32 of 48 (67%)	Homogeneous (26) Speckled (17) Antinucleolar (8)
Ritchie	1967	Immature rat liver	53 of 55 (96%)	Speckled (70%) or homogeneous (30%)
Burnham *et al.*	1968	Tumour imprint	Approx. 30%	Speckled 24% Speckle-like and thready 9%
Rothfield & Rodnan	1968	Mouse liver	28 of 47 (60%)	Speckled
McGiven *et al.*	1968	Rat liver	12 of 33 (36%)	Speckled
Burnham *et al.*	1969	Tumour imprint	72 of 95 (76%)	Not specified Thready in 17.
Ritchie	1970	Immature rat liver	21 of 24 (87%)	Not specified Antinucleolar in 13.
Bäumer and Brinkmann	1970	Mouse Liver	13 of 27* (48%)	Speckled in 11.
Jordan *et al.*	1971	Guinea pig liver	31 of 27 (48%)	Speckled

* Based on figures for patients in which A.N.F. was anti-IgG. (In some patients anti-IgM was also found).

twelve positive scleroderma cases, the antibody belonged to the IgG class. Others (Rothfield and Rodnan, 1968; Bäumer and Brinkmann, 1970) have found both IgG and IgM.

Other auto-antibodies are sometimes found in the sera of patients with scleroderma. The commonest is the rheumatoid factor which was found in fourteen of thirty-three patients by McGiven *et al.* (1968) and in ninety-two of 265 cases (35 percent) by Clark *et al.* (1971). McGiven *et al.* also found anti-thyroid cytoplasm antibodies in two cases, anti-gastric parietal cell in one and both these antibodies in two cases.

The auto-antibodies discussed above are detected by reacting the patient's serum with an extraneous antigen preparation, for example in the test for antinuclear antibodies with a source of nuclei from animal liver or tumour cells. It would be of interest to know whether antibodies in scleroderma patients reacted with the patient' own cells, particularly at a site of pathological change. Raskin (1964) found that sera from four patients with scleroderma (and immunological disturbance indicated by a positive antinuclear factor) failed to react with dermal vessels or connective tissue, although in two cases fluoresence was observed in eccrine sweat glands. McGiven *et al.* (1968) also were unable to demonstrate any antibody antigen reaction when sera from patients with scleroderma (including some with positive antinuclear factor) was applied to the skin of patients with scleroderma or control subjects.

Antigen-antibody complexes in tissue

As mentioned above, auto-antibodies are γ-globulins and their presence in tissues can be demonstrated by reacting the tissues with fluorescein-labelled antisera to the various human immunoglobulins. If auto-antibodies were responsible for pathological change one would expect to find them in the affected tissue.

However, Fisher and Rodnan (1960) could find no preferential localization of γ-globulin in the skin of patients with scleroderma and McGiven *et al.* (1968) obtained a similar negative result. Fennell *et al.* (1961) used the immunofluorescent technique for detection of the deposition of fi-

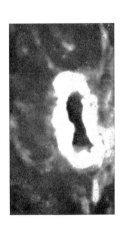 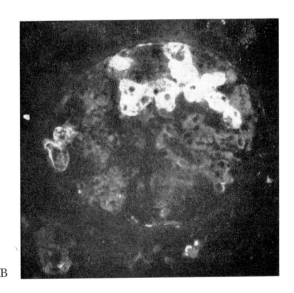

A   B

Figure 6–1. Fluorescent staining of (A) a small renal artery and (B) glomerular capillaries in sections of kidney from a patient with scleroderma dying in renal failure. The sections had been treated with fluorcein-labelled anti-human gamma globulin. Reproduced with permission from McGiven *et al.*, 1971, *Pathology*, 3:145–150.

brinogen and globulin in three patients with scleroderma dying from renal failure. Positive reactions were obtained for fibrinogen but not for globulin, the findings being the same as in three patients with malignant hypertension. However, McGiven *et al.* (1971) found accumulation of immuno-globulins (mainly IgM) and complement in glomeruli, small arteries and arterioles in two patients with scleroderma from my clinic, who died with renal failure (Fig. 6–1); albumin and fibrin were not found in these areas. However in a subsequent case from this clinic (unreported) also dying in renal failure, immunoglobulins were not detected.

Complement

The presence of an immune process may also be indicated by complement fixation. Kunkel (1964) found positive complement fixation reactions in a variety of diseases with auto-immune features, including scleroderma, in which there was a fifty percent incidence of positive results. Townes (1967) found a low complement level in only two of seventeen patients with progressive systemic sclerosis, and that the mean level of complement was normal. This suggests that antigen-antibody reactions involving complement are not taking place to any marked degree in this disease.

Plasma concentrations of immunoglobulins

If scleroderma is an immunopathy it might be expected that the concentrations of immunoglobulins would be raised, as manifested by an increase in concentrations of the total γ-globulins or of the individual immunoglobulins.

Zlotnick and Rodnan (1961) found an increased γ-globulin concentration (1.48 to 3.4 gm. percent) in eight of fifteen cases, Barnett and Coventry (1969) values over 1.6 gm. percent in thirteen of thirty-one cases (40 percent) and Clark *et al.* over 1.6 gm. percent in eighty-two of 313 cases (26 percent). Spencer and Winkelmann (1971) determined the levels of the individual immunoglobulins by the radial diffusion method in twenty-two patients with scleroderma. There was no consistent pattern, the means being close to the normal values. However two of five patients with *diffuse systemic sclerosis*, both very ill and dying within a few weeks of the determination, had markedly raised IgG levels. Three of the seventeen patients with acrosclerosis had definitely raised IgM levels.

The lack of consistent elevation of the total γ-protein levels or of individual immunoglobulins is not surprising in view of the variability in positive tests for auto-antibodies. There does not seem to have been a study on the relation between plasma levels of particular immunoglobulins and the presence of auto-antibodies. However no close relationship would be expected as the auto-antibodies probably only contribute a fraction to the total antibody content.

B. Cellular Immunity in Scleroderma

As outlined in the early part of this chapter, modern immunological theory recognizes a second major component of the immune response, cellular immunity, in which contact between the immunologically competent cells (lymphocytes) and antigen sets in action a train of events leading to tissue damage. Cellular auto-immunity is more difficult to demonstrate than humoral (or antibody) auto-immunity. Although methods have recently been established for studying cellular immunity in vitro, detailed studies of their use in scleroderma are not yet available.

As described in Chapter III accumulation of lymphocytes are common in tissues of the patients with scleroderma, but the view that these are immunologically active is only presumptive. Biggart and Nevin (1967) found hyperplasia of the thymus gland with numerous and greatly enlarged lymphoid follicles in a man with progressive systemic sclerosis dying from cardiac failure and suggested that this was indicative of an immunological disturbance.

Tuffanelli (1964) injected autologous leucocytes from thirteen patients with scleroderma into the volar aspect of the forearm, and recorded the response at twenty-four and forty-eight hours, as in the case of the tuberculin test which is regarded as the classical example of cell-mediated immunity, a positive result being an area of induration and redness of at least ten mm diameter. Positive results were obtained in all of the thirteen patients with scleroderma and negative results in all of twelve normal subjects. Biopsy of the test areas in the reactors showed leucocytic infiltration in the dermis and subcutaneous fatty tissue. The reaction was apparently specific for the leucocytes, as there was no reaction to plasma or red blood cells.

C. Experimental observations of possible significance

Animal experimentation has not been very helpful in the problem of immunity in scleroderma. Collagen is only a weak antigen and it has proved difficult to produce tissue injury by a collagen-antibody reaction. Rothbard and Watson (1959) found that when rabbit anti-rat collagen antiserum with Freund's adjuvant was injected into a rat, renal damage ensued. This did not occur when either the Freund's adjuvant or antiserum were injected separately. They suggested that a reaction between the rat's collagen and antiserum occurred in the kidney, but this did not result in damage. However in the presence of Freund's adjuvant, the collagen-antibody complex acted as a second antigen and a second antibody was produced in the rat and the resulting large antibody-antigen complex resulted in damage. The bearing of this experiment on scleroderma would seem remote. There is no evidence that the collagen in scleroderma is acting as an antigen and it has not been possible to demonstrate preferential accumulation of immunoglobulin attached to collagen fibres in the skin. Schmitt *et al.* (1964) suggested that the weak antigenicity of collagen might be due to the antigenicity residing in side chains which were mainly occupied in binding molecular units together to form collagen fibrils. They were able to produce antibodies (in the rabbit) to purified calf tropocollagen, presumably because these side chains had been exposed.

Stastny *et al.* (1963) suggested that *homologous disease* in the experimental animal might serve as a model for human auto-immune disease. Homologous disease was produced as follows. An intra-peritoneal injection of lymphoid cells from inbred donor rats was given to a recipient rat in the neo-natal period. This produced tolerance to the donor strain as evidenced by the fact that the recipient, when aged two months, would accept a graft from a donor strain animal. At four months, the recipient animal received an intravenous injection of spleen and lymph node cells from a donor strain animal. This produced *homologous disease*. Although the recipient rat was tolerant of the injected cells, the latter were not tolerant of the tissue of the recipient animal. Various skin lesions, acute and chronic, occurred in the recipient animal. There was histological similarity between the acute skin lesions and those of subacute lupus erythematosus and between the chronic skin lesions and scleroderma. These observation are of great interest and would fit in with the concept (see later) that the fault in auto-immune disease is in the immunocyte response rather than in the antigenic stimulus. In homologous disease the immunocytes are introduced from outside into an animal rendered tolerant to them, but which they (the immunocytes) regard as *foreign*. According to one modern theory (Burnet, 1969) abnormal immunocytes (forbidden clones) are somehow allowed to develop, and these immunocytes react against body tissues as if they were foreign. However caution should be exercised in accepting the skin lesions of homologous serum disease as the counterpart of scleroderma and as evidence that scleroderma is an auto-immune disease. Epidermal atrophy and dense collagen in the dermis are rather non-specific findings following damage. The story would be more convincing if the animals suffering from *homologous disease* followed for a longer time were found to develop visceral lesions similar to those in scleroderma.

D. Genetic Aspects

As explained in Chapter II, familial incidence is rare in scleroderma and it is therefore not considered to be a hereditary disease. There is, however, a familial relation in several so-called auto-immune diseases (Mackay and Burnet, 1963). It is therefore of interest to know if there is any evidence of auto-immune disturbance in relatives of patients with scleroderma.

Fennell *et al.* (1962) studied the occurrence of antinuclear factors in the relatives of patients with systemic rheumatic disease. They found an incidence of positive tests in twenty-nine of fifty (58 percent) in first degree relatives of twelve patients with progressive systemic sclerosis. This was surprisingly high, being more than in some series of scleroderma patients and more than in relatives of rheumatoid arthritis patients (47 percent) or patients with systemic lupus erythematosus (42 percent).

There have been occasional reports of the familial association of scleroderma with other diseases suspected of having an immunological basis. Thus Leonhardt (1961) reported a case in which the mother had scleroderma, mildly toxic goitre and Sjögren's syndrome and the son had dermatomyositis, two other near relatives had goitre and one had rheumatoid arthritis. Hagberg *et al.* (1961) recorded a case in which the mother suffered from scleroderma and Sjögren's disease and the daughter from systemic lupus erythematosus.

Burch and Rowell (1963) suggested "tentative partial interpretation of the genetic aspects" of four supposed auto-immune diseases (scleroderma, systemic lupus erythematosus, chronic discord lupus erythematosus and Hashimoto's thyroiditis) based on the known sex incidence and the relative frequency of occurrence in each sex for each decade. This however is highly speculative.

E. Scleroderma associated with other diseases with immunological disturbance

There have been various reports of association in the same patient of scleroderma and other diseases showing immunological disturbance, which comprise not only other connective tissue diseases, but also Hashimoto's thyroiditis and auto-immune haemolytic anaemia. One of our patients has features of scleroderma, Sjögren's disease and rheumatoid arthritis. Some of the reported associations are shown in tabular form below (Table VII).

Sharp *et al.* (1971) have described a group of twenty five patients with "mixed connective tissue disease" with features of scleroderma, systemic lupus erythematosus and myositis. Most had antinuclear antibody and five had a positive *L.E. test*. They had a high titre of antibody to extractable nuclear antigen (E.N.A.), whereas no patients with *classical* scleroderma showed antigen to extractable nuclear antigen. This and other overlap syndromes will be discussed more fully in Chapter XIV.

TABLE VII

REPORTED OBSERVATIONS OF ASSOCIATION OF SCLERODERMA WITH
OTHER DISEASES SHOWING AUTO-IMMUNE DISTURBANCE

Authors	Year	No. of Patients	Associated Diseases						
			Scl.	Sj.	DM	RA	SLE	Ha	AIHA
Fridenberg & Wintrobe	1955	1	+						+
Shearn	1960	2	+	+					
Burnim	1961	2	+	+					
Tuffanelli & Winkelmann *	1962	36	+		+				
		2	+				+		
		31	+			+			
		7	+	+					
		1	+					+	
Steiner et al. †	1967	1	+						+
Westerman et al.	1968	1	+						+
Chaves et al.	1970	1	+						+
Chlorzelski & Jablonska	1970	1	+			+	+		

Scl. = scleroderma, Sj. = Sjögren's disease, DM = dermatomyositis, RA = rheumatoid arthritis, SLE = systemic lupus erythematosus, Ha = Hashimoto's thyroiditis, AIHA = auto-immune haemolytic anaemia.

* The largest number of cases of scleroderma associated with other diseases in this Table, reported by Tuffanelli and Winkelmann, is based on review of 727 patients with systemic sclerosis (scleroderma) from the Mayo Clinic.

† Other features in this case included porphyria cutanea tarda, chronic leukopenia, hypogammaglobulaemia.

COMMENT: IS SCLERODERMA AN AUTO-IMMUNE DISEASE?

This chapter opened with a statement that scleroderma was considered by some to be an auto-immune disease. This proposition can now be considered in the light of the evidence presented above. It is necessary to define first what is meant by auto-immune disease. In their monograph Mackay and Burnet (1963) provisionally defined auto-immune disease as a condition in which structural or functional damage is produced by the action of immunologically competent cells or antibodies against normal components of the body. It will be noted that the definition does not include aetiology but lays the emphasis on *damage* by the immunological process. The authors recognize the possibility of extraneous causative factors, at least to the extent of an initiating process and state "auto-immune disease may arise spontaneously, but frequently there is an initiating or triggering process." These factors may be infection, chronic sepsis, pregnancy, minor injuries, drugs, cancer. However "once initiated, auto-immune disease tends to be self perpetuating." Mackay and Burnet discuss the two possibilities of whether the auto-immune state is due to an abnormal stimulus to antibody production or whether the abnormality is in the antibody-producing cells and reach the following conclusion: "Everything in fact points to auto-antibodies arising as a result of abnormal activities of the antibody-producing cells and not as a result of stimulating normal antibody-producing cells by an abnormal antigen."

Without being dogmatic on the point, they believe that the theoretical aspects of abnormal antibody production are best explained by the application of a *modified clonal selection* approach (that is, the appearance of forbidden clones of antibody-producing cells).

Mackay and Burnet recognize that it is usually impossible to establish the pathogenic role of either cells or antibody by direct methods and have enumerated certain *markers*, characteristics commonly observed in auto-immune conditions. These are listed in summarized form below:

1. Plasma γ-globulin level above 1.5 gm. per one hundred ml.
2. Presence of demonstrable *auto-antibody* against a body component.
3. Deposition of denatured γ-globulin or its derivatives, which probably include amyloid, at sites of election such as the renal glomerulus.
4. Accumulations of lymphocytes and plasma cells.
5. A significant transient or lasting benefit from treatment with cortico-steroid drugs.
6. Frequent occurrence of more than one type of auto-immune manifestation in the same individual.

While admitting that these *markers* are abitrary, it is of interest to note how scleroderma scores on this basis.

1. Raised γ-globulin is found in approximately one quarter to one half of the cases of scleroderma.
2. Auto-antibodies (mainly antinuclear factor) are commonly found, the frequency varying greatly from 35 percent to over 90 percent depending on the sensitivity of the technique. It should be remembered here that using a highly sensitive technique auto-antibodies of low titre may be found in a considerable proportion of normal people, in which case a positive result means a level about the normal range.
3. Deposition of *denatured γ-globulin* in renal tissue does not seem to be a feature of scleroderma. In fact the demonstration of immunoglobulin in glomeruli and renal vessels has only recently been reported, but further investigation along these lines is required.
4. Accumulations of lymphocytes are frequently observed in scleroderma, particularly in the oesophagus and skeletal muscle, but they do not appear to be prominent in other tissues showing marked damage, such as skin and kidney.
5. Treatment with corticosteroids has a marked beneficial effect on some of the acute manifestations such as joint pains and prolonged treatment is associated with some regression of the skin stiffness in the diffuse form. However no benefit has been demonstrated on the vascular or visceral manifestations.
6. There have been frequent reports of the association of scleroderma with other diseases showing auto-immune phenomena.

It will be seen that scleroderma scores moderately high in respect to some *markers* (1, 2, 6) and low in respect to others (3, 4, 5). Mackay and Burnet (1963) state "the evidence for immunopathy in scleroderma is circumstantial and rather meagre." Recent work has multiplied the reports of immunological disturbance in scleroderma, but the overall picture remains much the same.

Although the incidence of positive tests for antinuclear antibodies in scleroderma has increased with increasing sensitivity of the tests, there is usually no evidence that they are doing harm. In fact it has not been possible to demonstrate an antigen-antibody reaction in the dermis in this condition. One report of deposition of immunoglobulin in renal vessels and glomeruli in two patients dying in renal failure suggests that accumulation of antigen-antibody complexes at these sites may be a factor in the impaired renal function. However these observations have not been repeated, and fulminating renal failure is a rather rare complication in scleroderma.

In many of the reports on auto-antibodies in scleroderma, the authors have commented on the fact that their presence or concentration did not seem to correlate with the severity of the clinical condition. If one accepts the proposition that auto-immunity is an essential part of scleroderma, one encounters the difficulty of explaining the considerable proportion of such patients without auto-antibodies and, on the other hand, the presence of these antibodies in normal subjects, including relatives of scleroderma patients. After considering the evidence summarized above, we reach the conclusion that, although auto-antibodies are frequently demonstrated in scleroderma, there is no evidence in most cases that they are harmful and, accepting the criterion that there must be damage by the immune process to designate a condition as auto-immune, the evidence in the case of scleroderma must be considered inadequate.

Two observations not included in the immediately preceding discussion are the delayed (tuberculin-type) reaction produced by injecting leucocytes from a patient with scleroderma into his own forearm, and the production of scleroderma-like lesions in the skin of the experimental animal by the production of homologous disease. These observations, if confirmed, could prove a starting point for further investigation of immunological aspects of scleroderma, with special emphasis on cell mediated immunity rather than on humoral antibodies.

Chapter VII

CLASSIFICATION AND COURSE

PROBLEMS IN CLASSIFICATION

T HE DIFFICULTIES OF EARLY WORKERS in classifying scleroderma, aggravated by the use of numerous ill-defined terms, has been mentioned in the historical summary.

One of the notable attempts to classify scleroderma was made by Sellei (1931, 1934) who distinguished between *scleroderma verum, acrosclerosis,* and certain other conditions not included by him as scleroderma, but with somewhat similar skin changes or confusing names. *Scleroderma verum* as described by Sellei was a purely dermatological condition with no systemic involvement. The skin changes were asymmetrical and might be circular (*scleroderma circumscriptum*), ribbon-like (*scleroderma en bandes*) or irregular (*scleroderma diffusum*). Variations of this condition included *morphoea* (round plaques surrounded by a lilac ring) and *scleroderma papiraceum* (hard plaques like cardboard). In contrast with scleroderma verum he described *acrosclerosis* which comprised Raynaud's phenomenon, sclerosis of the fingers and face and was frequently accompanied by "involvement of the heart and aorta." He also discussed certain conditions sometimes confused with scleroderma, including *scleroedema adultorum* (a brawny oedema of the neck and dorsal region, sometimes following acute infections).

Scleroderma in which the skin changes affect predominantly the trunk, or the trunk equally with the extremities, associated with systemic disturbance, has been termed *diffuse systemic scleroderma*. This is *not* the same as the *scleroderma diffusum* of Sellei which referred to a subgroup of his *scleroderma verum*, a dermatological condition.

Possibly due to misreading of Sellei's paper and the term *diffuse* being applied to different conditions, there was uncertainty in the minds of some people for several years as to whether *acrosclerosis* and *diffuse systemic scleroderma* were separate diseases or varities of the same condition. In some reports Truelove and Whyte, 1951; Ramsey, 1951) it was considered that acrosclerosis was distinct from diffuse scleroderma. However the majority of workers, particularly those dealing with large series of cases, have held that acrosclerosis and diffuse systemic scleroderma are variants of the one disease (Leinwand *et al.,* 1954; O'Leary *et al.,* 1957). The problem was studied specifically by Jablońska *et al.* (1959) who found that similar visceral changes occurred in the acrosclerotic and non-acrosclerotic patients and concluded that "acrosclerosis is a variety of diffuse scleroderma preceded or accompanied by Raynaud's phenomenon." Farmer *et al.* (1960), following a study of 271 patients with generalized scleroderma (including acrosclerotic and generalized progressive forms), stated that they did not see any value in the separation of acrosclerotic and diffuse forms. Tuffanelli and Winkelmann (1962b) compared data from 288 patients with the acrosclerotic variety and thirty-eight with the diffuse variety from the Mayo Clinic and reached the same conclusion. The prognosis was generally worse in the diffuse type but individual cases of the acrosclerotic type could follow a rapidly downhill course.

Raynaud's phenomenon is a constant feature of acrosclerosis. This has to be distinguished from *primary Raynaud's disease* which is a vasospastic condition in which the digital arteries show increased sensitivity to cold in the absence of structural change or the presence of other underlying diseases, such as scleroderma (Allen *et al.*, 1955). Difficulty arises in that some patients originally presenting with Raynaud's phenomenon later develop sclerodermatous skin changes of the fingers, sometimes described as *Raynaud's disease with sclerodactylia.* Should such cases be classified with primary Raynaud's disease or with scleroderma?

Farmer *et al.* (1961) reported on seventy-one patients with Raynaud's phenomenon and sclerodermatous changes in the fingers but without systemic features after two years. In a follow-up ranging from one to thirty-one years, systemic scleroderma seemed to have developed in only three patients. The authors concluded that this finding did not support the view that systemic scleroderma and *sclerodactylia secondary to Raynaud's disease* are the same disease. However the fact that three patients developed features of systemic sclerosis would seem to point to an association and there is no indication that the writers looked for systemic disturbance by special tests.

Barnett and Coventry (1969a) included twenty such cases in a total of sixty-one patients with scleroderma. Of eight investigated intensively for systemic disturbance, reduced oesophageal mobility was observed in seven, skeletal abnormalities of the type found in other cases of scleroderma were fairly common, and other visceral disturbances characteristic of scleroderma were occasionally found. To avoid lengthy descriptive terms, with possible controversial implications, they referred to these cases as Type 1 scleroderma, Type 2 being the more usual type of acrosclerosis with skin changes involving the face as well as the hands and Type 3 the diffuse form with widespread skin changes including the trunk.

Winterbauer (1964) described seven cases of a *new* syndrome consisting of multiple telangiectases, Raynaud's phenomenon, sclerodactyly, and subcutaneous calcinosis (abbreviated to *CRST syndrome*) mimicking hereditary hemorrhagic telangiectasia (Rendu-Osler-Weber disease, R.O.W.). Further case reports followed (Dellipiani and George, 1967; Schimke *et al.*, 1967). It is of interest that a sister of one of the patients described by Schimke *et al.* had died with typical scleroderma, one of the rare reported instances of familial scleroderma. C.R.S.T. was regarded as a rare and relatively benign variant of the more common acrosclerotic type of scleroderma. Rowell (1968) criticized the term *C.R.S.T. syndrome* and the implication that it was benign. In his study of fifty-one patients with systemic sclerosis, telangiectasia was observed in thirty-six, calcinosis in twelve and seven had all four features of C.R.S.T.; all had some visceral involvement and one patient died of malignant hypertension. In a group surveyed by Barnett and Coventry (1969b) the proportions were similar with naevi in eighteen of thirty-one and calcinosis in seven of thirty-one cases. Oaks and O'Malley (1969) reported on two cases of C.R.S.T. syndrome each with systemic involvement of gastro-intestinal tract, lungs, joints and kidneys. It is apparent therefore that the C.R.S.T. syndrome does not differ in any important way from acrosclerosis in general.

Systemic sclerosis may vary in chronicity and any of the systemic manifestations may dominate the picture. The systemic disturbances may be more prominent than the skin changes and according to some reports (Crown, 1961, Rodnan and Fennell 1962) may even occur without them. This has led to the enumeration of numerous syndromes of scleroderma (Winkelmann, 1971). However, over-elaboration may lead to confusion. The main distinction is between the systemic and non-systemic types.

CLASSIFICATION ADOPTED

The following classification is in accord with modern views, but there are slight modifications in terms in order to prevent confusion.

A. *Scleroderma with systemic involvement* (= *progressive systemic sclerosis*).

1. Type 1 = Raynaud's phenomenon and sclerodactyly.
2. Type 2 = Acrosclerosis.
3. Type 3 = Systemic scleroderma with diffuse skin changes

B. *Scleroderma without systemic involvement* (= Scleroderma verum of Sellei; morphoea type).

1. *Scleroderma circumscriptum* (plaques).
2. *Scleroderma en bandes* (ribbon-like).
3. *Scleroderma disseminatum* (large irregular areas).
4. Variants

The classification is simple and does not attempt to include a variety of *syndromes*. In describing a particular case, a phrase could be added to indicate the extent or nature of the systemic involvement. For example, one could say "Scleroderma, Type 3 with widespread systemic involvement" or "Scleroderma, Type 2 with extensive gastro-intestinal involvement." The syndrome of visceral lesions characteristic of progressive systemic sclerosis but without skin changes ("visceral scleroderma without skin involvement" of Crown or "progressive systemic sclerosis *sine* scleroderma" of Rodnan) are not included as they are rare and only proven at autopsy. If diagnosed, Rodnan's term is preferable.

The subdivisions in *Group B* (scleroderma without systemic involvement) follow those of Sellei except that his *scleroderma diffusum* is replaced by *scleroderma disseminatum* to avoid confusion with diffuse systemic scleroderma. The term morphoea is sometimes used generally for the non-systemic type of scleroderma, sometimes for the sub-division with discrete round plaques.

There are various rare conditions including Hurler's syndrome and Weber's syndrome in which a scleroderma-like hardness of the skin occurs. These are not related to the two major types of scleroderma listed above and are not included. They will be described briefly when considering differential diagnosis (Chapter XIV).

DESCRIPTION OF TYPES WITH EXAMPLES

Type 1

In Type 1 cases, the earliest symptom is usually Raynaud's phenomenon without any disturbance of general health. If this occurs in a young woman, it may be impossible at first to make the differential diagnosis from primary Raynaud's disease. However, in many cases, the latter diagnosis is not feasible because the symptoms occur in a male or a patient over forty years. At the onset, skin changes are not diagnostic but the fingers may have a somewhat swollen, oedematous appearance. After several months, the skin over the terminal phalanges becomes tight and smooth and cornified patches develop on the finger-tips. Obvious sclerosis of the skin remains confined to the digits even after several years, however tightness of the skin of the neck may often be demonstrated by dorsiflexion of the head when the skin of the neck feels unduly taut to touch and tight vertical folds develop (Fig. 7–1). Raynaud's phenomenon persists and the patient may be subject to attacks of infection and ulceration of the digits. Dilated venules may appear on the neck and the face, but the skin of the face is not tight. Visceral disturbance is not a feature, but after many years the patient may develop dysphagia and barium swallow studies show impaired oesophageal mobility in most cases.

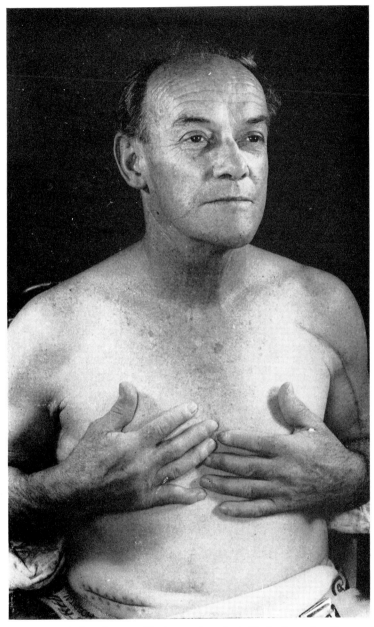

Figure 7–1. Type 1 Scleroderma. Obvious sclerosis is limited to the fingers. However tightness of the skin of the neck is apparent on extension of the head, and there are telangiectases on the face.

There is an uncommon subgroup (Type 1A) in which, although skin changes are limited to the fingers, there are severe systemic disturbances. One of my patients with such limited skin changes suffered from severe gastrointestinal features and two from respiratory involvement, proving fatal in each case.

Case Histories

The following case histories are illustrative of Type 1 scleroderma.

CASE 1: A wood-machinist, then aged forty-eight years, was seen in 1956 because of recurrent ulceration and pain in his fingers. During the past nine months he had repeated injuries to his fingers, resulting in ulceration and infection and also had experienced attacks of cyanosis of several fingers of each hand on exposure to cold. His general health was good.

On examination there was an area of necrotic skin at the tips of several fingers. The skin of his fingers was rather thick but it was considered that it was probably within normal limits for a man accustomed to hard manual work. Blood pressure was 120/70 mm. Hg. and no abnormalities were found on examination of his heart, lungs or abdomen.

Over the succeeding years he continued to attend because of recurrent ulceration of his fingers and ischaemic episodes. The skin of the fingers developed definite sclerodermatous changes and there was marked tightness of the skin of his neck demonstrated on extension of his head (Fig. 7–1). A brachial arteriogram showed marked obliterative disease of all the digital arteries. Electrocardiography showed partial right bundle branch block.

Vascular naevi appeared on his cheeks and tongue. There is no apparent sclerosis of his face, and his mouth and tongue are not small. However there is marked tightening and longitudinal ridging of his skin on extension of his head. He has had cholecystectomy for cholelithiases and has since developed mild angina, atrial fibrillation and obliterative arterial disease of the leg. Although he has no dysphagia, a barium swallow examination has shown hypoperistalsis of the lower end of his oesophagus. His current health at the age of 63 years is poor due to his cardiac and peripheral vascular problems, which are probably atherosclerotic in nature and not related to the scleroderma.

CASE 2: A single lady, then aged fifty-two, was seen in 1955, with a history that over the past five years she had suffered from stiff fingers and blanching of her fingers to the proximal interphalangeal joints in cold weather. There were no other significant symptoms. Apart from the statement that her mother had suffered from purple fingers in her latter years, there was no family history of vascular disease or of scleroderma.

On examination, the skin of her fingers was rather thick, but not particularly stiff. They were noted to be cyanotic on cold days. The resting heat elimination from her hands, as determined by calorimetry, was low and there was no increase from reflex heating.

Over the next ten years the skin of her fingers gradually became stiffer, she developed hardness of the skin and tenderness of the tips of her fingers, calcific nodules about her finger joints and red spots on her face. She also began to suffer from heartburn, a sensation of food sticking at the lower end of her sternum, upper abdominal discomfort after meals, a sensation of occasional thumping of her heart and swelling of her ankles in hot weather.

At a review examination, there was marked stiffness of the skin of her fingers, but not elsewhere and her mouth was normal. The skin of the tips of her fingers was cornified, there were tender lumps of her index fingers, non-tender swelling of each second metacarpo-phalangeal joint, and slight ulnar deviation of her fingers. Routine examination of her heart, lungs and abdomen gave normal findings. The only abnormalities detected by a series of tests was oesophageal hypoperistalsis and hiatus hernia on barium swallow examination and a positive latex agglutination test for rheumatoid arthritis.

The patient has continued to attend the clinic and is currently aged sixty-nine years. The fingers are markedly sclerotic, the ulnar deviation of the fingers has

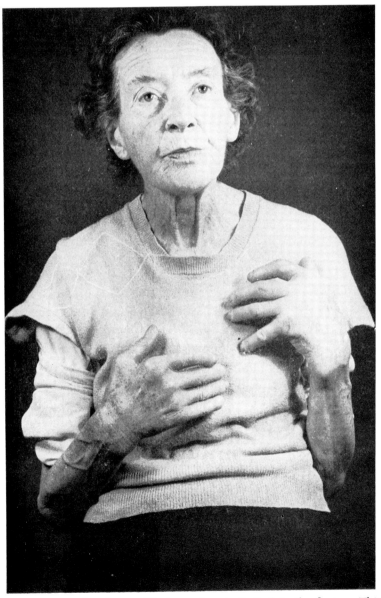

Figure 7–2. Type 1 Scleroderma. Obvious sclerosis limited to the fingers. This patient also showed telangiectases of the face and calcinosis of hands.

become more marked and there are telangiectases of her forehead and lips. There is no tightness of the skin of her face or smallness of her mouth and tongue (Fig. 7–2). She is very thin and has mild chronic congestive heart failure requiring treatment with digoxin and diuretics.

Summaries of the uncommon Type 1 cases (Type 1A) in which visceral manifestations predominate will be found in Chapter IX (Gastrointestinal involvement) and Chapter XI (Pulmonary Involvement).

Type 2

In Type 2 cases Raynaud's phenomenon occurs at the onset as in Type 1. However the sclerosis of the skin is not confined to the digits but extends on to the hands and forearms, the face appears smooth and the skin of the forehead becomes tight. The patient's features develop a *pinched* expression with a small beaked nose, and a small mouth. The tongue becomes pointed and resembles that of a bird. The neck sign is strongly positive and the sclerosis may extend to the upper sternal region, although the trunk generally is spared. The skin of the dorsa of the feet and ankles may be slightly tight, but the skin of the legs and thighs is not affected. Raynaud's phenomenon persists and the fingers are very subject to infections and ulceration. Telangiectases are common and affect the hands, face, upper sternal region and sometimes the tongue and buccal mucosa. Calcinosis of subcutaneous tissues occurs in some cases, and may cause painful lumps on the fingers which exude chalky material. (When both calcinosis and telangiectasia are found in the same patient, the designation *C.R.S.T. Syndrome* is applied). Flexion deformity of fingers develops giving a resemblance to rheumatoid arthritis, although the gross disorganization of joints, characteristic of the latter disease, does not occur.

Visceral disturbances eventually occur, affecting particularly the gastro-intestinal tract. They are generally of a chronic nature and although a source of great annoyance, may be endured for many years. However sometimes complications of the gastro-intestinal disease may lead to death. Cardiac or pulmonary symptoms may also occur and occasionally the patient may suddenly deteriorate and die from rapidly progressing systemic disease, particularly renal.

The following are illustrative case histories of Type 2 scleroderma.

CASE 3: A married woman, then aged forty-six, was seen in 1949, with a history that over the past three years she had experienced Raynaud's phenomenon of the fingers on exposure to cold and coldness and blueness of her feet and had noticed the skin of her fingers becoming harder and thicker. These symptoms occurred a few months after severe emotional upset caused by her husband being drowned in a boating accident, her struggle to pay for her home and support her two sons.

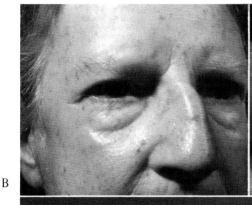

B

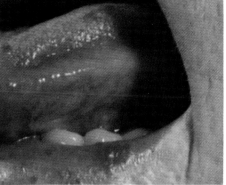

C

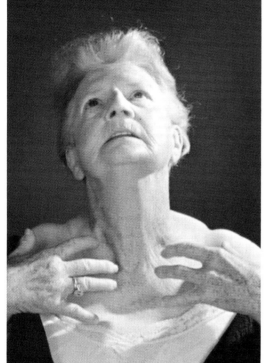

PLATE I. Type 2 Scleroderma. Sclerosis affects hands and face.

A. Picture showing face, neck and hands.

B. Close-up view of face showing telangiectases.

C. Tongue and lip showing telangiectases.

D. Fingers showing sclerosis.

E. Telangiectases of upper part of chest.

A

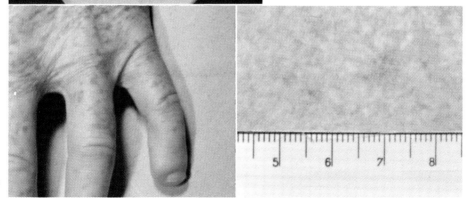

D

E

A bilateral cervical sympathectomy and right lumbar sympathectomy had been performed with improvement in her circulation in the sympathectomised areas, but she still experienced mild Raynaud's phenomenon in her hands in cold weather and developed small ulcers of her left foot.

On examination the skin of her fingers was smooth and relatively immobile. The skin on the back of her hands, forearms, and face seemed rather stiff and her forehead did not wrinkle well, but her mouth was normal in size. Both hands and the right foot (sympathectomised) were warm and pink. The toes of her left foot were cold and slightly cyanosed. The peripheral pulses were normal. Routine examination of heart, lungs and abdomen revealed no abnormality. Over the ensuing years the stiffness of the fingers increased and she developed calcific lumps on her hands which were not helped by a treatment course of disodium edetate (E.D.T.A.). She was troubled by intermittent diarrhoea and attacks of abdominal pain and vomiting and a barium enema examination disclosed *diverticulosis coli*. She was also troubled by rectal prolapse which was successfully treated by a suspension operation.

She was reviewed in 1965 with the following findings. Sclerodermatous changes were marked in her fingers, moderate in her face and slight on her hands and upper part of her chest. Vascular naevi were present on her face and lips. Her mouth was small and her tongue small and pointed (Plate I). There were large calcific lumps of her fingers and there was cornification of the tips of the fingers and small ulcers on some digits. There was a flexion deformity at the proximal interphalangeal joint of her left middle finger, and limited flexion at the terminal interphalangeal joints. Her blood pressure was 128/60 mm. Hg. The heart, abdomen and lungs were clinically normal. The major peripheral pulses were normal.

Abnormalities detected in a series of tests comprised: a moderate reduction in vital capacity, a slightly reduced creatinine clearance (seventy-seven ml. per minute), subcutaneous calcification and atrophy of the distal phalanges in radiographs of the hands, dilatation and aperistalsis of the oesophagus on barium swallow examination, a constant irregularity and narrowing in the left half of the transverse colon and large diverticula of the distal part of the colon on barium enema examination and a positive latex agglutination test for rheumatoid arthritis.

The patient has continued to attend the clinic. Her left middle finger, affected by chronic arthritis and calcinosis has been amputated. Currently she has reached the age of sixty-seven years and considers her health good. She has no dysphagia but regurgitates when lying flat. Her bowel symptoms are controlled by medication. The sclerosis of the skin, telangiectasia and calcinosis remain unchanged.

CASE 4: A man, then aged forty years, was seen in March, 1953 with the history that over the past seven months, while in the course of his job delivering milk on cold mornings, he developed *chilblains* of the tips of his fingers and since that time he had recurrent Raynaud's phenomenon and ulceration of his fingers, and his feet had been blue, cold and numb. Recently he had noticed swelling of his left hand and wrist.

On examination he appeared young for his stated age and the skin of his face was slightly tight. There was a gangrenous ulcer at the tip of his left index

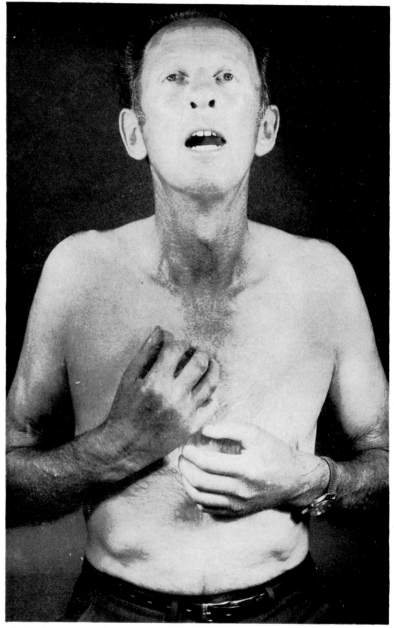

Figure 7–3. Type 2 Scleroderma. Sclerosis affects hands, forearms and face but spares
the trunk. In this patient there is marked stiffness and flexion deformity of the fingers.

finger, his hands were cold and the skin of his hands and forearms was stiff.
His blood pressure was 190/120 mm Hg. Examination of the heart and lungs
gave normal findings. The liver edge was palpable two cm. below the right
costal margin and enlarged, mobile, non-tender lymph glands were palpable
in his neck, axillae and groins.

Haematological examination showed a white cell count of 18,000 per c.mm due to a lymphocytosis, but was otherwise normal. Liver function tests were normal. Radiographic examination of his chest and hands gave normal findings. The electrocardiogram was normal. A skin biopsy showed changes consistent with scleroderma. The heat elimination from his hands, measured by calorimetry, was low and there was no response from reflex heating.

Pus was drained from his infected finger. Two months later he was readmitted for bilateral cervical sympathectomy but experienced little benefit. He was treated for several months with prednisolone twenty mg. per day and showed softening of his skin.

When he was reviewed in 1966, he stated he had developed dysphagia over the past two years. On examination the skin of his face was smooth and taut, his mouth was small, his tongue pointed and smooth at edges with limitation of protrusion. There was gross sclerosis of his fingers and moderate sclerosis of his hands, forearms and face (Fig. 7–3). His fingers were stiff and flexed. His blood pressure was 150/90 mm. Hg. The findings on clinical examination were otherwise normal. The *L.E. test* was positive but otherwise haematological test results were normal. The electrocardiogram was normal. The vital capacity and forced expiratory volume over one second were normal. Renal function tests were normal.

X-ray examination of his hands showed soft tissue atrophy over the terminal phalanges, early destruction of subungual tufts and early soft tissue calcification. A barium swallow examination showed the mid-portion of the oesophagus to be rather wide and with marked diminution of peristalsis. The stomach was radiologically normal, but the small bowel was rather more dilated than usual. The seventy-two hour faecal fat content was high (26.4 gm.). Liver function test results and plasma protein levels were normal. The latex agglutination test and the fluorescent antibody tests were negative.

Currently (1971) there is little change since his review in 1966. His general health at the age of 58 years remains good and he is able to continue with his work.

Further examples of Type 2 cases will be found in Chapters IX (Gastro-intestinal Involvement), X (Pulmonary Involvement) and XI (Cardiac Involvement).

Type 3

In Type 3 scleroderma, skin changes are diffuse from the onset and affect a large part of the body within a few weeks or months, as distinct from the slow progression affecting predominantly the extremities in Type 2. Characteristically the trunk and the limbs are affected simultaneously. The skin changes are symmetrical but not of the same intensity throughout. Thus the arms may be more affected than the trunk, and the dorsal region more affected than the front of the chest and the abdomen. The skin may be extremely hard and tight and is often markedly pigmented. The pinched expression and small mouth and tongue characteristic of Type two cases are not seen in early cases, but may develop in the rare patients who survive for several years. Raynaud's phenomenon may or may not be present, but if present, occurs concurrently with the skin changes rather than preceding them. Sometimes there are persistent cyanosis and coldness of the hands rather than the paroxysmal ischaemic attacks of Raynaud's phenomenon.

Severe systemic involvement is the rule and patients with Type 3 scleroderma usually die within five years of the onset, either suddenly (presumably due to cardiac arrhythmia) or from renal failure. Gastro-intestinal involvement, particularly oesophageal dysfunction, frequent in Type 2 cases, is less common in Type 3 cases.

The following are illustrative case histories of Type 3 scleroderma.

CASE 5: A woman then aged forty-six years, was admitted to hospital in April 1965. She had always been a nervous woman and had experienced dysphagia and heart-burn, diagnosed clinically as due to hiatus hernia for twenty years. Her recent illness began about fifteen months prior to admission to the hospital when, after using various chemical weed killers and garden sprays, she developed a rash of her eyelids, arms and legs which persisted for several months. About three months after the onset of the rash she contracted chicken pox and about two months later began to experience Raynaud's phenomenon of her fingers, coldness of her hands and feet and thickening of the skin of her arms, legs and face.

On examination she was a normally nourished, middle-aged woman. Her mouth and tongue were normal. Her blood pressure was 140/90 mm. Hg. The urine contained a moderate amount of albumin. There was sclerosis of the skin involving the whole body including extremities, face and trunk with slight oedema of the forearm and legs and pigmentation of her loins and groins. Examination of heart and lungs gave normal findings. Apart from a right upper paramedian scar (previous cholecystectomy) and a palpable liver edge just below the costal margin, the abdomen was normal. Reflexes were normal. The ankle pulses were slightly weak.

The only abnormal findings on a comprehensive series of tests were slightly reduced peristalsis and presence of coarse mucosal folds in the first part of the jejunum on barium meal examination, an abnormally high faecal fat excretion and minor changes consisting of infiltration with eosinophils and plasma cells in a jejunal biopsy specimen. The fasting blood urea concentration and creatinine clearance were both normal.

She was treated with prednisolone and discharged on a maintenance dose of twenty mg. per day. When seen in the outpatient clinic about two months' later she was complaining of abdominal bloating, heart-burn, passage of pink mucus *per rectum* and orthopnoea. The general appearance of her skin was unchanged. The blood pressure had risen to 170/110 mm Hg. Treatment with prednisolone was continued.

She was readmitted to hospital two month's later in a confused state with a letter from her local doctor that four weeks previously she had developed influenza from which she made a slow recovery, but on the previous evening prior to admission, had developed abdominal pain, had deteriorated mentally and was found to have a heart rate of 130 beats per minute and a blood pressure of 200/140 mm. Hg. On admission she was mentally confused with pulse rate of 140 per minute and tenderness in the epigastrium. The blood urea level was 140 mg. per one hundred ml. and the carbon dioxide content was reduced to thirteen vol. percent. She developed a neutrophilia with granulation of the neutrophils, reduction of platelets and red cell abnormalities indicative of severe toxemia. She was treated with intravenous therapy and antibiotics but continued to deteriorate, with marked peripheral vaso-constriction, and elevation of the blood pressure to 180/140 mm. Hg., anuria and, in spite of intensive intravenous therapy and peritoneal dialysis, she died in uremia six days after admission.

The main features on post-mortem examination were the widespread scleroderma, fibrotic changes and arterial thickening in the lungs, increased interstitial and submucosal fibrous tissue in the oesophagus, small infarcts studded with necrotic tubules in the kidneys and gross concentric thickening of the interlobular arteries resulting in severe obstruction of the lumen. The heart was enlarged mainly due to left ventricular hypertrophy but the coronary arteries were normal. The myocardium was edematous and there was mild infiltration with histocytes but otherwise nothing remarkable. The heart contained mural thrombi and there were multiple infarcts in viscera.

In summary this middle-aged lady developed her first symptoms of scleroderma approximately one year prior to admission and died of fulminating renal failure after another four months, the total duration of the disease being less than eighteen months.

CASE 6: Two years prior to presenting for examination, a man aged fifty-seven years began to notice attacks of numbness in his feet and legs and six months prior to attending, attacks of pallor and numbness in his hands. These episodes had become more frequent in the past three months, during which time he had become weak and fatigued, had lost one stone in weight, suffered from frequent headaches and had noticed that the skin of his face had become tight and shiny.

On examination there was generalized thickening and tightness of the skin, especially in the forearms and thighs (Fig. 7–4). His fingers were cold and cyanosed and the proximal phalanges and interphalangeal joints were swollen. Otherwise general examination revealed no abnormality. His blood pressure was 135/85 mm. Hg. /Lumbar puncture produced normal clear fluid and the Wassermann reaction in the blood and cerebrospinal fluid was negative. Renal function tests, haematological findings, plasma electrolyte levels were all normal. The erythrocyte sedimentation rate (Wintrobe) was nineteen mm. in oue hour; the L.E. phenomenon could not be demonstrated. A barium swallow examination showed oesophageal aperistalsis.

He was treated for several months with methyl prednisolone in an average dose of twenty mg. per day and believed that his skin became looser. However he continued to lose strength and weight in spite of a good food intake and also developed diarrhoea and marked generalized pigmentation. A malabsorption syndrome was suspected and on examination his faeces were found to contain

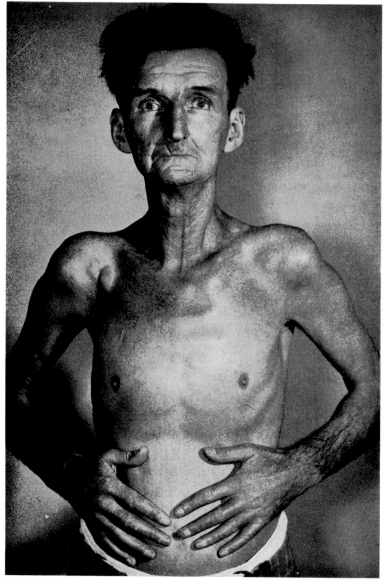

Figure 7–4. Type 3 Scleroderma. Sclerosis is diffuse, affecting face, trunk, arms and hands. The skin is pigmented.

undigested food, but the twenty-four hour excretion of fat was normal. Duodenal aspiration for the purpose of estimating the duodenal enzymes yielded practically no secretion. An attempt was made to improve the nutrition by administration of an anabolic hormone without appreciable effect. The pigmentation markedly decreased and the patient's general condition improved following the administration of pancreatin and various members of the Vitamin B group.

The patient has since moved to another area and it has not been possible to follow his condition but he was known to be alive in 1966, about nine years after presentation.

Summary: Man of fifty-seven years with recent onset of Raynaud's phenomenon, loss of weight and strength and fatigue; found to have widespread scleroderma and muscular wasting and absent esophageal peristalsis; developed features of malabsorption syndrome.

CASE 7: A young woman who had recently immigrated from Yugoslavia was admitted to hospital in January 1966, then aged eighteen years. The story was obtained through an interpreter that ten months previously she had noticed widespread thickening of the skin of her face, shoulders, arms and extremities associated with Raynaud's phenomenon of her fingers and toes, deformity of her fingers and, within a month of the onset, ulceration of the finger joints. She had lost weight and had noticed dysphagia.

Examination revealed a thin girl, with a high pitched nasal voice, and extensive thickening and tightness of the skin of face, trunk and extremities and diffuse pigmentation. Her mouth and tongue were not particularly small (Fig. 7–5A).

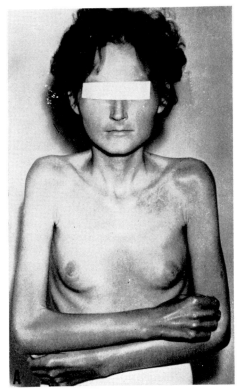 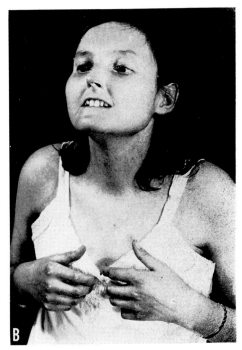

Figure 7–5. Type 3 Scleroderma. A. At presentation one year after onset. Sclerosis is diffuse, affecting entire skin. B. After treatment with adrenal steroids for six years. Note sclerosis is mainly in face and limbs; the mouth has become small. The latter features indicate a transition to Type 2 Scleroderma.

Ulceration was present over the elbows and there was hard subcutaneous plaques in the perineum. Her blood pressure was 105/70 mm. Hg. The cardiac rhythm was regular and routine examination of heart, lungs, abdomen and peripheral pulses revealed no abnormalities.

Abnormalities found in a comprehensive series of tests were as follows. There was an increase in the mature neutrophils with a total white cell count of 30,000 per c.mm. Her vital capacity was moderately reduced. There was a moderate proteinuria, slight reduction in creatinine clearance, but normal blood urea concentration. Barium swallow examination showed reduced oesophageal peristalsis and radiographic examination of her elbows, knees and buttocks showed marked soft tissue calcification. The serum glutamic oxalic transaminase (S.G.O.T.) was elevated and there was slight elevation of the plasma γ-globulin concentration. A skin biopsy showed increased collagen extending deep to the sweat glands indicative of scleroderma.

She was treated with prednisolone with a starting dose of sixty mg. per day reduced over the next two weeks to a maintenance dose of forty mg. per day and eventually over the subsequent months to fifteen mg. per day. When assessed two months after discharge, it was noticed that the skin was softer, the fingers more mobile, but she had developed a *moon face* characteristic of hyperadrenalism.

She continued to have ulceration over her elbows and pain in her buttocks on sitting, due to the calcium deposits. In July 1968 she was admitted for a treatment with disodium edetate (E.D.T.A.) but without benefit. Treatment with prednisolone has been continued.

Her main troubles have been stiffness of her fingers, Raynaud's attacks and the soft tissue calcification requiring, on one occasion, surgical excision. However, she has been able to do a secretarial course and find employment.

On review in 1970, the skin generally was softer than on her previous admission. She still had marked flexion deformity of her fingers. The appearance of her face has altered in that her nose was now pinched, mouth small and tongue pointed. (Fig. 7–5 B). Her blood pressure was 120/80 mm. Hg. A barium swallow examination again showed hypoperistalsis, but no other abnormalities. E.C.G. showed sinus tachycardia only. X-ray examination of her chest showed increased marking in the bases. Her creatinine clearance was further reduced, but the blood urea level was still normal. X-ray examination of her hands and other areas again showed soft tissue calcification. The plasma γ-globulin level was still elevated (1.8 gm. per one hundred ml.) but the immunoglobulin levels normal and the fluorescent antibody tests were negative except for a weakly positive anti-gastric parietal cell factor.

In summary, this young woman presented with diffuse scleroderma involving a widespread area of her body (Type 3). A rather unusual feature was the marked calcification. The skin condition has improved with treatment with prednisolone, but she has developed a small mouth and tongue suggestive of a Type 2 case. The major problems have been associated with ischaemic episodes of her hands and calcification. She remains reasonably well six years after presentation and seven years after the onset of her disease.

GENERAL CLINICAL PICTURE

It should be emphasized that patients with scleroderma present a wide spectrum in the extent of skin involvement, vascular disturbances and visceral involvement and the types represent only examples to which groups of cases more or less conform, but the divisions are somewhat indistinct and the groups tend to merge.

Age and sex Incidence and Frequency of Types

The sex distribution in the various types in one series (Barnett and Coventry (1969) is shown in Table VIII.

TABLE VIII *

SEX DISTRIBUTION IN A SERIES OF
PATIENTS WITH SCLERODERMA
SUBDIVIDED ACCORDING TO
CLINICAL TYPE

Type	Number of Patients		
	Male	Female	Total
1	8	12	20
2	3	29	32
3	6	3	9
Total	17	44	61

* From Barnett and Coventry: *Med J Aust, 1*:992–1001, 1969.

This shows that Type 3 (diffuse systemic sclerosis) is the rarest type comprising only nine of sixty-one (14 percent) of the patients. This is in accord with the large Mayo Clinic series where thirty-nine of 327 cases (12 percent) were of the diffuse type. In our series there were six men and three women, but the sex incidence cannot be judged from such small numbers. In the larger series the proportion of men and women is approximately equal. Type 2 accounted for thirty-two cases (53 percent) and showed a marked predominence of females (female to male ratio of

TABLE IX *

AGE OF ONSET † IN A SERIES OF PATIENTS WITH
SCLERODERMA SUBDIVIDED ACCORDING TO
CLINICAL TYPE

Type	Number of patients in stated age group					
	10–19 yr.	20–29 yr.	30–39 yr.	40–49 yr.	50–59 yr.	60 yr & over.
1	0	3	4	4	5	3
2	1	4	4	13	8	2
3	1	0	2	2	3	1
Totals	2	7	10	19	16	6

† Age of onset not determinable in one case.
* From Barnett and Coventry: *Med J. Aust, 1*:992–1001, 1969.

ten to one). Type 1 accounted for twenty cases (33 percent) with a female to male ratio of three to two. Considering the non-diffuse cases (Types 1 and 2) together the female to male ratio is approximately four to one. The age incidence is given in Table IX, which shows that most cases of scleroderma commence beyond middle age.

Visceral Involvement

Barnett and Coventry (1969a) analysed the extent of visceral involvement in sixty-one patients with scleroderma with the results shown in Table X.

TABLE X *

CLINICAL VISCERAL ABNORMALITY IN SIXTY-ONE PATIENTS
WITH SCLERODERMA

Method of Diagnosis of abnormality	*Type 1* (20 cases)	*Type 2* (32 cases)	*Type 3* (9 cases)	*Total* (61 cases)
Cardiac symptoms or signs	9	18	7	34
Radiography of the heart	4	5	1	10
E.C.G.	7	14	5	26
Pulmonary symptoms or signs	10	18	3	31
Pulmonary X-ray film	6	5	2	13
Upper gastro-intestinal symptoms or signs	16	19	9	44
Radiographic examination with barium bolus or meal	11	21	7	39
Renal symptoms or signs	4	5	1	10
Microscopic examination of urine	2	0	1	3
Renal function tests	10	20	4	34
Joint symptoms or signs	6	17	7	30

* From Barnett & Coventry: *Med J Aust*, 1:995–1001, 1969.

This shows that frequent visceral involvement occurs in all three types. It must be acknowledged that the frequency of involvement may be overestimated as not all the abnormalities found may be due to scleroderma. However it would be difficult to obtain a control population subjected to the same battery of tests. Even if some reduction is made on this account, the frequency of abnormalities is high for all types. Also the nature of the abnormalities, particularly in respect to gastro-intestinal findings, is similar. This confirms the thesis that all three types are variants of the one disease, systemic sclerosis.

Progress of Systemic Involvement

Barnett and Coventry (1969a) assessed the progress of severity of affection of various systems in nine patients who died within five years of presentation and in another thirty-one cases followed for five years or more with the results shown in Tables XI and XII.

These show that over the period of the study, in some cases the severity of affection of a particular system remained unchanged, but in

TABLE XI*

PROGRESS OF INVOLVEMENT OF VARIOUS SYSTEMS IN NINE PATIENTS
WITH SCLERODERMA WHO DIED WITHIN FIVE YEARS
OF PRESENTATION

Group	Systems	Initially Involved	Number of Patients Un-changed	Better	Worse †
Types 1 and 2 (4 cases: early, 1; late, 3)	Skin (extent)	4	2	0	2
	Cardiac (presence of symptoms)	4	3	–	1
	Pulmonary (presence of symptoms)	–	–	–	–
	Alimentary (radiological signs)	3	2	–	1
	Renal (results of tests)	1	1	–	1 (1)
	Joints	–	–	–	–
Type 3 (5 cases)	Skin (extent) ‡	5	4	–	1
	Cardiac (presence of symptoms)	3	1	–	3 (1)
	Pulmonary (presence of symptoms)	1	–	–	2 (1)
	Alimentary (radiological signs)	2	2	–	1 (1)
	Renal (results of tests)	0	–	–	2 (2) §
	Joints	5	3	–	–

† Figures in brackets refer to cases in which the particular feature has developed during the course of the study.

‡ Severity decreased in three cases of patients taking steroids (improvement was maintained in two cases; relapse occurred in one).

§ Terminal renal failure.

* From Barnett and Coventry: *Med J Aust,* 1:992–1001, 1969.

most cases worsened and rarely did it improve. Similar results were obtained when the patients were divided into those seen early and late (several years) after the onset, indicating that over the period of the study the disease did not burn itself out. The name progressive systemic sclerosis therefore seems appropriate.

PROGNOSIS

In a disease such as scleroderma in which the duration of illness is very variable and may last beyond the period of observation of one observer, it is difficult to obtain data on the prognosis.

O'Leary and Nomland (1930) regarded the prognosis of *generalized scleroderma* (that is, the systemic sclerosis type) as poor. Twenty-six of their forty-eight cases (54 percent) had had the disease for more than two years before being seen at the Mayo Clinic. Of the eight patients who died, the average duration of the disease was more than four years, with a maximum of twelve years and a minimum of one year. They also remarked on a tendency to remission and found that 1.4 percent were slightly improved, 10.5 percent decidedly improved and 6.3 percent almost completely cured. This spontaneous cure rate does not accord with views of

TABLE XII *

PROGRESS OF INVOLVEMENT OF VARIOUS SYSTEMS IN THIRTY-ONE
CASES OF SCLERODERMA FOLLOWED FOR FIVE YEARS OR MORE;
CASES SUBDIVIDED ACCORDING TO TYPE

| | | | Number of Patients | | |
| | | Initially | Un- | | |
Group	Systems	Involved	changed	Better	Worse †
Type 1 (11 cases: early, 7; late, 4)	Skin (extent)	10	9	0	2 (1)
	Cardiac (presence of symptoms)	3	2	0	2 (1)
	Pulmonary (presemce of symptoms)	3	0	0	4 (1)
	Alimentary (radiological signs)	2	2	0	6 (6)
	Renal (results of tests)	1	1	0	2 (2)
	Joints	1	1	0	1 (1)
Type 2 (18 cases: early, 13; late, 5)	Skin (extent)	15	4	0	14 (3)
	Cardiac (presence of symptoms)	6	3	0	6 (3)
	Pulmonary (presence of symptoms)	1	1	0	4 (4)
	Alimentary (radiological signs)	5	2	0	9 (6)
	Renal (results of tests)	4	2	1	4 (3)
	Joints	6	2	1	6 (3)
Type 3 (2 early cases)	Skin (extent)	2	2	0	0
	Cardiac (presence of symptoms)	0	0	0	0
	Pulmonary (presence of symptoms)	0	0	0	0
	Alimentary (radiological signs)	2	2	0	0
	Renal (results of tests)	0	0	0	1 (1)
	Joints	2	1	1	0

† Figures in brackets refer to cases in which the particular feature has developed during the course of the study.
* From Barnett and Coventry: *Med J Aust,* 1:991–1001, 1969.

subsequent writers. However, it is possible that some of the reported improvements with treatment may have been due to a spontaneous remission.

Tuffanelli and Winkelmann (1961) in their study of 727 cases, found a five-year survival rate from the time of diagnosis at the clinic of 70.3 percent and a ten-year survival rate of 58.9 percent. Again there was a tendency to remission as indicated in statements of 209 patients in follow-up letters: six considered their condition cured, fifty-nine considered it improved, ninety unchanged and fifty-four worse. The prognosis was worse for the diffuse type with a five-year survival of 17 percent and ten year survival of 15 percent compared with the acrosclerotic type for which the corresponding figures were seventy-four percent and sixty-two percent (Tuffanelli and Winkelmann, 1962b).

More recently (Medsger *et al.,* 1971) have made a life-table analysis of 309 patients obtained from combining subjects from two clinics (Pitts-

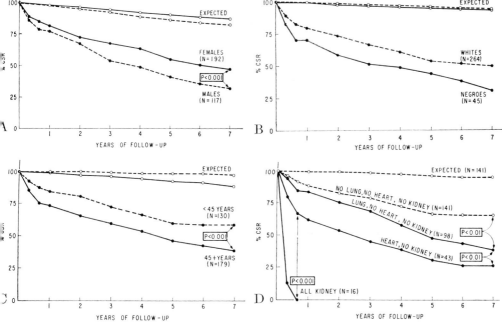

Figure 7–6. Cumulative survival rates for scleroderma patients, subdivided according to (A) sex, (B) race, (C) age at presentation, (D) organ involvement at presentation. CSR = Cumulative survival rate where 1.00 = 100% survival. Reproduced with permission from Medsger *et al.*, 1971, *Ann Int Med*, 75:369–376.

burgh and Memphis) and plotting survival rate from the time of first diagnosis at the respective clinics. Their graphs show a five-year survival of approximately fifty percent and a ten year survival rate of approximately 40 percent. They found that survival was worse in older patients, worse in males than in females and worse in negroes than in whites. As would be expected the presence of visceral involvement considerably worsened the prognosis which was particularly bad in cases with renal involvement (Fig. 7–6).

Our figures are insufficient for construction of meaningful survival curves but follow-up data on seventy-eight patients seen over approximately twenty years indicate the outlook in the various types of systemic scleroderma (See Tables XIII, XIV, XV, XVI).

In these tables, reference is made to the duration of illness (from the time of first symptoms judged to be due to scleroderma) rather than time followed, as the former is more significant in respect to course of the illness. In some patients not seen recently at the clinic, the current state of health is assessed from replies to follow-up letters.

Some points of interest which arise from the figures are as follows: In Type 1 and 2 survival may be considerable; nine of thirty-three survivors

TABLE XIII

PRESENT STATUS OF SEVENTY-EIGHT PATIENTS WITH SCLERODERMA SURVEYED IN CURRENT STUDY

		Patients		
Type	*Alive*	*Deceased*	*Lost from Survey*	*Total*
1	19	12	1	32
2	14	15	6	35
3	1	8	2	11
Total	34	35	9	78

TABLE XIV

INFORMATION ON THIRTY-FOUR LIVING PATIENTS WITH SCLERODERMA IN CURRENT STUDY

Type	*Number*	*Known Duration of Illness (Years)*			*Present Health* *		
		0–9	*10–19*	*>20*	*Good*	*Fair*	*Poor*
1	19	6	9	4	9	8	2
2	14	2	7	5	7	4	2
3	1	1	0	0	0	1	0
Total	34	9	16	9	16	13	4

* Current health of one Type 2 case not assessed.

TABLE XV

INFORMATION ON THIRTY-FIVE DECEASED PATIENTS WITH SCLERODERMA FROM CURRENT STUDY

Type	*Total Deaths*	*Probable Relation to Scleroderma*		*Age at Death (years)*			*Duration of Illness (years)*		
		Probable	*Unrelated or Unknown*	*0–39*	*40–59*	*60+*	*0–9*	*10–19*	*20+*
1	12	3	9	1	6	5	7	3	2
2	15	6	9	0	7	8	6	5	4
3	8	8	0	2	5	1	8	0	0
Totals	35	17	18	3	18	14	21	8	6

TABLE XVI

NATURE OF DEATHS RELATED TO SCLERODERMA IN SEVENTEEN CASES FROM CURRENT STUDY

Type	*Gastrointestinal*	*Cardiac*	*Pulmonary*	*Renal*	*Total*
1	1	–	2	–	3
2	1	1	3	1	6 *
3	–	3	1	4	8
Total	2	4	6	5	17

* In two additional cases, scleroderma was probably contributory.

have lived for more than twenty years from the onset. The prognosis is particularly bad in Type 3 cases. No patient had survived more than ten years. In Type 1 cases only a quarter of the deaths were related to scleroderma, in Type 2 half the deaths and in Type 3 all the deaths. Renal failure occurs predominantly in Type 3 cases. Approximately half of the survivors regard their current health as good.

SUMMARY

It is seen from the above that the primary classification of scleroderma is into a form with systemic involvement (progressive systemic sclerosis) and one without systemic involvement (*scleroderma verum* or morphoea type). Scleroderma with systemic involvement may be subdivided into various types. A classification is suggested based on the type of skin involvement: Type 1, skin involvement remaining localized to fingers; Type 2, skin involvement spreading slowly to involve hands, forearms and face; Type 3, skin involvement diffuse from onset or rapidly progressive. All types are associated with systemic involvement. The prognosis is variable and depends mainly on the extent of visceral involvement. Most Type 1 and Type 2 cases have a long survival rate in the order of 60 percent at ten years and may die from unrelated causes; most Type 3 cases have a short survival and die within ten years.

Chapter VIII

CUTANEOUS, VASCULAR AND SKELETAL INVOLVEMENT

THE CUTANEOUS, vascular and skeletal manifestations of scleroderma are best considered together as they are inter-related and together determine the characteristic features by which the disease is recognised.

CUTANEOUS

With the cutaneous features are included changes of the subcutaneous tissues which may be of equal or greater importance than those in the dermis in producing immobility or stiffness of skin. Also calcification, although usually considered as a skin manifestation (*calcinosis cutis*), in effect involves mainly the subcutaneous tissues.

The *extent* of the skin involvement has already been discussed and has been used as the basis for dividing scleroderma into Types 1, 2 and 3. In some Type 1 cases, there is a fairly abrupt transition between affected and apparently normal skin, but in others and in Type 2 cases the transition is gradual.

The *nature* of the change is more readily experienced than described. The term scleroderma means *hard skin* but this is not an adequate description as there are other more characteristic properties. The skin may be *hard* in other conditions, such as scars, which are not scleroderma. One of the characteristic features is smoothness of the skin both in appearance and in touch, so that the hands and face appear and feel smooth. The diagnosis of scleroderma may be made by greeting the patient and shaking hands. The skin is commonly considered to be thick but some workers maintain that this is an incorrect impression based on appearance and feel and that the skin, at least the forearm, is really thin (Black *et al.*, 1970). In fact, fingers of patients with scleroderma may be of normal thickness, thin or thick and the different degrees of thickness of the skin may be apparent on radiographs and in biopsy specimens. The most characteristic feature of the skin in scleroderma is its tightness. It is difficult to pinch it up from the underlying tissues, which may be due to its being stretched or bound down to underlying tissues. The lack of wrinkles suggest that it is in a stretched position. It is difficult to measure this property of immobility of the skin. Bachman (1961) has devised a clinical method in which the distance apart of dots on the skin is measured during compression and stretching by the

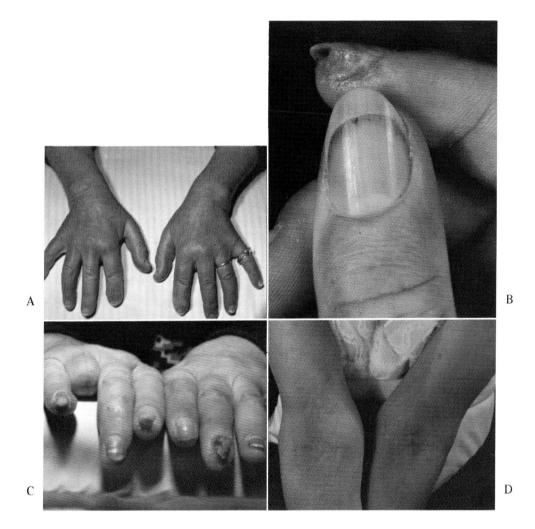

PLATE II.

A. Cyanotic, slightly swollen fingers of a patient with early scleroderma.

B. Fingers of a patient with early scleroderma showing splinter haemorrhages and superficial ulceration.

C. Fingers of a patient with Type I Scleroderma showing advanced ulceration.

D. Skin pigmentation in a patient with Type 3 Scleroderma.

observer's thumb and forefinger and the vertical elevation during pinching, but the method is not very precise. The tightness of the skin is the basis of a simple clinical test (neck test) valuable in the early diagnosis of scleroderma. A patient may exhibit Raynaud's phenomenon and the fingers may appear somewhat smooth. It may be doubtful whether this is outside normal limits. In such a case extension of the neck may cause the skin to tighten with the appearance of vertical ridges and the skin will feel tight (Fig. 8–1). This sign may be present even in Type 1 cases indicating that, although the obvious skin changes are limited to the digits, the tightness of the skin is more extensive.

Hyperkeratotic lesions (cornification) of the fingertips (Fig. 8–2) are a common feature, particularly in Type 1 and Type 2 cases, and are a frequent source of annoyance. The palms are often sweaty.

Other skin lesions of the digits are probably related to the vascular disturbance (Plate II,A). The fingertips are extremely prone to infections, and ulceration (Plate II,B and C) presumably due to the impaired blood flow. These troubles are often episodic, the patient being affected with repeated ulceration of fingers over several months and then free of them for months or years. They are often preceded by severe pain in the fingertip suggestive of a vascular incident, either a thrombosis or hemorrhage into the soft tissues. Sometimes a ring of splinter hemorrhages may be observed about the nail bed (Plate II,B) probably representing, on a somewhat larger scale, the hemorrhages from dilated capillaries observed by capillaroscopy.

Patients with scleroderma often show brown pigmentation. In Type 3 cases this is often widespread involving the affected skin and may give a superficial appearance of Addison's disease (Plate II,E). However pigmentation may also occur in Type 2 cases and may involve regions in which the skin is not appreciably thickened. Sometimes there are small areas (guttae) of depigmented skin in the midst of the pigmented areas (Fig. 8–3).

Calcification of the superficial soft tissues in scleroderma was apparently first described by a Swiss Physician Weber in 1878, but only became generally recognised following the publication of Thibierge and Weissenbach (1911) who collected eight cases from the literature and added one of their own. The condition was reviewed by Durham (1928) who found an additional thirteen reported cases and added another. The incidence and distribution of calcinosis in scleroderma was studied intensively by Muller *et al.* (1959) in the large series from the Mayo Clinic. They found no instance in twenty-three patients with diffuse scleroderma and fifty-three in 230 cases of the acrosclerotic form (13 percent), being about five times more frequent in the *severe* than *moderately severe* forms of the disease. It was practically confined to females (twenty-eight of the thirty-one cases). It was rare in the non-systemic (morphoea) type of sclero-

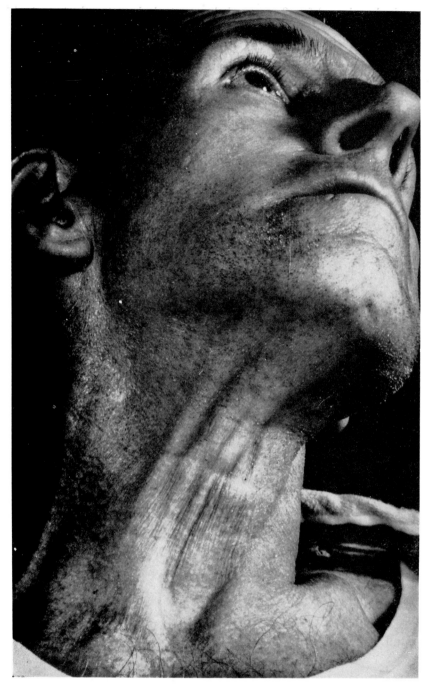

Figure 8–1. Neck test in patient with Type 1 Scleroderma. The skin of the neck, while apparently normal in the resting position, becomes tight and ridged when the head is extended.

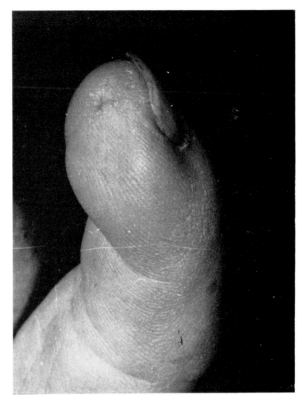

Figure 8–2. Fingertip from a patient with scleroderma showing pitting at a point where a hyperkeratotic nodule has been lifted off.

derma with only two instances in 128 cases. Calcinosis in acrosclerotic patients mainly involved the upper extremities, particularly the hands, and was uncommon in the lower limbs. It was a late sequel, the average time of appearance being eleven years from the onset of the disease. They considered that it probably indicated a favourable prognosis because it was associated with chronicity. Calcinosis had suggested to previous workers the possibility of parathyroid disease and Muller *et al.* list several reports of parathyroidectomy for scleroderma performed on this basis. However they could find no laboratory or clinical evidence of parathyroid disease in their cases. Tuffanelli and Winkelmann (1961), on reporting on a large series of 727 patients with scleroderma from the Mayo Clinic, found that in the 173 cases in which serum calcium determinations were done, these were all normal, except in one patient with co-existant hyper-parathyroidism. However, Samuelsson and Werner (1965) reported a case of scleroderma and calcinosis with histological and clinical features of mild hyper-parathyroidism and, from a study of the literature, concluded that this association was not uncommon. Barnett and Coventry (1969b) found

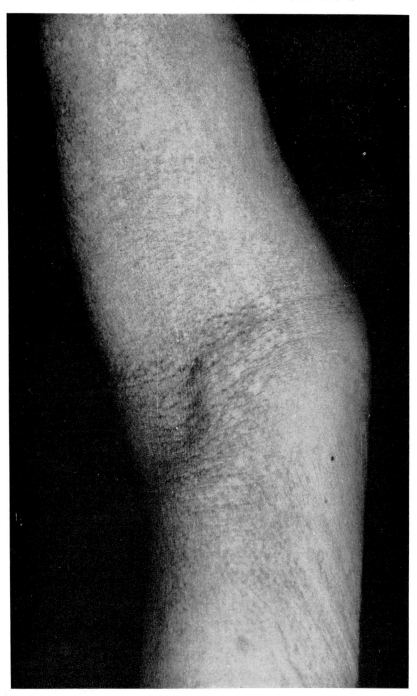

Figure 8–3. Pigmentation with areas of depigmentation in a patient with Type 1 Scleroderma. Although sclerosis was limited to the hands, pigmentation was extensive.

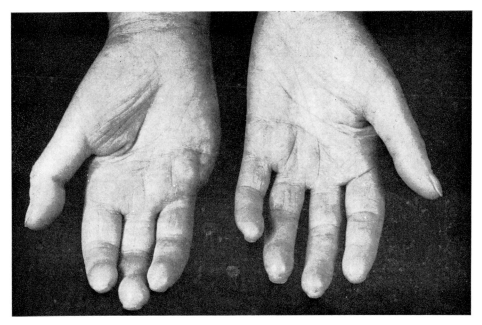

Figure 8–4. Lumpy hands due to calcinosis in a patient with Type 1 Scleroderma. The right little finger has been amputated because of ischemic ulceration.

calcinosis in seven of thirty-one patients, including one with Type 3 disease.

Calcification occurs most frequently in the hands where it produced a lumpy appearance (Fig 8–4) and is of great annoyance to the patient because of pain and recurrent discharge of chalky material. It is readily demonstrated by radiography (Fig. 8–5). Although calcinosis is most frequent in the upper limbs, large accumulations may sometimes be found in the lower limbs as in the following cases.

One elderly lady with Type 2 scleroderma had large masses below the patella requiring surgical excision.

Another elderly lady was referred because of recurrent ulceration of her legs considered to be stasis ulcers. There were no gross varicose veins. She gave the story of removing rock-hard material from the ulcers on several occasions. Radiological examinations showed marked calcification of the soft tissues of her legs. Inspection of her hands showed definite scleroderma (Type 1) and on questioning she gave a history of Raynaud's phenomenon over many years.

Since calcinosis is a late development, its virtual absence in diffuse (Type 3) cases is expected as death from this condition usually occurs in five years. In our one case of Type 3 disease with calcinosis (Case 7, Chapter VII), survival has been longer than usual (to date six years). However calcinosis became marked within three years of the onset and was particularly prominent in the buttocks, legs and feet (Figs. 8–6 and 8–7).

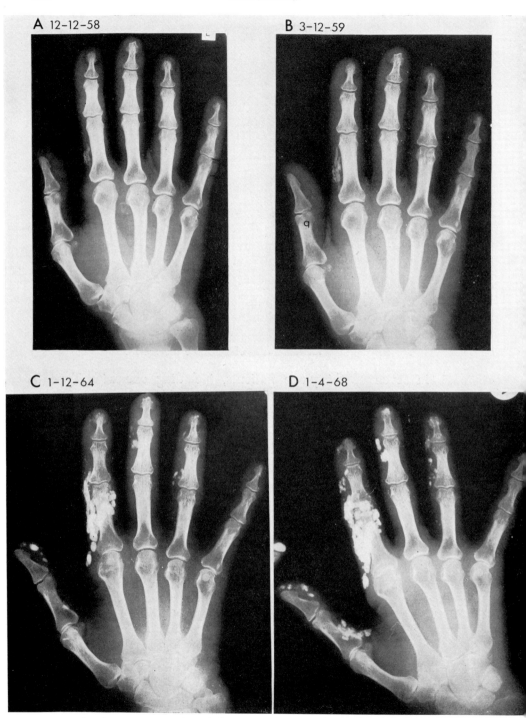

Figure 8–5. Serial radiographs of hands of a patient with Type 1 Scleroderma, showing gradual development of calcium deposits over a period of ten years.

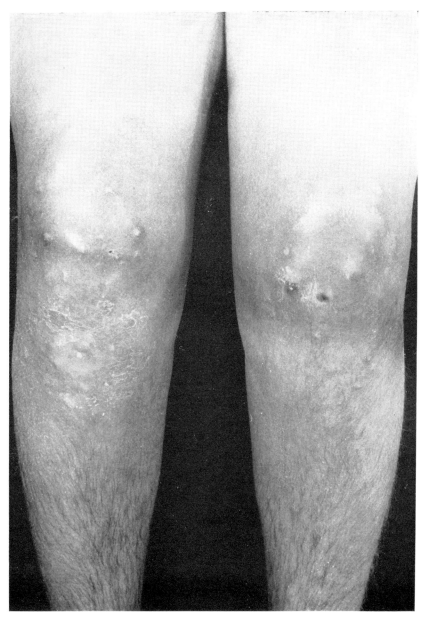

Figure 8–6. Subcutaneous nodules and ulceration over knees in a patient with Type 3 Scleroderma and extensive calcium deposits.

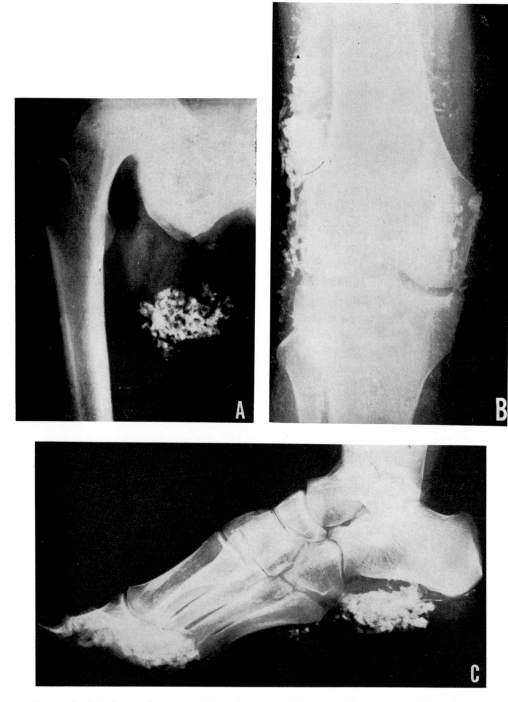

Figure 8–7. Calcium deposits: (A) in buttock, (B) around knees and (C) in foot in a patient with Type 3 Scleroderma. (Same patient as in Figure 8–10).

Telangiectasia

In view of their frequency and striking appearance in some cases, it seems curious that telangiectases, in association with scleroderma, did not appear to excite very much interest until comparatively recent times. Verel (1956) reported on nine women with Raynaud's disease, telangiectasia

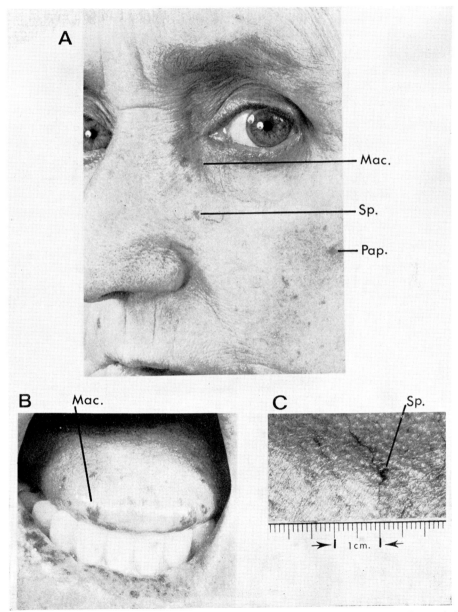

Figure 8–8. Telangiectases in patient with Type 1 Scleroderma (A) on face, (B) on tongue and (C) on upper part of chest. These may be flat macules (mac.), papular (pap.) or have the appearance of spider naevi (sp.).

and acrosclerosis (three of whom also had calcinosis). Winterbauer (1964) in his description of the *C.R.S.T. syndrome*, could only find eighteen reported cases of Raynaud's phenomenon associated with telangiectasia in the past ten years. In his paper based on seven cases (six of whom also had calcinosis), he gave a clear description of the telangiectasis as follows: "The macroscopic appearance of C.R.S.T. and R.O.W.* telangiectasia is identical. The C.R.S.T. angiomata vary from pin-point to five mm in size, have sharply demarcated borders, are purplish red in colour and maculo-papular with no central arteriole. The lesions blanch with pressure although blanching is frequently incomplete, and the lesions are non-pulsatile." They predominate on the upper extremities, face and mucous membranes. Epistaxis occurred in three of his seven patients, although this could not

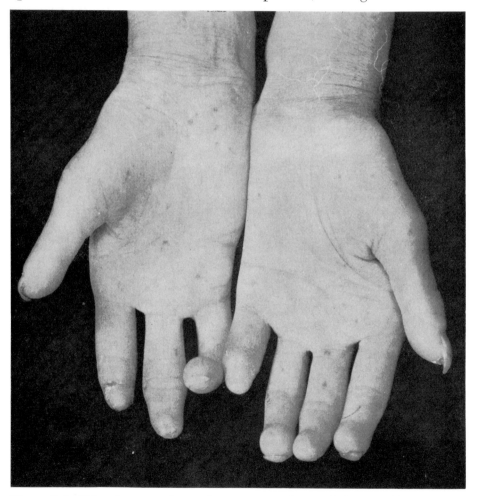

Figure 8–9. Telangiectases of macular type in palms and fingers of patient with Type 1 Scleroderma.

---

* R.O.W. = Rendu-Osler-Weber disease. See p. 73.

be attributed with certainty to the angiomata. One patient had telangiectases of the stomach and in another patient, not included in the report,
who suffered from repeated hematuria and hematemesis, telangiectases
were demonstrated in the bladder and rectum. Since Winterbauer's paper,
others have reported on telangiectasia in association with the acrosclerotic
type of scleroderma (Carr *et al.*, 1965, Berris *et al.*, 1967) and agree that
the telangiectases are quite similar to those found in the R.O.W. syndrome.

I have found angiomata very common in patients with scleroderma (in
eighteen of our thirty-one patients studied in 1969, including two with
diffuse (Type 3) scleroderma). They are of different types. One type
(described in detail by Winterbauer) is a discrete, circumscribed maculo-
papular lesion several millimetres in diameter, commonest on the face
but also occurring on the lips, palate and tongue (Fig. 8–8). Lesions on
the fingers are usually flat and of pin-head size (Fig. 8–9). Patients with
Type 2 scleroderma frequently have dilated venules somewhat like the
spider naevi of liver disease, most commonly about the clavicles and
blotchy macular erythematous patches frequently seen in elderly people
(Plate I). The lesions are mainly of cosmetic nuisance although some
patients are troubled by bleeding from lesions of the lips on brushing their
teeth.

PERIPHERAL VASCULAR DISTURBANCE

Peripheral vascular disturbance is almost universal in scleroderma.
Raynaud's phenomenon is always present in the Type 1 and Type 2 cases
and commonly precedes the skin changes by several months. In fact it has
been stated (de Takats and Fowler, 1962) that the Raynaud's phenomenon
may precede the skin changes by years, but in my experience, early skin
changes are usually visible after several months and, when they are
minimal, further confirmation of the diagnosis may be obtained by the
neck test. Occasionally patients have been seen in whom the initial
diagnosis was Raynaud's disease and who have returned several years
later with scleroderma. It is sometimes stated that Raynaud's phenomenon
is not a feature of the diffuse form, but this has not been my experience.
However, Raynaud's phenomenon may not be so prominent in these cases,
particularly if the onset is in the warmer months. Sometimes the circulatory disturbance may manifest itself more as a persistent coldness and
cyanosis rather than as paroxysmal ischaemic episodes.

The physiological and diagnostic aspects of the circulatory disturbances
in scleroderma have already been discussed in Chapter V.

The recurrent ulceration and infection mentioned when discussing the
cutaneous features no doubt have a vascular component but cannot be
explained completely on the basis of ischaemia. Extensive gangrene is uncommon and skin biopsies, even from apparently ischaemic digits, usually heal remarkably well. The commonest ulcers are superficial soggy

lesions which are extremely painful. Paronychia often occur in digits which are not particularly ischaemic. The lesions are frequently preceded by severe pain in the digit and it seems possible that they may originate as infection in a small hematoma such as have been demonstrated by capillaroscopy in the region of dilated capillary loops (See Chapter V).

Affection of the larger arteries is not commonly considered a feature of scleroderma. However, Barnett and Coventry (1969b) found absence of one or both ankle pulses in twenty-five of thirty-one patients. The popliteal pulse was absent in only four cases and this may have been coincidental.

SKELETAL

Skeletal involvement in scleroderma was recognized fairly early. Leontjewa (1924) and Klingman (1930) found skeletal involvement in about 25 percent and bone and joint involvement have since been described in the larger series.

Joints

Joint involvement of various types is fairly common in scleroderma. Tuffanelli and Winkelmann (1961) found that the onset of the disease was heralded by articular pain, swelling and redness in 12 percent and articular changes developed in the courses of the disease in 46 percent. The main problem was limitation of movement due to restriction of joints by sclerosis of surrounding tissues or secondary ankylosis.

Although flexion deformity of the fingers is common (Fig. 8–10) radiological changes of the joint surfaces are less common and usually of an osteo-arthritic nature (Fig. 8–11). It is often difficult to tell how much of the deformity is due to involvement of joint structures and how much to tightness of the surrounding skin. Other joints are less frequently involved. In Type 3 cases there may be marked limitation of extension of the elbows (Fig. 8–12).

There may be similarities to rheumatoid arthritis but classical rheumatoid deformity of spindle shaped joints and ulnar deviation is rarely seen, and when found is best interpreted as the association of the two diseases (See Chapter XIV).

Rodnan (1962) found histological abnormality of the synovial membrane in twenty-four of twenty-nine cases, comprising infiltration with lymphocytes and plasma cells in the acute stage and vascular sclerosis in the later stage. Others have also described infiltration with lymphocytes and plasma cells and vessel changes (Sokoloff, 1956, 1961; Mikkelsen *et al.*, 1958), or fibrosis and deposition of fibrin (Bennett and Dählenbach, 1951; Bywaters and Scott, 1965, Nice, 1966). Recently Clark *et al.* (1971) have reported on the histological findings in thirty-four cases and found that these correlated with the absence or presence of rheumatoid factor in the

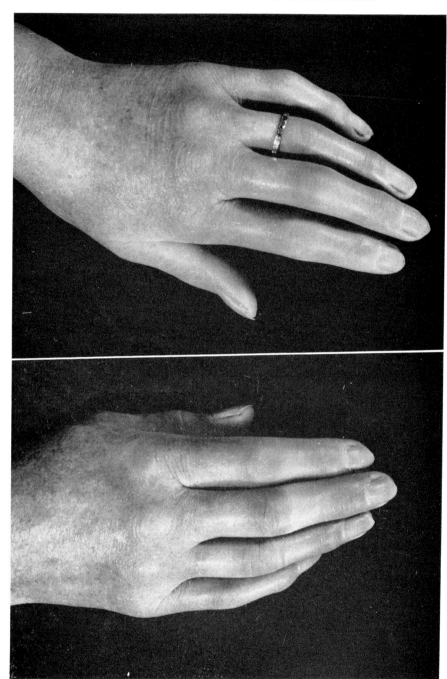

Figure 8–10. Flexion deformity of fingers in patient with Type 2 scleroderma giving appearance similar to that of rheumatoid arthritis.

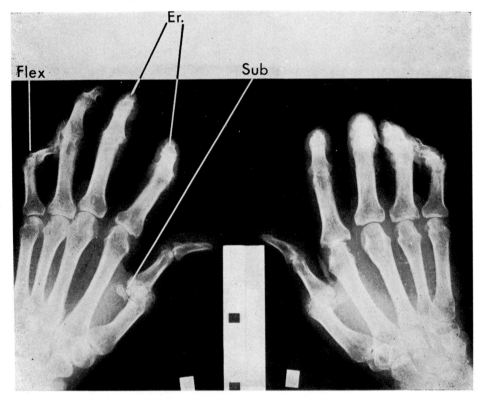

Figure 8–11. Radiograph of hands of a patient with scleroderma. Note: gross erosion of tufts of terminal phalanges (er.), flexion deformity of some interphalangeal joints (flex.), and subluxation of metatarso-phalangeal joints of the thumbs (sub.).

serum or synovial fluid. The characteristic features in the group of fourteen without rheumatoid factor was fibrosis, hyalinization of collagen, relative absence of inflammatory change and fibrosis of blood vessels and more than half of the specimens had marked fibrin deposition. The histological appearance of the specimens from the twenty patients with rheumatoid factor were variable: most showed moderate lymphocytic infiltration of the synovial and perivascular regions, sclerosis of blood vessels was not prominent, and fibrin deposition was present in only two cases. Two of the specimens were considered compatible with rheumatoid arthritis, but there were no instances of villous hypertrophy, pannus formation and plasma cell infiltration characteristic of rheumatoid arthritis.

Reports on examination of synovial fluid are scanty. Rodnan and Medsger (1966) reported that when synovitis is present clinically, the fluid is turbid, has a high protein content and contains polymorphonuclear leucocytes with inclusion bodies (*ragocytes*) similar to those in rheumatoid arthritis. Clark *et al.* (1971) found *ragocytes* in four of nine cases.

The limitation of joint movement in scleroderma is often secondary to

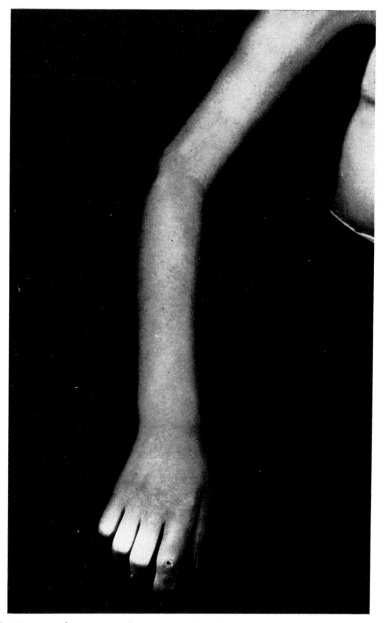

Figure 8–12. Arm of patient with Type 3 Scleroderma held in full voluntary extension of the elbow joint showing marked flexion contracture.

subcutaneous or peritendinous sclerosis. Tendon involvement is common and leathery tendon crepitus is a common sign (Shulman *et al.*, 1961; Bywaters and Scott (1965).

Karten (1969) has described a case of severe disorganisation of joints resembling neuropathic arthropathy in a patient with *C.R.S.T. syndrome.*

Bones

Erosion of the tufts of the terminal phalanges is common. In less severe cases, the tip of the terminal phalanx is tapering instead of tufted; in extreme cases the terminal phalanx is reduced to a mere nubbin of bone (Fig. 8–11).

The cause of the erosion is not clear. Ischaemia and compression by overlying tight skin have been suggested but neither of these explanations is completely satisfactory. Tuft erosion may be seen in fingers which are not remarkably ischaemic and is not a feature of other ischaemic conditions of the hands such as primary Raynaud's disease or in the ischaemic digits in elderly people due to atherosclerosis. However the ischaemia in these cases may not be as prolonged or as persistent as in the scleroderma cases. Also the skin in patients with resorption does not always seem particularly tight. Scharer and Smith (1969) made a curious observation that in a patient who had suffered a previous partial amputation of a finger which had been sewn back and who subsequently developed scleroderma, skin changes and bone resorption failed to occur in the previously damaged finger, while affecting the neighbouring fingers. They were unable to explain this phenomenon.

Other bones are rarely involved in scleroderma. Bjersand (1968) reported a case of scleroderma with bilateral carpal synostosis and new bone formation in the upper part of both femoral diaphyses and in both humeri. Wilde *et al.* (1970) reported a case of avascular necrosis of the femoral head in scleroderma and suggested it was due to an obliterative vasculitis.

Bone and joint changes are reported to be particularly common in children with scleroderma and affect the hands and feet and also the cervical spine (Szymańska-Jagiello and Rondio, 1970, Jakubowska *et al.*, 1970).

Skeletal Muscle

Involvement of skeletal muscles in scleroderma was recognized very early in the study of the disease. According to Medsger *et al.* (1968) the first report of muscular involvement in scleroderma was made as early as 1870 by Westphal. Histological changes of fibrosis and mild degenerative changes in muscle cells were described by Mery in 1889 and by Dinkler (1891). Lewen and Heller, in their monograph in 1895, reviewed twenty-six patients with muscle atrophy. Matsui in his pathological study (1924) gave a detailed account of the muscle changes. More recently, there have been detailed studies on the fine structure of muscle using both light microscopy and electron microscopy.

Hausmanowa-Petrusewicz and Koźmińska (1961, 1966) have described the electromyographic findings in *diffuse* (systemic) scleroderma and morphoea. In diffuse scleroderma there was a pattern similar to that in myositis and extending beyond the limits of the clinically affected skin. The severity of the muscle involved did not run parallel with the visceral involvement. In morphoea there was a similar pattern but much less severe even under the affected skin, and the distal muscles were affected less frequently.

The clinical aspects of muscle involvement do not seem to figure prominently in most of the general accounts of the disease. Slight generalized muscle atrophy and weakness are rather nonspecific and are apt to be overlooked or attributed to malnutrition or disuse.

Recently Medsger *et al.* (1968) have made a detailed study of the skeletal muscle involvement in scleroderma based on clinical and biochemical studies in fifty-three patients and histological examination of biopsy material in thirty-six. On the basis of muscle weakness, abnormal serum enzymes, disturbances or urinary creatinine they concluded that most patients with scleroderma had clinical and biochemical evidence of primary myopathy. Histological examination showed abnormalities of the muscle fibres (connective tissue or blood vessels) in all of the thirty-six patients.

SUMMARY

The characteristic skin changes in scleroderma are stiffness and tightness of the skin rather than hardness. The affection may vary in extent giving rise to the different types. Calcification of soft tissues is a common occurrence and may give rise to great annoyance by ulceration or production of tender nodules. Ischaemic features are the rule, giving rise to Raynaud's phenomenon and ulceration, although the latter is not completely explicable by simple ischemia. Telangiectases are common in all three types and not confined to one syndrome. They are of various types: flat or raised macules, spider naevi and blotchy erythematous patches.

Bone and joint involvement are common. Joint involvement may occur acutely at the onset or in the course of the disease. Although there are certain similarities to rheumatoid arthritis, the two diseases are distinct. Muscle involvement is probably common but is not frequently recognized clinically.

Chapter IX

GASTRO-INTESTINAL INVOLVEMENT

INTRODUCTION

IT IS NOW GENERALLY APPRECIATED that involvement of the alimentary system is frequent in scleroderma. As pointed out in Chapter One, description of the esophageal disturbance gave the first indication of visceral involvement in this disease. Subsequent studies have shown lesions extending from the oral cavity to the distal part of the colon.

Appreciation of the nature of the disturbances of the various parts of the alimentary tract in scleroderma is important for various reasons. These features are common, cause considerable distress and present problems in treatment. Gastro-intestinal features may dominate the clinical picture and the presence of scleroderma may be missed if the physician is not alert to the finer points of diagnosis.

This chapter will be concerned mainly with clinical and diagnostic aspects. Pathological features will only be mentioned in so far as they are related to clinical features, as they have already been discussed in Chapter Three.

FREQUENCY

It is probable that gastro-intestinal symptoms may have been over-looked in the early series, as some of the symptoms such as anorexia, weight loss and vomiting are rather non-specific and may occur in various illnesses. Thus in the series of O'Leary and Nomland (1930) including forty-eight cases of diffuse scleroderma there is no mention of gastro-intestinal disturbance. Leinwand *et al.* (1954), writing on 150 cases, state that fourteen patients who had dysphagia showed dilatation or stricture of the lower end of the esophagus on radiology. Although they refer to reports by others of disturbance of small bowel and colon, they do not cite any cases of their own. In the recent large series of 727 cases seen at the Mayo Clinic, reported by Tuffanelli and Winkelmann (1961) esophageal symptoms were present in forty-two percent and signs of esophageal dysfunction were found in seventy percent of 481 patients studied by radiography. However changes in the rest of the bowel were infrequent: delayed emptying of the stomach was demonstrated in only five cases, small bowel dysfunction in fifteen. Abnormality of the colon was found in two of fifty patients studied by barium enema. There were seven cases of cirrhosis of the liver, of which four were of an obscure nature and possibly related to scleroderma.

It is probable that the incidence of small bowel dysfunction was underestimated as this would not have been carefully looked for in the earlier part of the study period. Reinhardt and Barry (1962) were only able to find forty-two cases of small bowel involvement reported in the literature. However, in a series of 191 patients seen at the Duke University Hospital from 1930 to 1960, there was evidence of small bowel involvement in twenty-three of fifty-two cases who had radiological study of small bowel plus esophagus. This gives an incidence of 44 percent of the cases studied and 12 percent of the total series, indicating that involvement of the small bowel is more frequent than is suggested by the earlier reports.

Harper and Jackson (1965) in a paper on the radiological features based on a survey of fifty-two cases of systemic sclerosis, found abnormality of the esophagus in forty-one of forty-nine examined (84 percent), of the stomach and duodenum in seven of thirty-eight (18 percent), of the small bowel in eight of thirty-seven (22 percent) and of the colon in twenty of thirty-nine (51 percent). In the series reported by Barnett and Coventry (1969) upper gastro-intestinal symptoms or signs occurred in forty-four of sixty-one patients and abnormality was noted in radiological examination with a barium bolus or meal in thirty-nine. Some disturbance of small bowel function was found in twelve of thirty-one patients studied in detail (Barnett and Coventry 1969b). Most of these would not have been suspected clinically.

Oral Cavity

Oral manifestations of scleroderma, including small mouth, small tongue and telangiectases of mucosae, have already been mentioned in descriptions of the *types*. The small mouth may cause problems to the dental surgeon due to difficulty in retracting the lips. Widening of the periodontal membrane shown in dental radiographs (Stafne and Austin, 1944; Smith, 1958; Green, 1962) is a frequent finding when looked for routinely (Tuffanelli and Winkelmann, 1961). See Figure 9–1.

Esophagus

The first report of esophageal dysfunction in scleroderma is ascribed to Ehrman (1903) who reported on a patient who aspirated food into his esophagus on eating. The radiological picture of esophageal dilation was described by Schmidt (1916), Helm (1918) and Ochsner and DeBakey (1939). The case of Goetz and Rous (1942) showed esophageal spasm. Lindsay *et al.* (1943) found a stricture four to five cm. above the lower end of the esophagus in three of their five patients. Hale and Schatzki (1944)

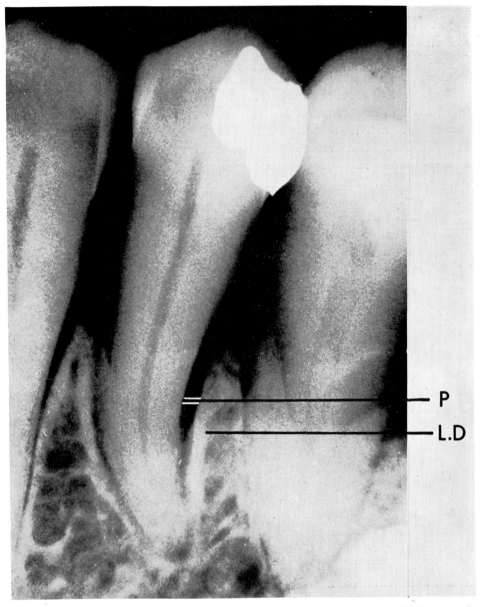

Figure 9–1. Dental radiograph of a patient with scleroderma showing thickening of periodontal membrane (P.) between the lamina dura (L.D.) of the socket and root of the tooth.

gave a detailed report on the radiological findings in twenty patients and found esophageal abnormality in fifteen. Although the usual picture was dilatation and diminished peristalsis, in one case the esophagus was narrower than normal. Olsen *et al.* (1945) found radiological abnormality of the esophagus (of the type previously described) in fifteen of twenty-four patients with dysphagia and reported the additional finding of hiatus hernia in some cases.

The pathological basis of this disturbance is not completely clear. Rake (1931) found thickening of submucosa and infiltration with cells. Goetz (1945) described inflammatory changes, hypertrophy of the muscle coat near the cardia and scarcity of ganglion cells in the myenteric plexus. More recent studies (Treacy *et al.*, 1963; Sackner 1967, d'Angelo *et al.*, 1969) have found muscle atrophy and/or fibrosis to be the main lesion.

The main clinical feature of esophageal involvement is dysphagia. This is usually of the *low type*, food seeming to stick at the sternal region, although the patient may indicate the site on the upper or middle portion of the sternum rather than the lower end. One of our patients had high dysphagia with difficulty in commencing swallowing and reflux of food into the naso-pharynx. Other common symptoms are due to gastro-esophageal reflux and comprise burning retro-sternal pain (*heart burn*) and regurgitation of fluid (*water brash*), particularly when lying down.

The radiological changes have been studied extensively (Hale and Schatzki, 1944; Harper, 1953; Lorber and Zarafonetis, 1963). They comprise aperistalsis (best shown in the recumbent position), dilatation, cobblestone appearance of the mucosa, tertiary contractions (fixed, non-peristaltic contractions), spasm, stricture, achalasia, hiatus hernia. Radiological abnormality is to be expected in those patients with symptoms, but also occurs in some without symptoms and there is only a loose correlation between the severity of the symptoms and the radiological signs.

During recent years one method of studying disturbed esophageal function is to measure intra-luminal pressures through fine tubes. In some studies the pressure change from the sphincter region is measured from a balloon and from more proximal regions from holes in the tubes (Code and Schlegel, 1958) and in others a series of fine tubes, each with a hole at a different level is used. Normally there is a relatively high pressure area at the cricopharyngeal sphincter region and in the lower sphincter region just above the diaphragm. During swallowing there is relaxation and then contraction of the sphincter regions when the bolus reaches them and then an orderly progression of the peristaltic wave.

Creamer *et al.* (1956) found that in nine patients with scleroderma the findings at rest were characterized by normal pressure of the pharyngo-esophageal sphincter, slightly increased pressure in the body of the esophagus and diminution of the tone in the gastro-esophageal sphincter at end of expiration. During deglutition the peristaltic wave failed a short distance below the pharyngo-esophageal sphincter and contractions throughout most of the esophagus were absent or inco-ordinated. The normal response of relaxation followed by contraction of the gastro-esophageal sphincter was feeble or absent. These findings have been confirmed and extended by

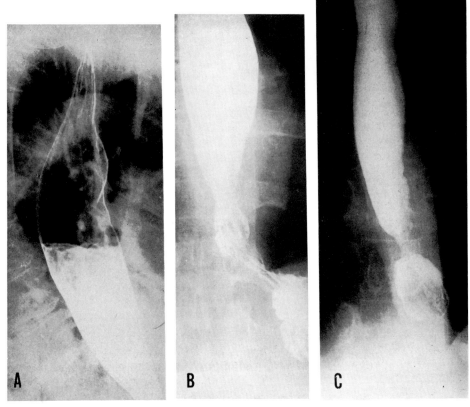

Figure 9–2. Examples of abnormalities of the esophagus found in patients with scleroderma. A. Grossly dilated esophagus with delayed emptying. B. Dilated esophagus and sliding hiatus hernia. C. Dilated esophagus with stricture near lower end.

subsequent workers (Kelly, 1963; Saladin *et al.*, 1966; Kaufman and Spiro, 1968). Esophageal pressure studies are a more sensitive method of detecting esophageal dysfunction than radiology and may show abnormalities in spite of normal radiological findings.

Abnormal esophageal patterns similar to, but less marked than, those in scleroderma have been reported in other connective tissue diseases and the specificity of the esophageal pressure findings to scleroderma has been open to doubt. Stevens *et al.* (1964) found aperistalsis in five of nine patients with *Raynaud's disease.* (However the series included four males, three patients with thickened fingers and six with telangiectasia and it is probable that they would have been classified by others as scleroderma with minimal skin changes.) The findings of Clark and Fountain (1967) suggest the pressure changes are specific for scleroderma. They found aperistalsis in five of seven patients with scleroderma, four of twenty-five patients with other collagen disorders (three of whom were later considered to have scleroderma) and none of thirteen patients with primary

Raynaud's disease. Recently Garrett *et al.* (1971) carried out progress pressure studies in 124 patients. They found that the severity of the esophageal involvement either remained static or progressed, but never improved. They described another abnormality of the esophagus in scleroderma, *diffuse spasm*, present in seven patients.

Esophageal disturbance has been common in my patients. Of thirty-one cases studied in detail (Barnett and Coventry, 1969b), fourteen had dysphagia, reduced esophageal motility was present in twenty-four, dilatation in eight, hiatus hernia in nine and esophageal stricture in two. The incidence of hiatus hernia of the sliding type is more frequent in this series than in others. Characteristic radiological pictures of esophagus in patients with scleroderma are shown in Figure 9–2. Manometric studies were carried out in ten patients with dysphagia. All showed abnormal tracings which correlated generally with the radiographic findings although in some the pressure tracings suggested a more severe disturbance than did the radiographic findings.

Stomach

The stomach seems to be affected only rarely in scleroderma. Tuffanelli and Winkelmann (1961) found only five cases of delayed emptying of the stomach in 727 cases, although the number studied by barium meal is not stated. Peachey *et al.* (1969) described a case with marked sclerosis of the stomach associated with involvement of small and large intestine, but the patient also had a pyloric ulcer. Apart from the gastro-esophageal reflux (considered under esophageal features), radiological gastric disturbance has not been observed in our series.

Gastro-intestinal Bleeding: This is not a common problem in scleroderma but has been reported in the *C.R.S.T. syndrome* due to gastric telangiectases (Binford, 1968).

Small Intestine (with or without Large Intestine)

Although Kraus had commented on dilatation of the stomach and duodenum at autopsy in 1924, clinical recognition of small bowel involvement in scleroderma was relatively late. Rake (1931) reported on a patient with scleroderma and a long history of abdominal pain and diarrhoea. X-ray examination showed dilatation of esophagus, small and large intestine and at operation the colon was enlarged and filled with a putty-like mass. Ileo-sigmoidostomy was performed but the patient died. At necropsy it was noted that, in spite of dilatation of the esophagus and colon, there was no hypertrophy of muscle in these organs.

Goetz and Rous (1942) drew attention to clinical features indicating intestinal involvement in scleroderma, and later Goetz (1945) described the pathological findings in detail. About the same time Hale and Schatzki (1944) described the radiological findings in four cases with gastro-intestinal symptoms. These comprised dilatation of loops of small intestine, predominantly the jejunum, and delayed passage of their contents. Bevans (1945) and Skouby and Teilum (1950) reported further cases.

Since 1950 there have been numerous reports of small bowel involvement in scleroderma but many of these have been of small numbers of cases (one to ten). In many of the reports the small and large bowel are affected together with an overall picture of atony and dilatation and will be considered together. The bowel features may be the presenting symptoms and skin changes inconspicuous (Drake *et al.*, 1964).

STASIS SYMPTOMS: The clinical picture is variable and comprises non-specific upper abdominal symptoms, weight loss, extreme atony progressing to ileus or pseudo-obstruction, and the malabsorption syndrome; these different features may be seen at various times in the same patient (Cullinan, 1953; Abrams *et al.*, 1954; Arcilla *et al.*, 1956; Sommerville *et al.*, 1959; Drake *et al.*, 1964). In some cases there is widespread atony of the bowel leading to stasis and in the extreme case resulting in death from paralytic ileus (Prowse, 1951) or faecal impaction and perforation of the colon (Hoskins *et al.* 1962). Greenberger *et al.* (1968) reviewed thirteen cases of intestinal atony in scleroderma, reported another of their own, and found that resection of the bowel had been carried out in five cases with improvement in three. Sometimes the clinical features (abdominal pain, distension, vomiting) had suggested mechanical obstruction leading to surgical exploration (Sommerville, 1959) although at operation no obstruction was found but flaccidity of the bowel (Weeks *et al.*, 1965).

The following case history is illustrative of some chronic bowel involvement in a patient with scleroderma.

CASE 1: The patient, aged 42 years, was admitted to hospital in July 1954, with a history that she had suffered from Raynaud's attacks of the fingers since teenage and painful fingertips for eight years. Other complaints were of *fainting turns*, frequent headaches, dyspnoea on exertion, palpitations and a feeling that her food tended to stick in the lower part of her chest. Examination revealed a small, thin woman with pinched features and tightness of skin of her face and hands, a small mouth and small tongue and cold cyanosed feet (Fig. 9–3). The skin of her fingers was tight and the terminal parts of the digits missing. X-ray examination of chest showed prominent markings of her left base and slight emphysematous changes. A barium swallow and meal examination showed a dilated, atonic esophagus, but with no hold-up of barium in the erect posture, and a hypotonic stomach. A bilateral lumbar sympathectomy was performed resulting in temporary improvement in the circulation of her feet.

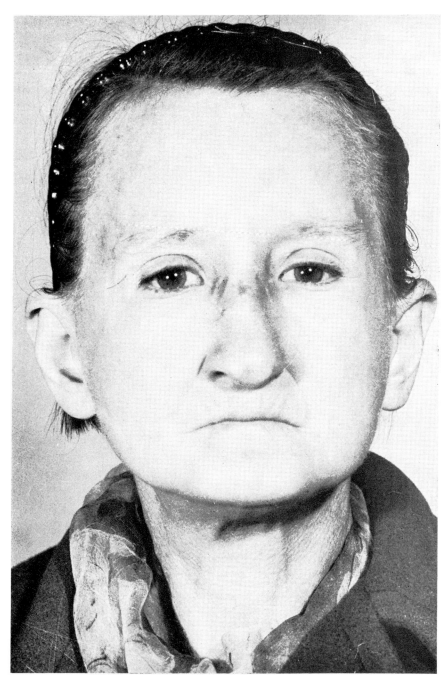

Figure 9–3. Photograph of a patient (Case One, Chapter IX), with long-standing Type 2 Scleroderma and severe gastro-intestinal involvement.

She was admitted to hospital again later in the year and commenced a course of cortisone treatment (maintenance dose of one hundred mg. per day). She was not improved by this treatment. The ischaemic symptoms in her hands increased necessitating digital nerve crush for relief of pain. The dysphagia increased and she obtained little help from the passage of mercury-filled dilators (Hurst's tubes).

She was again admitted to hospital in May 1962 because of considerable loss of weight, severe dysphagia and retrosternal pain, occurring two to three hours after meals and worse on stooping or lying. A barium swallow examination revealed, in addition to the previous findings, narrowing of the lower end of the esophagus and a sliding hiatus hernia. The stricture was dilated and the hiatus hernia was repaired via a thoracic approach. Her post-operative course was complicated by bowel obstruction due to inspissated barium in the sigmoid colon and by vertigo due to a post-operative course of streptomycin.

There was temporary improvement of the dysphagia and pain but the symptoms recurred, and eventually she was unable to pass Hurst's tubes. She was admitted to hospital in November 1963 and was treated by vagotomy and pyloroplasty and division of a fibrous band causing obstruction of the lower end of the esophagus.

She was not greatly helped by the treatment and was admitted to hospital again in May 1964 because of several weeks of intermittent constipation and diarrhoea, abdominal pain and vomiting. A barium meal examination was reported as showing an ulcer on the lesser curve just below the cardia. There was also very free gastro-esophageal reflux and delayed emptying of the stomach and duodenum.

A Bilroth Type 1 gastrectomy was performed. However there was only a small ulcer in the anterior wall of the stomach near the suture line of the old pyloroplasty and the radiological appearances of a lesser curve ulcer were attributed to extrinsic compression of the stomach by a loaded dilated colon. After the operation she continued to have abdominal pain radiating to her back and her abdomen became distended. Adequate emptying of the colon could not be obtained. About two weeks after the operation she complained of more severe abdominal pain and had signs of right sided peritonitis and later generalized peritonitis. A laparotomy revealed copious free purulent fluid in the peritoneal cavity with a perforation of her lower colon in the sigmoid region. A colonic resection was performed but after the operation she became hypotensive, had a poor urinary output, became oedematous and continued to discharge pus from the abdomen. In spite of intensive treatment with antibiotics and intravenous fluid, she died within two weeks with evidence of septicaemia.

At necropsy there was ulceration of the lower end of the esophagus and fibrotic change in the muscle; the small bowel was distended but there were no other obvious pathological changes; the large bowel had been removed. There were other widespread changes of systemic sclerosis: adhesive pericarditis, fibrosis and obliterative arterial changes in the myocardium, honeycomb lung with sclerotic changes in blood vessels, intimal thickening of interlobular arteries and fibrinoid necrosis of small vessels in the kidney. A bronchial adenocarcinoma was revealed in histological sections of the lungs.

In summary, this woman with a long history of scleroderma Type 2 developed visceral complications in heart, lungs, kidney and alimentary canal. The main clinical problems were associated with her alimentary system and comprised dysphagia, esophageal stricture, gastro-esophageal reflux, gastro-intestinal stasis and eventually death from perforation of the sigmoid colon.

MALABSORPTION: Malabsorption probably plays an important part in systemic sclerosis of the small bowel. There were features of malabsorption in many of the case reports discussed above, and in some there is a report of a flat glucose tolerance curve. Marshall (1956) reported on three patients with *collagen disease* with weight loss and abdominal symptoms treated surgically. One patient showed remission with treatment with phthalylsulphathiazole, later relapsed but was treated successfully by resection of the second and third parts of the duodenum and a segment of the jejunum. The other two patients died after operation. The first case in which malabsorption was demonstrated by increased fecal fat excretion seems to be that reported by Rosenthal (1957). Necropsy showed atrophy of the muscle of the small and large intestine and the mucosa of the small intestine was atrophic and infiltrated with lymphocytes. In several of the case reports the skin manifestations were minimal or absent (Horswell *et al.*, 1961, McBrien and Mummery, 1962, Leneman *et al.*, 1962). The administration of corticosteroids has not helped in malabsorption (Sonnenveldt *et al.*, 1962).

Recently cases had been reported in which malabsorption was the dominant symptom and investigations have been carried out to elucidate the mechanism. Salen *et al.* (1966) reported on a case with malabsorption, demonstrated by increased fecal fat excretion and decreased absorption of Vitamin B12 and xylose, in whom culture of jejunal contents showed increased bacterial flora and treatment with tetracycline resulted in fall in the jejunal bacterial count, clinical improvement and decrease in the fecal fat excretion. Kahn *et al.* (1966) reported on four cases with malabsorption in whom bacterial proliferation in the upper part of the small intestine was suggested by increased urinary excretion of indican and was confirmed by culture of duodenal aspirate. Three of the patients responded dramatically to long term treatment with antibiotic drugs. Atlas (1968) reported a similar case with E. Coli invasion of the duodenum and benefit from treatment with tetracycline. Radiography showed diffuse interstitial collections of gas in the wall of the small intestine (*pneumatosis intestinalis;* see later). Scudamore *et al.* (1968) reported on eight patients with systemic sclerosis with small bowel involvement and mild to severe steatorrhoea, but only minimal evidence of other defects in absorption. Although pancreatic function tests were generally normal, they considered that the normal absorption of ^{131}I labelled oleic acid (which does not require splitting by pancreatic lipase prior to absorption) and a favourable therapeutic response to treatment with pancreatic enzyme suggested that relative pancreatic insufficiency might play a part in the impaired absorption of fat.

The following is a summary of one of my cases in which malabsorption dominated the clinical picture.

CASE 2: A man, then aged 54 years, was admitted to hospital in October 1964 for investigation of chronic diarrhoea with two to eight bowel actions per day and loss of two stones in weight over the past two months. Apart from occasional swelling of his legs he had no other complaints about his health. Although he had poor circulation in his fingers, he did not give a history of typical Raynaud's phenomenon. He attributed the hardness of his fingers to his work as a truck driver and the ulceration at the tips of the fingers to his hobby of banjo playing.

On examination he was a pale, emaciated middle-aged man. The skin of his fingers was hard and there was some chronic ulceration of the tips of some fingers. His blood pressure was 100/80 mm. Hg. His heart, lungs and abdomen were clinically clear. Rectal examination and sigmoidoscopy to fifteen cm. revealed no abnormalities. Significant findings in a comprehensive series of tests were as follows. The serum potassium concentration was very low (2.6 m.eq. per liter), the calcium concentration was also low (3.0 m.eq. per liter) but the other electrolyte values were normal and blood urea level was normal. Radiography of his hands showed considerable soft tissue loss and a loss of tufts of some phalanges. A barium meal examination showed no abnormality in the esophagus, stomach or duodenal cap, but the small bowel was abnormally dilated. A jejunal biopsy specimen appeared normal under the dissecting microscopy and there were minor histological changes only (slight blunting of the villi and increase in the plasma cells in the lamina propria). His fecal fat excretion while on a 100 gm. fat intake was very high (ninety-four gm. per seventy-two hours). Malabsorption of xylose and vitamin B12 was also demonstrated and the glucose tolerance test revealed a flat curve. Liver function tests were normal except for a slightly low prothrombin level. He was treated with potassium and calcium supplements, vitamins B, D and K, folic acid, reduction of fat intake and diuretics. He kept fairly well with this regime and gained some weight.

He was reviewed in 1966. The clinical findings were much the same as previously. The serum calcium concentration was still low (2.6 m.eq. per liter). The bone and soft tissue changes shown in radiographs of the hands had progressed. Barium meal examination again showed dilatation of the small bowel and the barium swallow now showed reduced esophageal peristalsis. The fecal fat excretion was still high (sixty-eight gm. per seventy-two hours). The prothrombin level was still slightly low and in addition the serum glutamic oxalic transaminase (SGOT) was raised, although the other liver function tests were still normal. The previous treatment was continued with the addition of a course of tetracycline, but this had little effect on his diarrhoea and increased fat excretion.

He was admitted to hospital again in September, 1968 for further assessment. On examination he was a thin middle-aged man, rather slow mentally, with an irregular pulse of eighty-eight per minute and blood pressure of 105/75 mm Hg. The skin changes of scleroderma in his hands were similar to the previous examination. There were widespread rhonchi audible over his chest. The results of the special investigations were as follows: Haemoglobin was 9.9 gm. per one hundred ml., white cell count 8,000 per c.mm. An electrocardiogram showed sinus rhythm with premature atrial beats and premature ventricular beats, a radiograph of the chest showed mild cardiomegaly, but the lungs were relatively clear. A barium meal examination showed grossly dilated large and small bowel loops but without any obstruction. See Figure 9–4. The blood urea level was 44 mg/100ml., total plasma protein was 6.9 gm per one hundred ml. with an albumin of 3.9 gm per one hundred ml. and elevation of the β and γ fractions of the globulin. The serum folate level was raised as expected from his folate therapy and the vitamin B12 level was normal. The faecal fat content was 34.9 gm for 72 hours. The antinuclear factor in his serum had become strongly positive. He was discharged taking the same treatment.

He was finally admitted to the hospital in November 1968 with increasing fatty diarrhoea and general malaise. He was noted to be very thin and mentally vague and there were crepitations at his lung bases, but no other features of note. The following day he suffered a grand mal fit and became collapsed with a very weak pulse. The electrocardiogram showed frequent multifocal ventricular extrasystoles which were abolished with treatment with intravenous xylocaine. Blood chemistry showed a low potassium level (2.6 m.eq. per liter) and a low calcium (2.6 m.eq. per liter), a low bicarbonate level (total CO_2 12 m.eq. per liter) and a blood urea level of 62 mg per one hundred ml. In spite of intravenous fluid and electrolyte therapy his general condition continued to deteriorate and died after a few days.

At necropsy, the esophagus was found to be dilated and showed mucosal ulceration and fibrosis in the wall. The loops of small and large bowel showed gross dilatation. However histological examination was unsatisfactory because of autolytic changes. Both layers of the pericardium were thickened by fibrosis. The coronary arteries showed atheroma but were widely patent. The myocardium showed patchy interstitial fibrosis. There were bilateral pleural effusions and the lungs showed emphysema, fibrosis and honeycomb change. The kidneys showed mild granularity and mild arteriosclerotic changes. Immunofluorescent staining showed deposits of globulin in glomeruli and small arteries.

In summary, this middle-aged man was admitted to the hospital because of gastro-intestinal symptoms, mainly diarrhoea and weight loss. Although sclerodermatous changes were noted in the skin, these had not been considered of importance by the patient. He continued to have severe bowel disturbance and malnutrition and was shown to have grossly dilated bowel and features of malabsorption. His response to treatment was poor and he died four years after presentation. Other systemic manifestations were not prominent during his life, but at necropsy there was evidence of systemic sclerosis in heart and lungs and deposits of globulin in his renal vessels.

Patients with long standing scleroderma are commonly underweight and it would seem possible that there may be an element of malabsorption

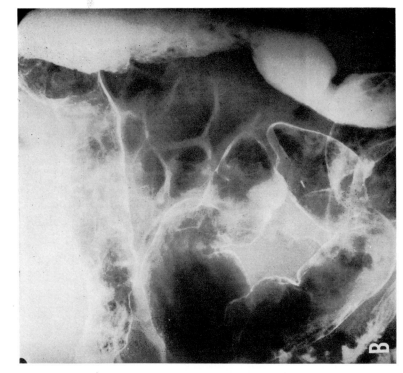

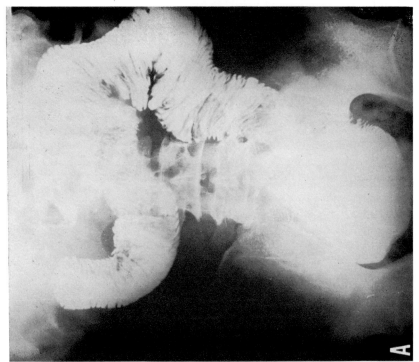

Figure 9–4. Radiographic appearances of the bowel following barium meal study in a patient with scleroderma. (Case Two, Chapter IX). A. Small bowel pictures. Note marked dilatation of the duodenum. B. Large bowel pictures. Note dilated colon lacking in normal haustra.

short of a full-blown malabsorption syndrome. Bendixen *et al.*, (1968) studied ten patients with scleroderma but without gastro-intestinal symptoms, using a range of gastro-intestinal absorption tests, including serum vitamin B12 and folate levels, D-Xylose absorption and fecal fat excretion, and found that the results were normal except in one patient with increased fecal fat excretion. However, Barnett and Coventry (1969b) found increased fecal fat excretion (above the upper limit of normal of seven gm. per twenty-four hours) in seven of thirty-one patients studied.

SURGICAL ASPECTS: Bowel involvement in systemic sclerosis may present as a surgical problem as in some of the cases already mentioned (Arcilla *et al.*, 1956; Marshall, 1956; McBrien and Mummery, 1962). Herrington (1959) reported on a patient presenting with symptoms of small bowel obstruction and relieved by excision of dilated jejunum and upper part of ileum. Treacey *et al.* (1962) reported on a further two cases with symptoms of obstruction of the small bowel, both dying after operation (biopsy only in one, colostomy in one). Nash and Fountain (1968) reported on surgery in two cases with acute abdominal symptoms. In one case there was inflammation of the terminal part of the ileum with the appearances of Crohn's disease; no resection was performed and the patient recovered. The other patient had a perforated stercoral ulcer of the caecum with fecal peritonitis and died. They reviewed the literature and found that laparotomy had been performed seventeen times for symptoms due to systemic sclerosis: for features of intestinal obstruction in eleven, signs of peritonitis in two, gas under the diaphragm in one, and gastric or esophageal symptoms in three. McMahon (1972) has reported on a case presenting with an acute abdominal catastrophe due to massive infarction of the intestine and liver.

Various reports on the operation findings give a rather characteristic picture: dilated and sometimes edematous small bowel, sometimes *white streaks* in the wall of the gut or mesenteric lymph glands. It appears from a study of the case reports that obstructive bowel symptoms in systemic sclerosis are not due to organic obstruction but to *pseudo-obstruction* due to inability of the bowel to propel its contents past an atonic segment. It is difficult to decide from the various reports concerning the correct treatment. Some patients have died following resection, but others have survived and obtained relief. Although there are no recorded cases of organic obstruction, one of my patients developed obstructive symptoms and was relieved by resection of a stenosing lesion of the small bowel. It would seem that if the patient develops marked obstructive symptoms, surgery should be considered and if there is a localized segment of affected bowel the best prospect of relief is by excision.

RADIOLOGICAL FEATURES: The radiological features of systemic sclerosis of the small bowel described by Hale and Schatzki (1944) have been confirmed and amplified by various subsequent reports (Harper 1953, Sommerville *et al.*, 1959; Heinz *et al.*, 1963; Harper and Jackson, 1965; Swischuk and Welsh, 1968, Peachey *et al.*, 1969). The prominent features are dilatation and atony affecting duodenum or jejunum or both associated with prolonged transit times. When a localized segment is involved this is most commonly the duodenum, although it may extend into the proximal part of the jejunum. Peachey *et al.* have emphasized the presence of *straightened loops* of duodenum and jejunum. Sometimes the whole of the small bowel is involved and the process may extend into the colon. Radiological features of the small bowel of a normal subject and of a scleroderma patient are compared in Figures 9–5 and 9–6. It has been claimed by some (Swischuk and Welsh, 1968) that the dilated bowel in systemic sclerosis with malabsorption can be distinguished from that in other malabsorption syndromes such as adult coeliac disease: in systemic sclerosis the valvulae conniventi, although thin and stretched, are usually close together and not widely separated as in adult coeliac disease. However differential diagnoses on radiological grounds may be difficult.

PATHOLOGICAL CHANGES: The pathological changes in systemic sclerosis of the small bowel have been described in detail by Goetz (1945) who found atrophy of muscle, replacement by fibrosis and decrease in the ganglion cells in the myenteric plexus. The fibrosis and muscle atrophy have been confirmed in the various cases described above in which histological examination has been made. The mucosa is relatively unaffected and shows normal leaf-like villi with the result that the findings on peroral duodenal biopsy have not been remarkable. However Rosson and Yesner (1965) described collagenous encapsulation (periglandular sclerosis) in peroral duodenal biopsies from six patients.

It is seen that small bowel disturbance in scleroderma may be localised or generalised and present a varied picture. The main abnormality is disturbed motility resulting in delayed transit and obstructive symptoms. Atony and dilatation of the bowel may be associated with bacterial overgrowth as in the *blind loop syndrome*. This is followed by malabsorption, the main features of which are steatorrhoea due to bacterial interference with bile salt metabolism, vitamin B deficiency due to bacterial consumption, and general features of malnutrition. Structural changes in the bowel wall are not marked.

PNEUMATOSIS INTESTINALIS: *Pneumatosis intestinalis* (or intramural gas) is a rare condition in which there are collections of gas in the intestinal wall showing as cystic areas or linear streaks in radiographs of the abdomen,

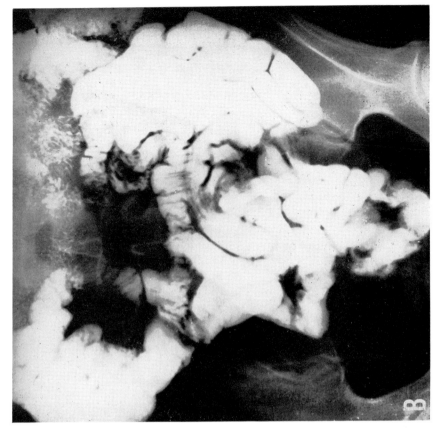

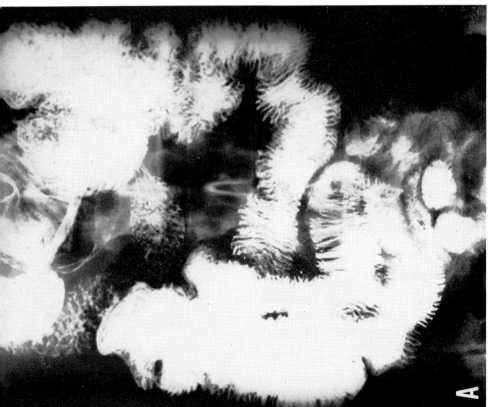

Figure 9–5. Radiographic appearance of normal small bowel following a barium meal. A. Early phase; B. Late phase.

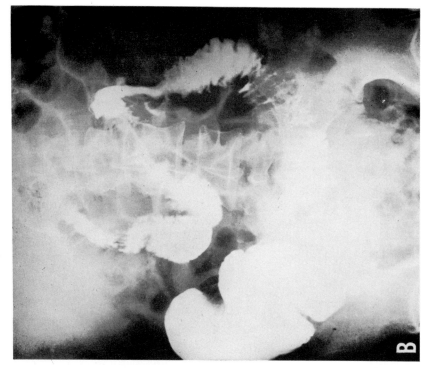

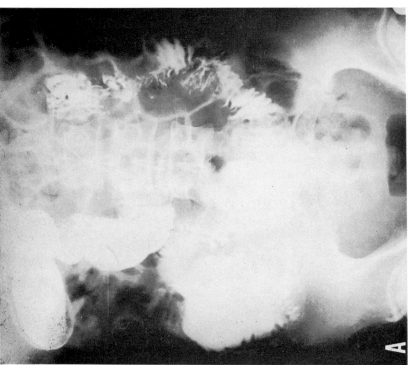

Figure 9–6. Radiographic appearance of small bowel following a barium meal in a patient with scleroderma. A. Early phase. Note the marked dilatation of the duodenum. B. Late Phase. The dilated bowel in the right iliac fossa is jejunum.

particularly when the bowel contains barium. The cause of the condition is not known and the theories comprise (1) bacterial infections, (2) dietary deficiency, (3) mechanical break in the intestinal wall and (4) leakage of gas from the air passages due to respiratory disease. It may occur under various conditions and the mechanism may not be the same in all cases. Aspiration of a cyst in one case (not systemic sclerosis) yielded an admixture of gases of blood and intestinal origin. The mechanism in systemic sclerosis is not clear but it usually occurs in association with other features of bowel involvement. Respiratory disturbance presents another possible factor. The five cases described by Hughes *et al.*, (1966), one included a patient with systemic sclerosis with small bowel symptoms and pneumoperitoneum. There have since been several further reports of this condition in systemic sclerosis with bowel involvement usually with malabsorption or pseudo-obstruction (Fallon, 1967– one case; Meihoff *et al.*, 1968– three cases; Atlas, 1968– one case; Miercort and Merrill, 1969– three cases; Gompels, 1969– one case). Pneumoperitoneum has been present in several of the cases. Where operation has been performed it has not been helpful. Meihoff *et al.*, considered that the condition carried a bad prognosis, as two of their three patients with this condition died within six months and the third was going rapidly downhill. White *et al.* (1970) reported a patient still alive after five years, although the patient was then in a poor state of health due to malnutrition.

Colon

Dilatation and stasis of both the small bowel and colon in systemic sclerosis has already been mentioned. However, in one report (Lushbaugh *et al.*, 1948) death was due primarily to colonic involvement. The patient presented with abdominal pain, constipation and distension of the abdomen and collapse. Necropsy showed peritonitis secondary to a ruptured diverticulum and a dilated, dark red colon, in which there was fibrous replacement of smooth muscle and the fibrosis and thrombosis of small arteries.

The frequency of colonic involvement is difficult to assess as barium enema examinations are not commonly done without clinical indications. In the series Tuffanelli and Windelmann (1961) comprising 727 patients, only fifty were studied by barium enema and only two of these were abnormal. However in patients with bowel symptoms, a high proportion have colonic involvement. Thus Harper (1953) reported colonic abnormality in eight of eleven patients with gastro-intestinal symptoms. If the colon is involved there is likely to be involvement of the alimentary canal elsewhere (Meszaros, 1958). The characteristic radiographic finding is broad mouthed diverticula (Fig. 9–7) and the main symptoms constipation and

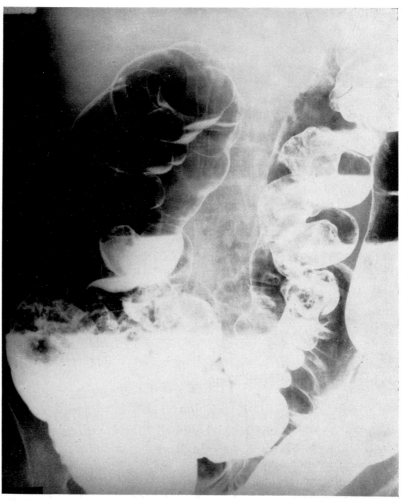

Figure 9–7. Radiographic appearance following a barium enema in a patient with scleroderma showing large diverticula on the antimesenteric border of the colon.

diarrhoea (Harper, 1953). The pathological basis is atrophy of the muscle, and oedema and fibrosis of submucosa. The diverticula consist of all layers of the bowel wall (Rake, 1931, Heinz *et al.*, 1963; Goldgraber and Kirsner, 1957). Rarely large diverticula may lead to obstruction as in a case reported by Monroe and Knauer (1962) and two cases reported by Comptom (1969) successfully treated by resection. Lockhart-Mummery and Jones (1960) reported a case of infarction of the colon (treated by hemicolectomy) associated with systemic sclerosis, believed to be due to ischaemia of the bowel due to obliterative changes in the arteries. Ulcerative colitis has occasionally been reported in association with systemic sclerosis (Harper, 1953, Bicks *et al.*, 1958; DeLuca *et al.*, 1965) but is probably coincidental.

Liver

Serious affection of the liver in scleroderma is apparently uncommon. Abnormality of so-called liver function tests is not unusual. In fact, using as tests raised serum bilirubin level (over 1.2 mg/100ml), raised alkaline phosphatase level (over twelve King Armstrong units/100ml), raised S.G.O.T. level (over forty-five units) and low prothrombin level (less than fifty percent of normal), Barnett and Coventry (1969b) found evidence of possibly disturbed function in sixteen of thirty-one patients tested. However these tests are non-specific and do not indicate primary liver pathology.

Hepatosplenomegally in association with scleroderma was observed by Milbradt (1934) and the case reported in detail by Goetz (1945) had chronic biliary cirrhosis as an autopsy finding. There have since been sporadic records of liver disturbance in association with scleroderma (reviewed by Murray-Lyon *et al.*, 1970) but the significance of these is obscure, particularly as there were usually no detailed histological studies. Calvert *et al.* (1958) reported on two cases of systemic sclerosis with portal hypertension. In one of these, fine hepatic cirrhosis was seen at operation but no biopsy was taken and in the other, biopsy showed "cirrhosis with hyperplasia and mild round cell infiltration."

Bartholomew *et al.* (1964) reported on the only eight patients with serious liver disease found in the large Mayo Clinic series of 727 patients. Biopsy was obtained in five of these, the diagnosis being post-necrotic cirrhosis (two cases), cholangiolitic hepatitis (two cases), chronic hepatitis with periportal fibrosis (one case). Of the other three cases, two had a clinical diagnosis of *cirrhosis of the liver* and the remaining one disturbed liver function tests. They stated that the low incidence of serious liver disease in scleroderma hardly suggested a significant relationship. In two of the cases the histology and results of tests are suggestive of primary biliary cirrhosis. Grilliat *et al.* (1967) reported on a case of hepatosplenomegaly and portal hypertension in association with the Thibierge-Weissenbach syndrome. Biopsy of the liver showed periportal fibrosis with cellular infiltration, mainly polymorphs, new bile cannaliculi, preservation of liver cells with absence of fatty change or accumulation of iron pigment. In contrast to most other workers Aprosina *et al.* (1970) have found a very high clinical occurrence of liver disturbance in scleroderma and frequent fibrotic lesions at necropsy.

Recently there have been several reports of primary biliary cirrhosis in scleroderma, often with features of *C.R.S.T. syndrome*. Reynolds *et al.* (1971) * have reported six cases all of whom had telangiectases and calci-

* Although not published until 1971, the paper by Reynolds *et al.* was submitted for publication in 1970 and is referred by Murray-Lyon *et al.* 1970.

nosis. O'Brien *et al.* (1972) have reported one case without features of C.R.S.T. The patients have shown the characteristic biochemical abnormalities, histological picture and, when determined, a positive mitochondria antibody test, which is reported to be found in about ninety percent of patients with primary biliary cirrhosis. The scarcity of previous reports is surprising. However it must be remembered that reports of bowel involvement were also rare in the early literature, although they are now recognized as being frequent in scleroderma.

SUMMARY

Gastro-intestinal involvement is a most important form of visceral disturbance in scleroderma.

Certain manifestations, particularly esophageal dysfunction are common and an important diagnostic feature. Although the dysphagia and gastro-esophageal reflux symptoms may occasion considerably annoyance to the patient, they are usually able to be managed medically and do not provide a threat to the patient's life.

Small and large bowel disturbances are less common but more serious. The main abnormality is loss of tone of the wall of the bowel. This is recognized radiologically as a dilated segment with delayed passage of contents. It may produce a variety of clinical features, ranging from upper abdominal pain and distension to severe stasis and malabsorption syndrome. The patient may develop acute abdominal symptoms simulating intestinal obstruction. The characteristic large bowel involvement is the presence of wide-mouthed diverticula demonstrated radiologically. They are usually symptomless but may give rise to symptoms by fecal impaction and perforation. The rare condition of *pneumatosis intestinalis* has recently been recognized in association with scleroderma. The association of hepatic disease with scleroderma has been conjectural but recent reports indicate that there may be an association between scleroderma and primary biliary cirrhosis.

Chapter X

PULMONARY INVOLVEMENT

HISTORICAL SURVEY

ALTHOUGH THE FREQUENCY AND IMPORTANCE of pulmonary involvement in scleroderma has only been appreciated in relatively recent years, it is possible to find isolated references to respiratory disturbance in patients with this disease in the older literature as detailed in an excellent review article by Weaver *et al.* (1967). Early clinical reports include those of Day (1870) of a case with dyspnoea and râles at the left apex (attributed to subcutaneous induration), Harley (1877) of a case with increased breath sounds (attributed to fibrous degeneration of the lung), Hoppe-Seyler (1889) of diminished vital capacity and accentuated pulmonary second sound, Finlay (1889, 1891) of a patient with impaired respiration and pulmonary infection attributed to limitation of chest expansion due to tight skin over the thorax. In the absence of pathological confirmation, none of these can be claimed to be definite reports of scleroderma lung.

Dinkler (1891) found necropsy evidence of pulmonary fibrosis in a sclerodermatous patient with severe dyspnoea, but still attributed the dyspnoea to restriction of the chest wall. Lewen and Heller (1895) in their review of 509 cases of scleroderma found two in whom fibrosis of the lung had been noted post-mortem. (They also found six patients in whom dyspnoea had been a prominent symptom but attributed this to involvement of the chest wall). Notthafft (1898) described pulmonary fibrosis and thickening of the walls of pulmonary arteries. Kraus (1924) described similar changes plus emphysematous changes, alveolar proliferation in a glandular fashion and right ventricular hypertrophy. Matsui (1924) also found pulmonary fibrosis, arterial changes and right ventricular hypertrophy and, in addition, pleural effusions and pleural adhesions. Rake (1931) described metaplasia of the bronchial epithelium. Masugi and Yä-Shu (1938) described more acute changes of fibrinoid necrosis, proliferative endarteritis and perivascular inflammatory cell reaction.

The recognition of pulmonary involvement in scleroderma as a clinical entity followed the description of the radiological changes by Murphy *et al.*, (1941) who reported on the findings in a chest radiograph in a thirty year old woman with scleroderma as follows: "Within the pulmonary fields, with exclusion of the apices and lateral aspect of the bases, there was a diffuse network-like shadow extending from the cardiac border to the periphery." They proved that the shadow was due to an abnormality of the lung by observing that it disappeared after a diagnostic pneumothorax. Linenthal and Talkov (1941) reported a further three cases in the same year, Jackman (1943) two cases and Lloyd and Tonkin (1948) another four cases. Getzowa (1945) gave a detailed account of the pathological changes in two cases and subdivided them into *cystic pulmonary sclerosis* and *compact pulmonary sclerosis* (see later). Baldwin *et al.* (1949) included three patients with scleroderma in a group of patients with pulmonary fibrosis and arterial oxygen desaturation on exercise whom they studied by pulmonary function tests. They concluded that the evidence indicated a veno-arterial shunt or diffusion defect or both (see later). Spain and Thomas (1950) correlated the results of pulmonary function tests in one patient with the necropsy findings. Church and Ellis (1950) surveyed the literature on fibrosis of the lungs in scleroderma and reported two cases with cysts.

INCIDENCE

The apparent incidence of pulmonary involvement in scleroderma varies according to the method of detection used: clinical, radiological or special tests. The main symptom is dyspnoea which may not be complained of until the late stages or may be attributed to other causes, with the result that in the early series of reported cases of scleroderma the condition was overlooked. Since the recognition of the radiological changes, pulmonary involvement has been found to be relatively common. In the large Mayo Clinic series (Tuffanelli and Winkelmann 1961, 1962b) radiological changes were found in 137 of 555 patients who had X-ray examination of the chest (25 percent), with approximately the same incidence in those with the acrosclerotic and diffuse form of the disease. In the series of Barnett & Coventry (1969a) positive radiological features were found in thirteen of sixty-one cases (21 percent), giving approximately the same incidence as in the large series. Pulmonary symptoms or signs were found at some stage in thirty-one patients (50 percent) but these were probably not all due primarily to the specific lung disease of systemic sclerosis. Using special lung function tests, an even higher incidence is found. Ritchie (1964) investigated twenty-two patients (who belonged to the series of sixty-one later reported by Barnett and Coventry) and found some abnormality in twenty-one, although it is doubtful that all of these were attributable to systemic sclerosis. De Muth *et al.* (1968) investigated ninety-eight unselected patients with scleroderma and found some objective manifestation of pulmonary involvement in sixty-one (62 percent). It is apparent therefore that pulmonary involvement in scleroderma is common, approaching in frequency that of the esophagus.

RADIOLOGICAL FEATURES

The commonest radiological abnormalities are those originally described by Murphy *et al.* (1941) consisting of a reticular pattern of opacity affecting particularly the basal regions and sparing the apices. These have been reported on numerous occasions. The disease progresses to diffuse symmetrical pulmonary fibrosis, most marked at the bases. Both lungs are usually involved, but, if one lung only is affected, this is most frequently the right. Less frequently there is a nodular type of fibrosis simulating pneumocomosis. Systemic sclerosis is one cause of honeycomb lung (Opie 1955). Cysts are most often subpleural, are situated in the basal and paravertebral areas and are usually bilateral. Although they are usually small (five mm in diameter), large cysts may sometimes occur and may rupture to produce a pneumothorax. Occasionally there may be disseminated pulmonary calcification, difficult to distinguish from the calcification of the soft tissues of the thoracic case, also sometimes found in scleroderma (Ashba and Ghanem 1965). The radiological picture may be complicated by the presence of pleural effusion, pleural thickening and by enlargement of the pulmonary artery and right heart chambers in patients developing pulmonary hypertension.

PATHOLOGY

The main pathological changes consist of thickening of alveolar walls by collagenous tissue and narrowing of the lumina of small pulmonary arteries. The severe grades of the disease have been described in detail by Getzowa who found two types of lesion, *compact pulmonary sclerosis* where there was much overgrowth of collagenous tissues in the interalveolar spaces and *cystic pulmonary sclerosis* where avascular interalveolar walls had broken down to form cystic spaces. In some advanced cases, the cystic change may be very marked leading to a type of honeycomb lung. Pimental (1967) studied the pathogenesis of honeycomb lung in various diseases including scleroderma by cutting serial sections, staining, mounting in layers and constructing three-dimensional models. He concluded that the fundamental changes consisted in dilatation of bronchioles associated with obliteration or rigidity of the corresponding ducts and alveoli and peribronchial fibrosis. Bullous development was due to distortion of bronchioles resulting from valve-like arrangements which permitted the entrance of air but hindered its exit. A most comprehensive report on the pathological changes in the lung in scleroderma has been given by Weaver *et al.* (1968) based on a study of twenty-eight necropsy cases over forty years. Histological changes were found in all cases. Changes in the alveoli and interstitial tissue included interstitial fibrosis (all cases) and lining of alveoli with cuboid epithelium. Changes in the blood vessels included increased collagen in their walls, intimal proliferation, medial hypertrophy, myxomatous change, P.A.S. positive material in the wall, occlusion of small vessels and increase in elastic tissue. Changes in bronchi and bronchioles included an apparent increased number of bronchi and bronchioles, increased thickness of basement membrane, lining of bronchioles with cuboidal epithelium, acute and chronic bronchitis. Cysts were of two types: sub-pleural cysts lined with cuboidal epithelium and cysts due to rupture of avascular and acellular alveolar walls. Pleural changes included thickening and increased vascularity.

Caplan (1959) reported on two cases with cystic fibrosis of the lung associated with pulmonary adenomatosis of which one was probably malignant and the other definitely so. Batsakis and Johnson (1960) reported a further case and there have since been several further reports of this rare tumour in association with honeycomb lung in scleroderma. It presumably arises in the metaplastic cuboidal alveolar epithelium.

CLINICAL FEATURES

It is difficult to obtain a reliable estimate of the frequency of respiratory symptoms in scleroderma. Respiratory infections are common in the community and symptoms such as cough and sputum can only be ascribed to systemic sclerosis of the lung if persistent. The commonest symptom is dyspnoea but this is often insidious in onset and its presence may not be appreciated unless elicited by questioning.

In patients with cardiac disturbance it is difficult to distinguish between dyspnoea and cough due to primary lung disease and that secondary to heart disease. However cardiac failure in scleroderma is usually secondary to lung disease and increased pulmonary vascular resistance and it is justifiable to attribute the initial dyspnoea in these cases to pulmonary disease. DeMuth *et al.* (1968) found respiratory symptoms or signs in forty-seven of ninety-eight patients (50 percent) and Barnett and Coventry (1969b) a similar proportion. DeMuth *et al.* found the commonest symptoms to be dyspnoea (thirty-nine patients), cough (twenty-five patients). Dysphonia was present in three cases. The commonest signs were fine râles (twenty-eight cases) and limited expansion (twenty-three cases). Clinically, hyperpnoea was only noted in three cases but the authors considered this to be probably an underestimate. Weaver *et al.* (1968) found a higher incidence of dyspnoea on exertion (eighteen of twenty-eight cases) but lower incidence of cough (only four of twenty-eight). Other uncommon symptoms were recurrent pneumonitis, hemoptysis and pleural pain. With the onset of cardiac involvement secondary to lung involvement, the symptoms and signs of cardiac failure are added, as described in Chapter XI.

A potentially dangerous complication of cystic fibrosis in scleroderma is the occurrence of spontaneous pneumothorax, which, presumably because of valvular openings in the cyst, may progress to tension pneumothorax and cause death (Israel and Harley, 1956). Dines *et al.* (1967) suggest that the correct treatment for spontaneous pneumothorax with honeycomb lung is closed tube thoracostomy with suction and, if rapid expansion does not occur, open thoracostomy and abrasion of the parietal pleura.

Pulmonary involvement usually occurs late in the disease by which time skin signs are usually definite, but sometimes pulmonary disturbance occurs early and may dominate the picture.

Case Histories

The following case is illustrative of pulmonary involvement occurring after a long history of scleroderma.

CASE 1: A woman then aged forty-eight years, was first seen in November 1958, with a complaint of episodes of coldness and pallor of fingers and toes in response to cold over the previous six months and recently an infection of her left index finger, treated with antibiotics. Otherwise her health had been good.

On examination she was a healthy looking, middle-aged lady with a blood pressure of 140/70 mm. Hg. Routine examination revealed no abnormality apart from atrophy of the tip of the left index finger and pallor and coldness of some of her toes. Calorimetry gave a normal resting heat elimination but there was poor response to reflex heating. Within a few months she developed sclerodermatous changes of her fingers. She continued to suffer from painful ulceration in her fingers necessitating on one occasion a nerve crush and later amputation of her left index finger.

The circulatory trouble in her fingers continued over the next few years but her general health remained good. When reviewed in 1965, she stated that sometimes food tended to stick both at the pharyngeal level and at the lower end of the sternum and that she experienced retrosternal discomfort on stooping and after meals, relieved by an antacid. On examination she was found to have vascular naevi of her forehead and face and her body skin was slightly pigmented and sclerosis of the skin was still limited to the fingers.

A comprehensive series of tests revealed the following abnormalities. The erythrocyte sedimentation test was slightly elevated (twenty-one mm. in one hour, Wintrobe method). A chest radiograph showed increased markings at the bases. Her vital capacity was normal, but the forced expiratory volume over one second (FEV_1) was slightly reduced. Radiography of her hands showed loss of soft tissue and of the subungual tufts of her fingers, and a little soft tissue calcification of her thumbs. A barium swallow examination showed minor esophageal dilatation, almost complete lack of persistalsis and a small hiatus hernia. The fecal fat excretion was twenty-one gm. per seventy-two hours (upper limit of normal). The latex agglutination test was positive but the immunofluorescent tests were negative.

Over the succeeding years the dysphagia and symptoms of gastro-esophageal reflux became more marked. She lost weight and showed evidence of malabsorption in raised fecal fat excretion and impaired xylose absorption. Her pigmentation increased and she developed numerous naevi of her chest and face, but the sclerosis of the skin remained confined to her fingers (Fig. 10–1). Chest radiograph showed opacities consistent with fibrotic changes of the right lower lobe (Fig. 10–2).

In April 1972, in addition to her other symptoms she complained of shortness of breath on exertion, occasional pain in the precordial region and swelling of the ankles. On examination she had signs of congestive cardiac failure with slightly raised jugular venous pressure, crepitations at lung bases, enlarged liver and some oedema of the ankles. The second sound in the pulmonary area was duplicated. An electrocardiogram showed ST-T changes and peaked P waves in Lead II indicative of right atrial enlargement. Radiography of the chest showed more marked opacities at the lung bases and slight cardiac enlargement. She was also slightly anemic with a hemoglobin of nine gm. per one hundred ml. She was treated with digoxin, diuretics and iron therapy and lost her signs of cardiac failure but remained dyspnoeic on mild exertion.

Comment: This is a history of a patient with Type 1 scleroderma who has, over the years, developed features of gastro-intestinal and pulmonary involvement. She eventually had an episode of congestive cardiac failure, probably mainly due to pulmonary involvement.

The following cases are illustrative of lung involvement occurring early in the disease in the absence of marked skin changes and dominating the clinical picture.

CASE 2: A man aged forty years, was seen in 1951 with a history that over the past five months he had experienced Raynaud's attacks in the fingers on exposure to cold and over the past month he had a sensation of swelling of the fingers. He had been a foundry worker for twenty years but was currently employed as a maintenance laborer with the Board of Works, a job requiring attention to water pipes in the cold.

Examination gave normal findings apart from his hands which were cold and slightly cyanosed and some fingers were rather thick. His lungs were clinically and radiologically normal. The Raynaud's attacks continued over the ensuing months and he did not get any great benefit from stopping smoking.

In June 1952 he was admitted to hospital because of an infection in one finger requiring antibiotic treatment. The skin of the fingers was stiff, thick and smooth, indicative of scleroderma and the hands were frequently cold and blue.

In May 1954, he developed a respiratory infection associated with pain in the chest and difficulty in breathing. A radiograph of his lungs showed fine mottling. Over the ensuing three years he steadily became more dyspnoeic and lost weight. In view of the history of having worked in a foundry, he was accepted by the Health Department as suffering from silicosis. He died out of hospital from respiratory failure.

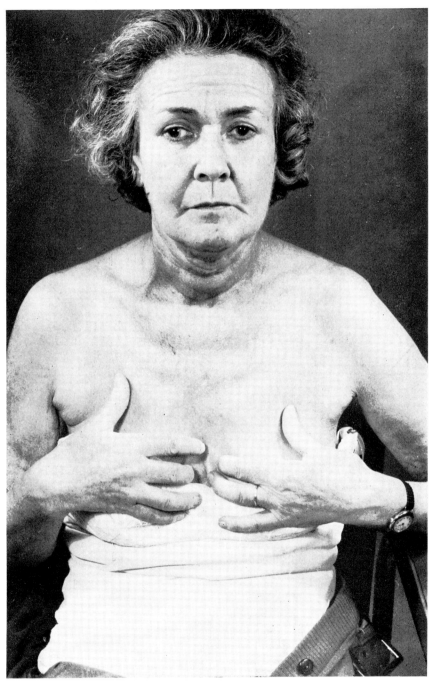

Figure 10–1. Photograph of a patient (Case One, Chapter X) with clinical and radiological lung involvement. Note that the sclerosis is limited to the hands (Type 1 Scleroderma).

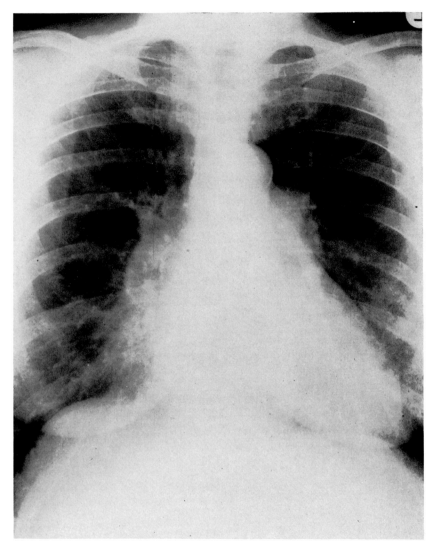

Figure 10–2. Radiograph of chest of a patient (Case One, Chapter X) showing decreased translucency at both lung bases.

Comment. This man presented with Type 1 scleroderma. His lungs at that time were clinically and radiologically clear. Over the ensuing years he developed progressive dyspnoea and mottling of his lung fields. Although he was accepted for compensation for silicosis it is more likely that the respiratory impairment was due to scleroderma.

CASE 3: A physician aged fifty-one years, was seen in August 1966 with a history that twelve months previous he had developed shortness of breath on exertion and an irritating cough followed a few days later by a headache and white mucopurulent nasal discharge. A chest radiograph had shown an elevated right hemidiaphragm and an opacity in the right lung. He was treated with bed rest and achromycin but his shortness of breath and cough had continued.

Esophagoscopy and bronchoscopy were normal but a bronchogram showed some crowding of the bronchi of his right lower lobe. He later developed mild dysphagia and some retrosternal burning pain, but barium swallow and barium meal examinations and electrocardiogram were normal. Before the onset of his symptoms he had noticed that his right forefinger would go numb and white while washing his car, but he did not have any other ischaemic symptoms until mid-June 1966 (winter-time) when he began to experience Raynaud's phenomenon of all his fingers on exposure to cold and shortly after this paraesthesia of his fingers and pain and weakness of his wrists. His fingers and hands had become swollen and he had difficulty in making a fist.

On examination he was a somewhat undernourished, middle-aged man with cold sclerodermatous fingers. There was no sclerosis of other parts and the mouth and throat appeared healthy. His blood pressure was 150/80 mm. Hg. There was a short systolic murmur at the cardiac apex but no other cardiac abnormality. There was prolongation of expiration at the lung bases and crepitations at the right base. His feet were cold and slightly cyanotic and the dorsalis pedis pulses could not be found.

He was commenced on treatment with prednisolone forty mg. per day, later reduced to twenty mg. per day and following this the joint symptoms and appetite improved. However there was no improvement of his dyspnoea which in fact became somewhat worse. A chest radiograph showed diffuse opacities of both lungs (Fig. 10–3). Respiratory function tests showed a reduced vital capacity (2.4 liters compared to normal 3.8 liters) and maximum breathing capacity seventy-six liters (compared to normal one hundred liters per minute). Arterial oxygen tension at rest was slightly reduced (eighty-four mm. Hg.) but rose to a normal value when breathing oxygen. The alveolar-arterial oxygen gradient was increased (twenty-two mm. Hg. compared with a normal ten mm. Hg.). The carbon monoxide diffusing capacity was at the lower limit of normal (fifteen ml. per minute per mm. Hg. with a normal range fifteen to twenty-five ml. per minute per mm. Hg.). He continued treatment with prednisolone but there was no improvement in any of his symptoms. In addition to his other troubles, he became very weak and also suffered from severe constipation. Azathioprine was added to the prednisolone therapy but without benefit.

In July 1968, he developed influenzal bronchopneumonia and was admitted to hospital where he required treatment with continuous inhalation of oxygen and antibiotics. Following discharge he remained confined to bed with continuous oxygen inhalation. He complained of painful areas in his intercostal region, relieved by injection of procaine. Friction rubs were heard from time to time over both lungs. He was readmitted to hospital where a tracheostomy was performed and he was returned to home with continuous oxygen therapy. With careful home nursing he lingered on until he died in respiratory failure in May 1969, less than four years from his initial symptoms.

Comment: This is a case of a middle-aged man with initial onset of respiratory disturbance, Raynaud's phenomenon and sclerodermatous changes in the fingers occurring shortly afterwards. Although the skin changes were never extensive he suffered from marked respiratory embarrassment and died in respiratory failure.

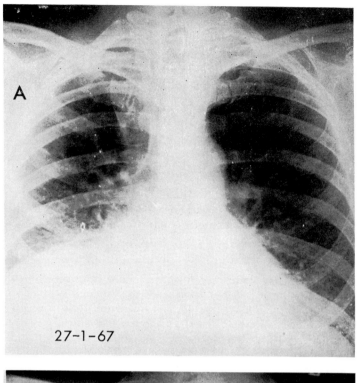

27-1-67

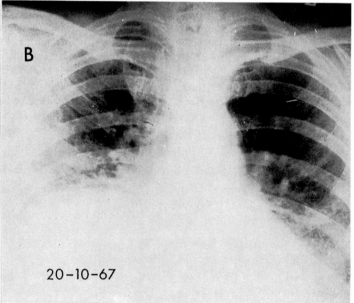

20-10-67

Figure 10–3. Radiographs of a patient (Case Three, Chapter X) showing marked reticular opacities of lung bases. There is marked progression in the nine months between the early picture (A) and the subsequent picture (B).

PULMONARY FUNCTION STUDIES

To facilitate further discussion of disturbed pulmonary function in scleroderma, it may be helpful to outline briefly the types of respiratory disturbance which may be present and which may have been looked for by various workers. The patterns are as follows: (1) *restrictive ventilatory defect* in which there is limitation of full expansion of the lungs due to one or other of the following factors: diseases hindering movement of the chest wall, limitation of lung expansion by pleural disease, stiffness of the lungs from venous congestion or changes in the lungs themselves; (2) *obstructive ventilatory defect* in which there is increased resistance to gas flow from narrowing of respiratory passages at any level from the bronchioles to the large bronchi; (3) *defect of gaseous diffusion* or *impaired gas transfer*, in which there is limitation of diffusion of oxygen from alveoli to the pulmonary capillary blood; (4) *uneven distribution of ventilation and perfusion* or *ventilation-perfusion mismatching*, in which some alveoli, although ventilated, are poorly perfused, and others, although well perfused, are inadequately ventilated. The extremes of this defect occur when there is no effective perfusion of the air sacs (wasted ventilation) and when there is no ventilation of perfused alveoli (pulmonary artery to vein shunting). The various patterns listed above frequently occur together and this is particularly so in a condition such as systemic sclerosis producing diverse pathological changes in the lungs.

The different types of respiratory disturbance are distinguished by various tests of respiratory function. Thus a *restrictive ventilatory defect* is characterized by decreased vital capacity, mainly from decrease in the inspiratory capacity; the frequency of respiration is increased and ventilation may be normal (or even increased) until the late stage, although the work of breathing is increased. An *obstructive ventilatory defect* is characterized by a decreased expiratory volume over a specific time (usually one second), decreased maximum expiratory flow rate or some other index of obstruction to gas flow, together with hyperinflation as evidenced by an increased residual volume, and in moderate or severe cases, an increased functional residual capacity and total lung capacity. *Impaired gaseous diffusion* results in arterial hypoxemia, which may become apparent only during exercise when the increased cardiac output results in decreased transit time of the blood in the pulmonary capillaries. It is determined by measuring the diffusing capacity for carbon monoxide. *Ventilation-perfusion imbalance* results in hypoxemia at rest. If there is ventilation of poorly perfused alveoli (wasted ventilation) there is increased dead-space/tidal volume ratio, the hypoxemia worsens on exercise, but is corrected by breathing pure oxygen. If there is perfusion of blood through non-ventilated units, there is similarly anoxemia at rest, worse on exercise, but in this instance not corrected by breathing pure oxygen. Usually both types of abnormality occur together resulting in anoxemia which is only partially corrected by breathing pure oxygen.

Baldwin *et al.* (1949) studied thirty-nine cases in whom there was radiological evidence of pulmonary fibrosis, absence of evidence of ventilatory obstruction in the spirogram and no increase in residual air. A subgroup of those in whom the arterial oxygen on exercise was less than ninety-two percent included three patients with scleroderma. The chief findings in this group were a marked reduction in lung volumes, with vital capacity and total lung capacity about half normal, and residual volume/total lung volume slightly raised, maximum breathing capacity relatively normal, hyperventilation at rest and on exercise, impaired intrapulmonary mixing, arterial oxygen saturation only slightly reduced at rest, but markedly reduced on exercise, normal arterial carbon dioxide pressure at rest and on exercise. They argued that in view of the normal blood carbon dioxide pressure, inadequate alveolar ventilation was ruled out and that the arterial oxygen desaturation must be due to a veno-arterial shunt or a diffusion defect or both.

Since these initial observations, there have been numerous studies of varying degrees of complexity of pulmonary function in scleroderma. It is not possible in a reasonable space to discuss these individual studies. A representative list is given in Table XVII with an indication of the types of tests performed and the chief conclusions. Only studies involving more than ten patients have been included in the Table. A general picture of the disturbance of pulmonary function will be given based on these various studies.

Disturbed pulmonary function is common in scleroderma. Ritchie (1964) found some abnormality in twenty-one of twenty-two patients. Sackner *et al.* (1964) found normal lung volumes in only five percent. The type of disturbance varies from patient to patient but the two main types of abnormality are restrictive and diffusion defects. One or other may dominate the picture or even be present alone, but there is commonly a combination of both types. Ventilation at rest is normal or slightly increased with a slightly increased frequency of respiration. Except in severe disease, maximum voluntary ventilation is normal. Patients may hyperventilate on mild exercise. Except in severe cases, the blood gas levels (content and pressure) are normal at rest, but there may be oxygen desaturation on exercise. The blood partial pressure of carbon dioxide (P_{CO_2}) may fall on exercise, instead of rising as normally would occur. This may be associated with a rise in the blood lactic acid, possibly due to anaerobic metabolism associated with muscular abnormality (Godfrey *et al.*, 1969).

Although most series contain occasional patients with an obstructive

TABLE XVII

REPORTED LUNG FUNCTION STUDIES IN SCLERODERMA

Authors	Date	Subjects	Lung Volumes	Ventilation (Freq., Basal, MVV)	Breathing Mechanics: Airways Factors (FEV₁, Airways Resist.)	Breathing Mechanics: Tissue Factors (Compliance)	Distribution of Gas (Single Breath)	Diffusion (DLco)	Blood Gases	Exercise	Haemodynamic	Main Patterns	Other Comments
Miller *et al.*	1959	28-Pulmonary symptoms in 18 graded according to degree of fibrosis.	+	+	+				+			Restrictive	
Adkihari *et al.*	1962	13-Subdivided according to presence or absence of skin changes over thorax.	+	+	+	+		+				Restrictive + Diffusion defect	Diffusion defect not due to skin involvement.
Catterall & Rowall	1963	16-Subdivided according to degree of dyspnoea.	+		+			+				Diffusion defect in all. Restrictive in some.	Diffusion defect greater in those with symptoms.
Hughes & Lees	1963	12-Unselected; pulmonary symptoms not prominent.	+	+				+				Restrictive Diffusion defect	Treatment with steroids did not improve the diffusing capacity.
Ritchie	1964	22-Unselected	+			+		+		+		Restrictive Diffusion defect	Test results not related to duration of symptoms or extent of skin involvement. Related to radiological involvement.
Sackner *et al.*	1964	38-Unselected; subdivided according to presence or absence of right ventricular enlargement or heart failure.	+	+	+	+	+	+	+	+	+	Restrictive Diffusion defect Increased vascular resistance	No close relationship between increased vascular resistance and pulmonary hypertension and results of pulmonary function tests. Fall of arterial carbon dioxide content on exercise. Tightness of skin over chest wall not related to disturbed respiratory function.
Wilson *et al.*	1964	19-Unselected (8 had radiographic abnormality).	+	+		+	+	+	+			Diffusion defect mainly. Restrictive (3) Venous-arterial admixture (4)	

TABLE XVII (Continued)

Authors	Date	Subjects	Lung Volumes	Ventilation (Freq., Basal, MVV)	Breathing Mechanics: Airways Factors (FEV₁, Airways Resist.)	Breathing Mechanics: Tissue Factors (Compliance)	Distribution of Gas (Single Breath)	Diffusion (DLco)	Blood Gases	Exercise	Haemodynamic	Main Patterns	Other Comments
Catterall & Rowell	1965	31-Unselected	+	+				+	+	+		Restrictive (5) Diffusion defect (22)	
Ashba & Ghanem	1965	15-All had respiratory symptoms. 10 had radiographic abnormality.	+	+	+	+			+			Restrictive + Diffusion defect (5) Restrictive + obstructive (4). Diffusion defect only (3)	Diffusion defect deduced from oxygen saturation studies.
Huang, C. T. & Lyons	1966	13-Unselected	+	+	+				+	+		Restrictive Diffusion defect	
DeMuth et al.	1968	61-Unselected	+	+	+		+	+				Restrictive Diffusion defect	Changes more marked if radiological changes.
Godfrey et al.	1968	11-Unselected	+	+	+			+	+	+		Restrictive Diffusion defect Venous-arterial admixture (4)	Abnormal elevation of blood lactate on exercise in six.

"+" indicates that some tests in the particular category have been performed. MVV = Maximum voluntary ventilation. FEV₁ = forced expiratory volume over 1 second. DLco = diffusing capacity of lung for carbon monoxide.

defect and sometimes clinical emphysema, it is probable that these are incidental, as this disturbance is common in the community and the patients concerned are usually smokers. In fact in many patients with scleroderma the residual volume is decreased and the airways conductance increased beyond normal. There are several reports of veno-arterial admixture, usually superimposed on a diffusion defect, indicated by the fact that the arterial anoxia cannot be completely eliminated by breathing pure oxygen.

Of the various defects, diffusion defect is apparently the earliest and may occur in the absence of pulmonary fibrosis. Abnormal tests are more likely if there are symptoms or radiological evidence of pulmonary fibrosis (Catterall and Rowell, 1963; Ritchie, 1964; DeMuth *et al.*, 1968). Ritchie (1964) could find no good correlation between the duration of symptoms of scleroderma or the localization of the skin changes with the changes in the respiratory functions. DeMuth *et al.* (1968) also found that pulmonary disease was not related to the duration of the disease but tended to be associated with cutaneous involvement of the head and neck and with Raynaud's phenomenon.

Some workers have attempted to analyze further the nature of the particular abnormal pattern of respiration. A restrictive defect may reside either in the lungs or the chest wall. Most observers (Adhikari *et al.*, 1962; Ritchie, 1964; Sackner *et al.* 1964; Ashba and Ghanem, 1965) have found a decrease in lung compliance, although Wilson *et al.* (1964) found normal values. Ritchie (1964) found that the ratio "compliance/functional residual capacity" was also low indicating that the decreased compliance was not due simply to small lungs but each unit of functioning lung tissue was stiffer. Sackner *et al.* (1964) determined, in addition to the lung compliance, the total thoracic compliance and the thoracic wall compliance. The total thoracic compliance was slightly reduced but the thoracic wall compliance was normal, indicating that the suggestion by some of the early writers that the respiratory troubles in scleroderma were due to constriction by tight skin over the chest wall was incorrect.

All workers who have measured the diffusing capacity in scleroderma are agreed that it is reduced. Diffusing capacity depends on two components: the membrane diffusion and the capillary blood volume. Adhikari *et al.* (1962) found that both of these were decreased, the former more than the latter. It is perhaps worthy of comment that decreased diffusing capacity of carbon monoxide may not be due only to these two factors but, for diffusion to occur, the gas must enter alveoli perfused with capillary blood, and the measured diffusing capacity may be reduced because of ventilation-perfusion imbalance. It is probable that it is because it is affected by more than one pathophysiological abnormality that the diffusion capacity of carbon monoxide is such a sensitive indication of pulmonary involvement in scleroderma.

SUMMARY

Although general recognition came rather late, it is now appreciated that pulmonary involvement is common in scleroderma, being the second most common type of visceral involvement, following esophageal. Clinically obvious pulmonary involvement is usually a late manifestation, although occasionally it may occur early and dominate the clinical picture. The radiological findings are characteristic although not entirely specific, consisting of bilateral mottled opacities and sometimes a cystic appearance most marked at the bases and sparing the apices. Pathologically there is interstitial fibrosis and thickening of walls of pulmonary arteries. In its severe forms it is divisible into compact sclerosis where the alveolar spaces are decreased by fibrosis of their walls and cystic fibrosis where the alveolar walls are disrupted to form cysts. Clinical disturbance may be of two main types: cardiac failure due to increased pulmonary resistance, and respiratory symptoms (dyspnoea and cough) due directly to the lung involvement.

Pulmonary function tests have shown two main types of defect: restrictive defect and diffusion defect. These are extremely common and may be demonstrated before there are clinical symptoms or radiological signs. Respiratory symptoms and signs in scleroderma are due to pulmonary involvement and not to sclerosis of the skin overlying the thoracic cage.

Chapter XI

CARDIAC INVOLVEMENT

PATHOLOGICAL CHANGES in the hearts of patients with scleroderma were described before their clinical importance was recognized. Possibly the first report is that of Hektoen (1897) who included in his pathological findings of one case *interstitial myocarditis* and hypertrophy of the heart, but as there is no detailed description and the patient also had arteriosclerosis, a diagnosis of scleroderma heart disease cannot be accepted without reservation.

Kraus (1924) and Heine (1926) observed enlargement of the right side of the heart in their cases. Brock (1934) described extreme "diffuse increase of connective tissue in the heart with hypertrophy of the muscle fibres" in one case. However, the establishment of scleroderma heart disease as a clinical entity was due to Weiss *et al.* (1943) who reported a study of nine patients with scleroderma and cardiac symptoms of whom eight died (six with congestive cardiac failure) and post mortem studies in two. The latter showed fibrotic changes in the heart in the absence of coronary artery disease. East and Oram (1947), Mathisen and Palmer (1947) and Hurly *et al.* (1951) each presented single cases with cardiac features in life and necropsy findings of interstitial fibrosis. Goetz (1951) gave a detailed report with pathology findings in three cases and referred to the clinical aspects of twelve others. Gil (1951) in a report on the clinical study of eight cases of diffuse scleroderma found cardiac symptoms in seven and cardiac enlargement (clinical and radiological) in five. Baritt and O'Brien (1952) reported on the clinical features in two cases.

INCIDENCE

There have been widely differing views concerning the frequency of scleroderma heart disease. Rossier and Hegglin-Volkmann (1954) found clinical cardiac involvement in seven of twenty-six patients with generalized scleroderma and Bourel *et al.* (1966) in nine of fourteen, suggesting frequent involvement. On the other hand, Windesheim and Parkin (1958) found abnormal electrocardiograms in only five of sixty-three patients suggesting that cardiac involvement was infrequent. In the large Mayo Clinic series Tuffanelli and Winkelmann (1961) found congestive cardiac failure in twenty-one of 727 patients (3 percent) and abnormal electrocardiograms in 9 percent. Barnett and Coventry (1969a) found cardiac symptoms or signs in thirty-four of sixty-one patients but do not claim that these are all due to systemic sclerosis. Pathological studies also give varying results. Thus Helwig and Piper (1955) found cardiac involvement in twenty-eight of thirty patients (90 percent) whereas Sackner *et al.* (1966) found only three cases of scleroderma heart disease in twenty-five patients (12 percent).

Difficulties in estimating the frequency of scleroderma heart disease arise from the fact that many of the features are not specific and heart disease generally is common in middle-aged persons. D'Angelo *et al.* (1969) compared the incidence of various pathological features in fifty-eight patients dying from scleroderma and fifty-eight matched controls. They found an incidence of myocardial fibrosis of 81 percent in the scleroderma patients compared with fifty-five percent in the controls, giving an excess incidence of 26 percent in the scleroderma patients. Pericarditis (but not pericardial effusion) was more common in the scleroderma patients but valvular lesions were not more common.

PATHOLOGY

The pathological changes in the heart in scleroderma have already been discussed and will be briefly mentioned. They were described in detail by Weiss *et al.* (1943) and consist of accumulations of connective tissue of unusual character containing numerous fibroblasts and capillaries in the absence of any marked arterial changes and with myocardial fibres preserved in the centre of lesions. Similar changes have been described by other workers (Rottenberg *et al.*, 1959; Fletcher and Morton, 1967). Likewise, pericarditis has been noted (see later). Although a verrucous endocarditis has been described (Oram and Stokes, 1961), this probably is coincidental (D'Angelo *et al.*, 1969).

CLINICAL ASPECTS

General Clinical Picture

The general clinical picture of involvement of the heart in scleroderma, particularly in its severe form, is given by Weiss *et al.* (1943). Their nine patients were all suffering from cardiac symptoms and eight died, six following congestive cardiac failure. The main symptoms were dyspnoea (exertional in nine, orthopnoea in five and paroxysmal in two), cardiac chest pain, not related to excretion in four, ankle oedema in nine, and cough with mucoid sputum in several cases. Cardiac signs included clinical cardiac enlargement (all cases), faint heart sounds, arrhythmias (atrial fibrillation in one, extrasystoles in two), pericardial friction rub in one, systolic murmurs in five, accentuation of pulmonic second sound in four, triple rhythm and basal crepitations. Radiological abnormalities comprised cardiac enlargement, triangular shape of heart shadow, poor movement of the heart border, a prominent pulmonary conus and increased lung markings. The electrocardiogram was abnormal in all cases, the changes being atrial fibrillation in one, extrasystoles in three, low voltages in three, conduction defects in two and left axis deviation in two.

Subsequent reports have included some or other of these features. Oram and Stokes (1961) presented a study based on forty-nine patients comprising twenty-eight reported cases with both clinical and autopsy findings and twenty-one cases observed personally, with four autopsies. They listed the modes of presentation of cardiac involvement in scleroderma which were with (1) heart failure either due to (a) primary myocardial involvement or (b) secondary to chronic cor pulmonale, mitral valve incompetence or hypertension resulting from renal involvement or steroid therapy, (2) pericarditis, (3) cardiac pain resembling cardiac ischaemic pain or myocardial infarction, (4) arrhythmia, (5) syncope or (6) an incidental finding on clinical examination, electrocardiography or radiography.

Sackner *et al.* (1966) described the cardiological features in sixty-five hospitalized patients, presumably with severe disease, but not necessarily cardiac features. Cardiac symptoms or signs were present in a remarkably large number. Thus dyspnoea during the course of the disease occurred in fifty-two (80 percent), at rest in thirty-four, on exertion in eighteen, and chest pain in nine. Cough was uncommon. Inspiratory râles were heard in forty patients, enlarged liver was found in eighteen and ankle oedema in fourteen. Auscultation of the heart revealed accentuated pulmonary second sounds in thirty-three, gallop rhythm in twenty-eight, apical systolic murmurs in thirteen. The heart was radiologically enlarged in forty of sixty cases, although the enlargement was usually not distinctive in type. Electrocardiograms were abnormal in fifty-seven of sixty patients (see later). Abnormalities were also demonstrated by ballistocardiography and phonocardiography. Necropsies were obtained in twenty-five of the forty-three patients who died. Using as diagnostic criteria fibrosis, edema or inflammation of the myocardium in multiple sections unassociated with coronary artery disease, *scleroderma heart disease* was diagnosed in only three cases. However cardiac enlargement was found in eighteen cases (right ventricular in seven, left ventricular in six and combined in five) and pericardial disease in eighteen (acute in five of whom four had uremia, chronic in nine, and effusions in four). They conclude that scleroderma heart disease (as strictly defined) is an uncommon clinicopathological entity but abnormalities of cardiac function in scleroderma are often of major clinical significance because myocardial function is affected secondarily to pulmonary hypertension, systemic hypertension associated with *scleroderma kidney,* pericarditis and hypoxia associated with restrictive pulmonary disease.

Myocardial disease and pulmonary heart disease in scleroderma have been confirmed in various reports. Other aspects requiring further discussion are pericardial involvement, endocardial involvement and conduction defects.

Hemodynamic Findings

Sackner *et al.* (1964) compared the hemodynamic findings determined by cardiac catheterisation in twenty normal subjects with those in thirty patients with scleroderma. In the scleroderma patients there was increase in the right atrial pressure, right ventricular pressure, pulmonary arterial pressure, reduction in the cardiac index and stroke index and increase in the calculated right ventricular work and pulmonary vascular resistance. These changes were present not only in patients with clinically apparent right ventricular enlargement, but also (to a lesser degree) in those without clinical right ventricular enlargement.

Pericardial Involvement

A pericardial friction rub was observed in one of the nine cases in the classical paper of Weiss *et al.* (1943) but otherwise there is no reference to pericarditis in their report. However there have since been scattered references to pericarditis associated with scleroderma.

In two of the early reports mentioned above, there is mention of pericardial effusion (East and Oram, 1947, Mathisen and Palmer, 1947). Beigelman *et al.* (1953) in their autopsy report on five cases of progressive systemic sclerosis, included pericarditis, pericardial effusion, pleuro-pericardial adhesion and pleuro-pericardial thickening (each one case).

Meltzer (1956) reported on two cases of generalized scleroderma with pericardial effusion confirmed by aspiration. One patient died suddenly but the other was still alive eight months later without objective signs of congestive cardiac failure. The fluid was similar in the two cases with a high protein content, low cell count, absence of blood and negative culture. Steinberg and Rothbard (1962) reported two cases of scleroderma with pericardial effusions demonstrated during life by angiocardiography and later reported a further three cases (Steinberg and Rothbard 1964). One of the latter patients died following rupture of a stomach ulcer and at necropsy the effusion was confirmed, in the absence of marked changes in the myocardium. They regarded the condition as an "isolated effusion due to scleroderma pericarditis."

Sackner *et al.* (1966) found only three patients with clinical pericarditis in sixty-five patients with scleroderma but pericardial disease was found in eighteen of twenty-five necropsy cases (see above). More recent reports of pericarditis associated myocardial involvement have been made by Nasser *et al.* (1968) and Dilke and Richardson (1971). It would seem from a study of the literature that pericardial affection of various types is not uncommon in scleroderma, but may be missed clinically.

Endocardial and Valvular Involvement

Systolic murmurs, probably functional, are common in patients with scleroderma, but diastolic murmurs are rare. Oram and Stokes (1961) from their study of reported cases with necropsy included occasional *non-bacterial endocarditis* as part of the cardiac involvement. Jones (1962) found four cases of valvular disease in thirty-four patients but each of these could be attributed to previous rheumatic disease. Roth and Kissane (1964) described a patient who died with acute heart failure and at necropsy was found to have pan-aortitis, aortic valvulitis and perforated valve cusp. Sabour and Mahallawy (1966) reported a case of mitral and aortic valve disease in a patient with scleroderma but in the absence of any pathology data this cannot be accepted as due to this disease. Sackner *et al.* (1966) found mitral valvulitis producing minor valvular deformity in four of twenty-five hearts from patients with scleroderma. As previously mentioned D'Angelo *et al.* (1969) found valvular involvement in necropsy reports in patients with scleroderma no more frequent than in matched controls. It would appear that valvular disease of the heart is not common in scleroderma and when present is probably coincidental.

Conduction Abnormalities

Reference has already been made to the observation of partial heart block and bundle branch block in the report of Weiss *et al.* and other subsequent reports on scleroderma heart disease. There have been several reports of complete heart block (East and Oram 1947, Bocardelli and Fabri, 1956, Glück and Humerfelt, 1957; Escudero and McDevitt, 1958, Lev *et al.*, 1966; Raynaud *et al.*, 1967; Barr *et al.*, 1970), with Stokes Adams attacks in several patients. Usually the complete heart block has been preceded by other conduction defects. In all but one of the fatal cases (six of the seven listed), there was myocardiac fibrosis which, in the more recent cases, was shown to involve the bundle of His . The one surviving case (Barr *et al.*, 1970) was successfully treated with an implanted pace-maker.

Arrhythmias

Arrhythmias (atrial fibrillation, paroxysmal atrial tachycardia, atrial extrasystoles, ventricular extrasystoles) have been mentioned in various series (e.g. Weiss *et al.*, 1943; Oram and Stokes, 1961; Sackner *et al.*, 1966) and have been seen from time to time in my patients. Wren and Govindaraj (1968) reported on a case with nodal rhythm and A. V. dissociation which reverted to normal with atropine.

Electrocardiographic Changes

In the series reported by Weiss *et al.* (1943) the electrocardiogram was abnormal in all of the eight patients tested. Mustakallio and Sarajas (1954) also found abnormalities in all of seven patients, and abnormalities are usually reported in most of the individual case reports. These however are selected and it is of interest to know the frequency of electrocardiographic abnormalities in scleroderma generally and for this information it is necessary to turn to fairly large series in which electrocardiograms have been particularly studied. The findings are surprisingly inconsistent. Escudero and McDevitt (1958) found abnormal electrocardiograms in thirty of sixty patients (50 percent); Windesheim and Parkin (1958), nine of ninety (10 percent); and Sackner *et al.* (1966) in fifty-one of sixty patients (85 percent). Not surprisingly Escudero and McDevitt found a higher incidence of abnormality (75 percent) in patients with evidence of visceral involvement and a lower incidence (25 percent) in those without visceral abnormality. Also there is divergence of opinion concerning the types of abnormalities. Escudero and McDevitt found the commonest abnormalities to be notched P waves, left ventricular hypertrophy, low voltage, incomplete right bundle branch block and subpericardial ischaemia. On the other hand, Sackner found notched P waves in only twelve percent of cases, being exceeded by P pulmonale (15 percent), right ventricular hypertrophy (15 percent). Low voltage was rare (5 percent), right bundle branch block not mentioned, but first degree heart block was present in 15 percent.

The last available electrocardiogram in each of sixty-two patients in my series was analysed using the standard diagnostic criteria * and some abnormality was found in thirty-four, *i.e.* fifty-five percent (Silberberg, 1972). Abnormalities were varied in nature, the most common being ST-T changes suggestive of ischaemia (24 percent), prolonged QT_c interval (20 percent) and low voltage (18 percent). Arrhythmias were uncommon, the most frequent being ventricular ectopic beats, although these may have been underestimated as only the last tracing was studied. Five tracings (8 percent) showed an infarct pattern. Obviously more work needs to be done on the electrocardiogram changes in scleroderma using precise diagnostic criteria.

Case Histories

The following case summaries illustrate some of the cardiac problems in my series, probably attributable to scleroderma.

---

* As contained in Goldman's *Clinical Electrocardiography* (1967).

CASE 1: right heart failure secondary to scleroderma lung disease.

A lady aged forty-seven years, was admitted to hospital in February 1954, with a history that shortly after a cholecystectomy four years previously she began to experience episodes of blanching and numbness of her hands and four months before admission she developed an indolent ulcer on her right ankle. On examination she was a thin, tanned, middle-aged lady with widespread tightness of the skin, most marked on the face and hands (Fig. 11–1). Her blood pressure was 125/80 mm. Hg. Her feet were oedematous and toes cyanosed. There was an infected ulcer at the base of her left fifth toe, her left femoral pulse was weak, and the popliteal and ankle pulses were absent on both sides. Chest radiography showed prominent pulmonary arteries, small aorta, but otherwise normal cardiac shadow and a fine reticulate pattern of decreased translucency in the lower half of the chest (Fig. 11–2). Bilateral lumbar sympathectomy was performed but produced little effect and it became necessary to amputate three toes on her left foot.

Cortisone treatment was commenced on three occasions, but withdrawal was necessary because of recurrent infection of her feet and development of hypertension. During one course of cortisone treatment the patient developed a headache and transient disturbance of vision in her left eye associated with the disappearance of pulsation in the left superficial temporal artery. Cortisone was later recommenced at a lower dosage. In April 1956 she developed a sudden onset of lower cramping abdominal pains and vomiting, and had abdominal distension. Laparotomy revealed perforation of the bowel proximal to the region of fibrotic constriction. The affected part of the bowel was resected and she made a satisfactory recovery.

Over the subsequent years the circulatory symptoms persisted and she also developed dysphagia, dyspepsia and dyspnoea on exertion. She was readmitted to hospital in February 1961, when she was found to be a very thin woman with tight skin over the whole body, flexion deformity of the fingers and a blood pressure of 200/120 mm. Hg. She was treated with digoxin and thiazides with some improvement. She was again admitted to hospital in April 1961 because of a respiratory infection and increased shortness of breath. Examination showed, in addition to the features described above, a pulse of 120 per minute, presystolic triple rhythm over the right ventricular impulse and signs of pneumonia at the right base. The electrocardiogram showed marked right axis deviation. Her respiratory infection responded to treatment with tetracycline, but she developed frank cardiac failure requiring increased dose of diuretics. She was very sensitive to digitalis and at one stage developed a complete heart block. The cortisone treatment was discontinued during the phase of heart failure, but later recommenced. She appeared to be improving, but died suddenly one night.

At necropsy the cause of death was shown to be a pulmonary embolus. She had the findings associated with cardiac failure and also a widespread visceral systemic sclerosis. The sphincter muscle of the esophagus was largely replaced by collagenous tissue and also there were areas of fibrosis in the stomach and duodenum. The kidneys showed arteriosclerosis and pyelonephritis. In the heart there was fibrosis in the myocardium in a somewhat diffuse distribution but

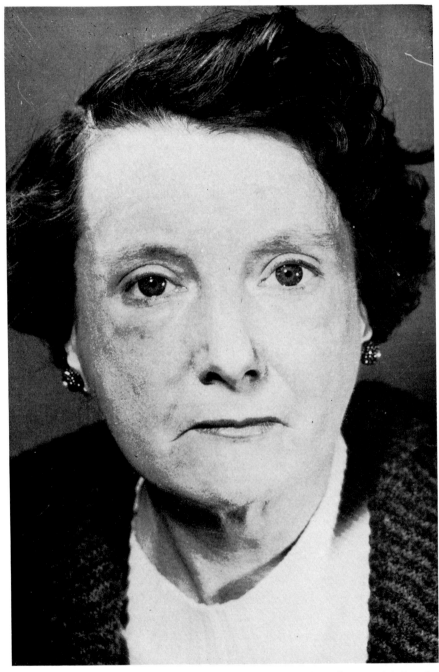

Figure 11–1. Photograph of a patient (Case One, Chapter XI) with Type 3 Scleroderma and severe pulmonary and cardiac involvement.

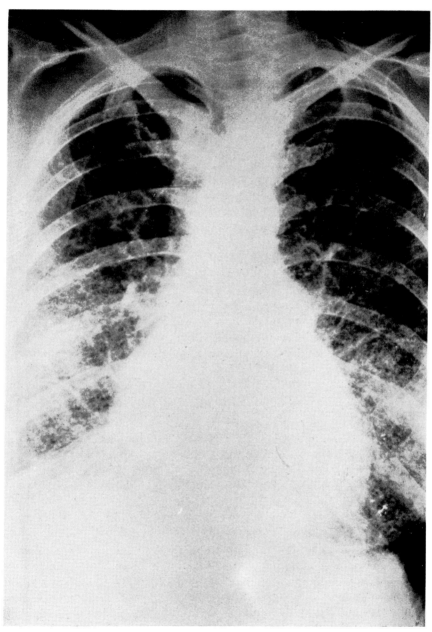

Figure 11–2. Radiograph of chest of a patient (Case One, Chapter XI) shown in Figure 11–1. Note the marked reticular type basal opacities and the prominent main pulmonary artery.

more definite in perivascular regions. The coronary arteries were moderately thickwalled, but patent, with marked intimal fibrosis. The lungs showed dense interstitial fibrosis in all sections.

In summary, this woman suffered from scleroderma Type 3. During the course of her illness she developed visceral complications, particularly gastrointestinal and pulmonary. Her final illness was due to right heart failure, secondary to the pulmonary involvement.

CASE 2: probable scleroderma cardiomyopathy.

A man then aged sixty years was referred because of recurrent ulceration of his right ankle over an old fracture site during the past ten years. However it was noted that the skin of his hands was quite stiff and his face was somewhat smooth. On further enquiry he gave the history that over the past two to three years he had suffered from rheumatic pains, particularly in his shoulders and thumbs and the skin of his hands had become thicker. He had not noticed any ischaemic episodes. He had been short of breath on exertion over the past eighteen months. On examination there was marked thickening and stiffness of the skin of his fingers and the skin of his neck became tight on extension of the head. Blood pressure was 140/80 mm. Hg. Examination of the heart revealed extrasystoles, and a loud split pulmonic second sound. He had a large sloughing ulcer and stasis pigmentation of his right ankle.

He was admitted to hospital for various tests with the following results. Chest X-ray showed mild cardiomegaly, prominent pulmonary arteries, fine opacities throughout the lungs, more prominent at the bases (Fig. 11–3). Hematological examination was normal apart from an elevated erythrocyte sedimentation rate (twenty-seven mm per min.). The *L.E. cell* test was negative. The fluorescent antibody test was positive for anti-smooth muscle cells, but others were negative. A barium swallow examination and meal showed a dilated, aperistaltic esophagus and hypomotility of the small bowel. X-ray examination of the hands showed cystic lesions in the carpal bones and metatarsals and atrophy of the tufts of the phalanges. An electrocardiogram showed sinus bradycardia, ventricular extrasystoles, T wave flattening in AVF lead. Pulmonary function tests showed a mild obstructive defect. Although the blood urea concentration and creatinine clearance were normal, a renal biopsy showed small vessel changes "consistent with hypertension" and minimal areas of mucinous change in the intima of some vessels. Local treatment was given for the ulcer of his ankle, but no specific treatment for scleroderma was instituted at this stage.

In October 1972, following an attack of *bronchitis*, he developed shortness of breath and signs of congestive cardiac failure with blood pressure of 130/100 mm. Hg., pulse rate 120 per minute, elevation of jugular venous pressure to three cm. above the sternal angle, cardiac enlargement, crepitations and enlarged liver. An electrocardiogram showed atrial flutter with two to one block. He was treated with digitalis and diuretics and improved rapidly. The atrial flutter reverted to atrial fibrillation and then to sinus rhythm. Respiratory function tests were repeated and again showed a mild obstructive defect only. He was able to return to his work on maintenance cardiac failure treatment.

In June 1972, after another attack of *bronchitis*, he again became dyspnoeic and developed signs of congestive cardiac failure. An electrocardiogram showed

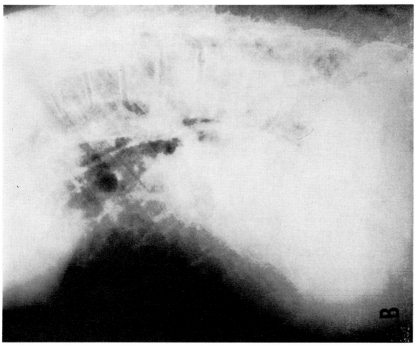

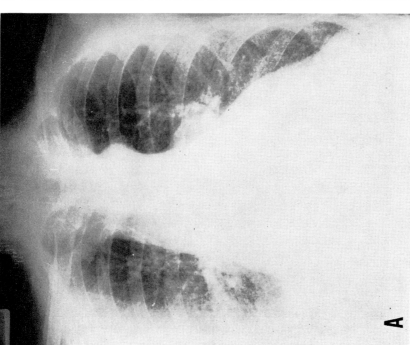

Figure 11–3. Radiograph of chest of a patient (Case Two, Chapter XI) showing basal pulmonary opacities. A. Anterior projection. B. Lateral projection.

multiple ventricular extrasystoles. His digoxin was stopped and intravenous
xylocaine was given for the extrasystoles which were eventually controlled
with quinidine therapy. The serum potassium level was 3.9 m.eq.per liter and
a serum digoxin concentration of only 0.8 ng. per ml. excluded digitalis toxicity.
He has since been able to return to light work, but his electrocardium con-
tinues to show frequent extrasystoles, sometimes in runs. (Fig. 11–4).

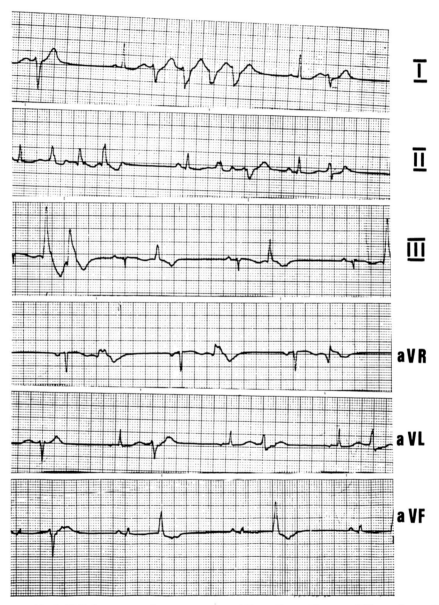

Figure 11–4. E.C.G. tracing from a patient (Case One, Chapter XI) with cardiac
involvement. There is a basic sinus rhythm with minor ST-T changes in the normally
conducted complexes. There are numerous ventricular extrasystoles of varied pattern,
sometimes occurring in *runs.*

Comment: This patient has Scleroderma Type 2. There is evidence of involvement of gastro-intestinal tract, lungs and heart. However the cardiac features seem disproportionate to the pulmonary involvement and it is suspected that he may have a scleroderma myocardiopathy. Arrhythmias (extrasystoles, artrial flutter, atrial fibrillation) have played a prominent part in his cardiac symptoms.

CASE 3: arrhythmias and sudden death.

A man aged thirty-four was first seen in December 1955 with a history that ten months ago he began to suffer from paraesthesia, thickening of the skin and stiffness of his fingers and later attacks of pallor or cyanosis to the metacarpophalangeal joints and stiffness of various joints. The skin of his face became thick and immobile and he suffered from lack of energy and shortness of breath on exertion. He had used a pneumatic drill for many years.

Examination revealed a well developed young man, with thick skin on his face, hands and wrists and ulceration of the tips of his middle fingers. Peripheral pulses were normal, blood pressure was 140/80 mm. Hg. and heart, lungs and abdomen were all clinically normal. The results of the special tests were as follows: haematological examination normal, electrocardiogram normal, *L.E. test* negative, barium swallow no abnormality, blood urea concentration twenty-five mg. per one hundred ml. and urea clearance normal.

He was treated with cortisone one hundred mg. daily, and over the next three months improved symptomatically and his skin became softer. He had an episode of dyspepsia associated with loose stools and experienced regurgitation on bending. A barium swallow and meal examination showed that the esophagus was atonic, and there was also very little peristaltic activity in the duodenal loop. However, the condition of his skin continued to improve.

In January 1957, he developed attacks of tachycardia and an electrocardiogram showed atrial flutter. He was admitted to hospital but the heart had reverted to sinus rhythm without specific treatment and he was discharged on treatment with quinidine. However he continued to have further attacks of rapid heart action associated with faintness for which he was admitted to hospital on several occasions. Electrocardiograms showed either atrial flutter or sinus rhythm. Treatment with digoxin was not helpful and quinidine was continued, although he still had occasional attacks of tachycardia. He also developed difficulty in swallowing and sometimes vomited large amounts of brownish material. In April, 1957 (sixteen months after presentation), he died suddenly when changing the wheel of his car.

Necropsy revealed a heart weighing 465 grams, but the coronary arteries showed only minimal atheroma. Histological examination showed areas of fibrosis, particularly in the sub-endocardial region and small focal collections of lymphocytes. Other significant features in the post mortem examination were typical features of scleroderma in the skin, collections of lymphocytes and fibrosis in the esophagus, interstitial fibrosis and areas of metaplasia of the lining of the alveoli and moderate medial hypertrophy of the small arteries in the lungs. The kidneys showed no significant changes.

Comment: This patient had scleroderma with marked visceral involvement. In the absence of other cause and the post mortem demonstration of myocardial involvement, it is probable that the arrhythmias were due to scleroderma and he probably died from an arrhythmia.

CASE 4: pericarditis, myocardial fibrosis and sudden death.

A man, then aged forty-five years, was admitted to the hospital in March 1954 with a history of pain in his wrists for several years and that two and a half years before admission he began to develop pain and stiffness in many joints. He also noticed thickening of the skin of his body, particularly his arms and face, and had also lost weight.

On examination there were widespread sclerodermatous changes present involving face, chest and limbs. There was pigmentation over his abdomen and hips. Most of his joints were stiff and his fingers were fixed in a claw position. His blood pressure was 140/90 mm. Hg. The cardiac apex was slightly displaced to the left being twelve cm. from the mid-sternal line and there was a soft systolic murmur heard over the precordium. An electrocardiogram showed changes interpreted as septal ischaemia. Chest radiography was normal. A radiograph of the hands showed degneration of joints, particularly of the interphalangeal joints with flexion and osteoarthritic changes in the larger joints. He was treated with cortisone with an initial dose of two hundred mg. per day decreasing over a fortnight to one hundred mg. per day on discharge from hospital. In three months it was noticed that there was obvious improvement in the suppleness of his skin, especially his face and upper arms and his joints had become less stiff.

He was again admitted to hospital in November 1954 complaining of chest pain over the past two days. His blood pressure was 170/100 mm. Hg. The cardiac apex beat was impalpable and a gallop rhythm and a pericardial friction rub were audible. An electrocardiogram showed sinus rhythm, small Q waves in Leads II and III and flat T waves in all leads. A radiography of the chest showed a heart of a triangular shape and moderately enlarged. It was noticed in the barium swallow examination that the barium persisted in the esophagus for a longer period than normal. There was a neutrophil leucocytosis and his temperature was slightly elevated on admission, but this soon settled. A Mantoux test was negative. The signs of pericarditis subsided and the patient was discharged home after about one month. His cortisone treatment, which had been discontinued, was started again with a smaller maintenance dose of thirty-five mg. per day. However, after about one year his blood pressure rose again and cortisone was eventually discontinued. He died suddenly at his home in June 1956, approximately two years after his first admission.

At necropsy, the heart was enlarged (weight 660 grams), with hypertrophy of the left ventricle. The two layers of the pericardium were adherent with fibrosis extending into the chest wall. There was an area of old myocardial infarction with fibrosis and calcification at the apex of the heart. However, in addition there was diffuse fibrosis of the myocardium, particularly the posterior wall of the left ventricle. Although there was marked coronary atheroma and occlusion of one branch of left descending artery near the apex, the major coronary arteries were patent. Histological sections showed patchy fibrosis throughout the heart with surviving muscle cells in the fibrosed areas.

Comment: This is a patient with scleroderma Type 3 with marked arthritic features who later developed features of pericarditis and died suddenly. Although necropsy revealed coronary atheroma, this did not seem adequate to explain all the features, particularly the widespread pericarditis and myocardial fibrosis, which were probably attributable to the scleroderma.

SUMMARY

Some cardiac abnormality in scleroderma is fairly common. However this is usually secondary to involvement of other organs, particularly the lungs, leading to pulmonary heart disease or the kidneys resulting in left ventricular failure and uremic pericarditis. Direct pathological involvement of the heart is rare, the main type of lesion being a patchy fibrosis resulting in chronic cardiac failure (scleroderma cardiomyopathy). Pericarditis of various types (acute, chronic, fibrous with effusion) may occur separately (isolated scleroderma pericarditis). Valvular involvement probably does not occur in scleroderma.

There are several reports of complete heart block in scleroderma and in some studies have been shown to be associated with a lesion of the bundle of His. Arrhythmias of various types have been described but do not appear to be of any specific type. Electrocardiographic abnormalities in scleroderma are common, but are varied and non-specific.

Chapter XII

RENAL INVOLVEMENT

HISTORICAL SURVEY

THE FIRST CASE of acute renal failure in association with scleroderma was reported as far back as 1863 by Auspitz who described a patient with tightness and pigmentation of the skin and who died following symptoms of rapidly progressing uremia. At necropsy the kidneys were small and their surface uneven with scattered small yellow areas. Meyer (1887) reported on a case in which the kidneys showed interstitial nephritis and endarteritis. Osler in his text-book (1892) stated that patients with scleroderma were apt to succumb to pulmonary complaints or nephritis. However these writers apparently regarded the renal involvement as another superadded disease. The recognition of renal involvement as part of the pathological process in progressive systemic sclerosis has come rather late in the study of this disease. Matsui (1924) observed increased connective tissue around the tubules, but none of his cases had shown the florid vascular changes associated with the acute renal failure sometimes observed in scleroderma. These were first described by Masugi and Yä-Shu in 1938 in the case of a young woman dying with diffuse scleroderma in whom they found severe vessel changes not only in the skin and subcutaneous tissue but also in most of the internal organs. In the kidney they found hyperplasia of the intima of interlobular arteries, with resulting narrowing of the lumen, and fibrinoid in the intima of these vessels and of some afferent arterioles sometimes extending into the glomeruli. In the following year * Talbott *et al.* described similar changes and also described changes in the interlobular arteries and cortical infarcts in a young woman dying from diffuse scleroderma.

Acute renal failure due to scleroderma did not receive clinical recognition until the description by Moore and Sheehan in 1952 of three patients whose renal function was satisfactory until a few weeks before their death in acute renal failure. None were severely hypertensive. At necropsy the kidneys from these patients showed similar changes: normal sized kidneys with irregular surface due to pale and dark nodules and, on microscopic examination, intimal thickening of intralobular arteries, producing a narrowed lumen, fibrinoid change in the distal part of these arteries and

---

* At the time of writing their report, Talbott *et al.* were unaware of the study by Masugi and Yä-Shu.

afferent arterioles and regions of ischaemia and infarction. They listed seven cases from the literature believed to show similar changes, but apart from those of Masugi and Yä-Shu, Talbott *et al.* (see above), Bevans (1945), and Platt and Davson (1950), the vessel changes did not show the full picture. Calvert and Owen (1956) discussed previous reports and coined the term *true scleroderma kidney* for the condition described by Moore and Sheehan and their own case in which the lesions comprised concenteric mucoid thickening of the intima of interlobular arteries, fibrinoid necrosis of afferent arterioles and renal cortical infarcts.

ACUTE RENAL FAILURE

Incidence

Acute renal failure in scleroderma is uncommon. There were only fifteen in the 727 cases of scleroderma reported from the Mayo Clinic by Tuffanelli and Winkelmann (1961). We have experienced only eleven cases in a series of seventy-eight patients. Most of the case reports are of single or a few cases.

Pathology

The findings of Moore and Sheehan, as outlined above, have been confirmed by various other reports, including more recently those of Rodnan *et al.* (1957), six cases; Fisher and Rodnan (1958), eleven cases; Rottenberg *et al.* (1959), three cases; and Tange (1959), three cases. Other features described by the later workers in certain cases include hyaline droplet degeneration of tubules, thickening of the basement membrane of glomerular capillaries producing a *wire-loop* appearance, and increased interstitial connective tissue. The pathological changes are very similar to those in malignant hypertension and there has been discussion as to whether the pathology of the two conditions is identical. This question was specifically studied by Fisher and Rodnan (1958) who compared sections from kidneys of eleven patients dying in renal failure from progressive systemic sclerosis with those of twelve patients dying from accelerated, or malignant, hypertension. They concluded that the renal lesions encountered in nine of the eleven patients with progressive systemic sclerosis were indistinguishable morphologically or in staining properties from the kidneys in twelve patients with malignant nephrosclerosis. (In the other two cases no renal lesions were seen.)

D'Angelo *et al.* (1969), in their necropsy series of fifty-eight patients with scleroderma, found that renal lesions were common. The three most specific lesions, hyperplasia of the interlobular arteries, fibrinoid necrosis of the afferent arteriole or in the glomerular tuft and thickening of the basement membrane or *wire looping*, were each found in approximately one third of the patients and only rarely in the controls.

Vascular changes in the kidneys have been studied in a novel way by Urai *et al.* (1961) by injection of a renal artery with a polyvinyl chloride solution in a mixture of cyclohexanone and acetone, precipitation of the polymer with alcohol and then removal of the parenchyma by corrosion in concentrated hydrochloric acid. In a normal kidney this shows the renal vasculature up to and including the glomeruli. In the kidney from a patient with scleroderma and renal failure there was reduction of the intra-lobular arteries to about one-third, decreased size of lumen of many of the remaining arteries, almost complete absence of afferent arterioles and glomeruli with almost all the remaining glomeruli in the cortico-medullary zone, and a crowded appearance of aglomerular arterioles. Sections from the other kidney showed a remarkable lack of tubular necrosis in spite of almost complete lack of afferent arterioles and glomeruli. The authors suggested that the post-glomerular capillary system may receive anastamoses for the maintenance of the circulation from the aglomerular arterioles. They also noted the discrepancy between the reduction of glomeruli in the injected specimen (by 98 percent) and in the histological specimen (by 40 percent) and suggested that in many places the obstruction of the afferent arterioles is not complete, but they are so narrow that the polymer used in the injection preparation cannot penetrate them.

Mechanism of the Changes

The mechanism of the renal changes is not known. The various theories have been reviewed by Fisher and Rodnan (1958). One is that they are due to the same pathological process in scleroderma which causes pathological changes elsewhere. However intimal mucoid change as found in the interlobular arteries is not seen in other viscera in this disease and fibrinoid necrosis is rarely seen in other sites without renal involvement. Spasm of vessels has been suggested as a cause of secondary vessel changes, both in the skin and renal vessels. However it is not conclusively shown that the ischaemic episodes of the fingers in scleroderma are due to spasm; they are more likely to be due to physiological response to cold in small vessels with reduced intraluminal pressure due to structural arterial disease. Severe hypertension may result in vascular damage and the similarity of the vascular lesions in the scleroderma kidney to those in malignant hypertension has been noted. However in several instances it has been recorded that hypertension is absent, as in the three cases of Moore and Sheehan (1952), one patient of Levine and Boshell (1960), the patient of Calvert and Owen (1956). In most cases where the blood pressure is raised, this is not to the degree found in malignant hypertension. McGiven *et al.* (1971) found deposits of immune globulin in arterioles and glomeruli in two patients with scleroderma dying in uremia and suggested the deposition of immune complexes in the walls of the vessels might play a part in the renal failure, but they could not demonstrate these complexes in another such patient (unpublished).

A.C.T.H. or cortisone has been used in many of the recent cases prior to the onset of the renal failure and has led to a suspicion that this may be a precipitating factor. There are some reports where the administration or steroids or A.C.T.H. seems to have precipitated or accelerated renal failure (Lunseth *et al.*, 1951, Sharnoff *et al.*, 1951, Calvert and Owen, 1956). Adrenal steroids are commonly used in the treatment of scleroderma and are more likely to be used in patients with the more diffuse or rapidly progressive forms and it is probable that these are the patients most likely to develop renal failure.

Clinical Features

A study of the published cases indicates that there is no age or sex predeliction of acute renal failure in scleroderma, the incidence in respect to these factors being similar to that for scleroderma generally. However renal failure tends to occur early in the course of the disease. Thus in all of nine cases reported by Rodnan *et al.* (1957) the renal failure occurred three years or less from the onset of the disease, in a series of eleven cases reported by Fisher and Rodnan (1958) within five years in eight (other times being sixteen years in two and seven years in one), and in the five cases reported by Levine and Boshell (1960) within two years in four but after twenty three years in one.

The extent of skin involvement is often not given in detail in the reports, but the impression is gained from the necropsy descriptions that the skin involvement is usually widespread and would respond to Type 3 of Barnett and Coventry (1969a). The term *acrosclerosis* is notably absent from the descriptions. In the five cases reported by Levine and Boshell the skin involvement was described as *severe* in all.

Commonly there is associated involvement of the heart, lungs or esophagus (Rodnan *et al.*, 1957; Fisher and Rodnan, 1958) and sometimes also of other viscera (Levine and Boshell, 1960).

The clinical features are non-specific and are those of rapidly progressing renal failure terminating in uremia and death. The duration of the acute illness is usually less than one month and may only be a matter of days. The clinical features based on nine cases have been described by Rodnan *et al.* (1957). Initial symptoms were headache, visual disturbance and convulsions. Eight of nine patients were hypertensive but the elevation of blood pressure was usually not gross. The ocular fundi showed narrow vessels, hemorrhages and exudates, and four patients also had papilloedema. Cardiomegaly and pulmonary congestion were the rule. The urine usually contained albumin and casts, but elevation of the urinary red cells and white cells occurred in a minority. The blood urea level rose steadily until the patient's death in uremic coma or convulsions. Salient features in our cases are shown in Table XVIII. Eleven patients died in renal failure and two others had characteristic arterial changes at necropsy. The two patients without characteristic proliferation of the intima died in a state of collapse and probably had pre-renal uremia.

CASE HISTORIES: The following are illustrative case histories of patients with scleroderma developing acute renal failure.

> CASE 1: A man aged fifty-nine years presented with complaints that over the past six months he had developed poor circulation in his hands and feet, stiffness of his hands, swelling of his ankles, burning of his tongue and numbness over his lower jaw. He also gave a history of ulcer-type dyspepsia over about eight years. Two months prior to attending, his ulcer pain became worse, with abdominal pain and vomiting and he was admitted to the hospital and an operation was performed: partial gastrectomy for penetrating gastric ulcer, cholecystectomy for gall stones, excision of a Meckel's diverticulum and appendectomy. Following this procedure his dyspepsia and vomiting ceased. The skin of the face was firm and smooth, giving him an appearance of being younger than his real age. His mouth was not unduly small. His tongue was coated, but otherwise appeared normal. The skin of the hands was smooth, tight and somewhat brown; the fingers were swollen and could not be fully flexed. His blood pressure was 120/80 mm. Hg. The heart and lungs were clinically normal. Apart from dullness to percussion for two cm. below his right costal margin and the presence of an upper midline scar, the abdomen was also clinically normal. Enlarged lymph glands were palpated in the groins and the left side of his neck. There was slight edema of the ankles.
>
> Electrocardiography, radiography of the chest, microscopic examination of the urine and renal function tests gave normal results. A barium swallow examination showed slow passage of the bolus but was otherwise normal.
>
> The patient was treated with prednisolone (average dose of twenty mg. per day) and during the early weeks of treatment experienced subjective improvement. He felt stronger, his hands were less swollen and fingers more mobile, the swelling of his ankles disappeared and the attacks of cyanosis of his fingers were less troublesome; however the burning sensation in his tongue and paraesthesia of his lower jaw were not relieved. He developed a hyperkeratosis of the skin of his hands and the skin of his body generally became dark and scaly. It was suspected that these symptoms might be due to a malabsorption syndrome. Some support for this was obtained by findings of the fecal fat content of ten gm. per twenty-four hours, and an abnormal xylose absorption test.
>
> Approximately one year after the onset of the features of scleroderma he was admitted to hospital with symptoms and signs of pneumonia. His blood pressure was 180/90 mm. Hg. and blood urea concentration 105 mg. per one hundred ml. He appeared to respond at first to antibiotic treatment but later rapidly became ill with severe dyspnoea and hemoptysis. A clinical diagnosis of pulmonary infarction was made and anticoagulant therapy was instituted.

TABLE XVIII
CASES OF SEVERE RENAL INVOLVEMENT IN CURRENT SERIES OF SCLERODERMA PATIENTS

A. Cases with Acute Renal Failure

Case	Age	Sex	Type	Duration of Scleroderma	Blood Pressure (mm. Hg.) Prior to Acute Phase	During Acute Phase	Blood Urea (mg./100ml.) Prior to Acute Phase	During Acute Phase	Treatment with Adrenal Steroids	Arteriosclerosis	Intimal proliferation of small arteries	Fibrinoid	Infarcts	Other pathol.* involvement	Comment
1	60	M	3	1½ yrs.	130/80	180/90	—	105	YES	+	+	+		H., L.	
2	67	F	2	12 yrs.	180/90	230/100	65	60 85	YES	+	+		+	L.	
3	58	M	1	4½ yrs.	105/75	110/80	44	62 85	NO	+				H., L.	Long history malabsorption syndrome.
4	44	F	2	4 yrs.	130/110	225/125	45	125 335	NO		+	+	+	Oes., L.	Also diabetic.
5	46	F	3	4 m.	140/90	130/100 180/140	24	140	YES		+		+	Oes.	
6	53	F	3	1 yr.	—	105/60	—	195	NO	+				Oes., H., L.	Admitted in state of shock and died within three days.
7	45	F	3	2 yrs.	160/90	170/125	30	206 578	NO		+	+	+		
8	63	M	2	4 yrs.	160/90	160/90	22	65 144	NO		+			Oes., H., L.	
9	73	F	3	2 yrs.	190/80	190/95	50	100 344	NO		+			Oes., L.	

B. Other Cases with Intimal Fibrosis of Small Arteries

Case	Age	Sex	Type	Duration of Scleroderma	Blood Pressure (mm. Hg.) Prior to Acute Phase	During Acute Phase	Blood Urea (mg./100ml.) Prior to Acute Phase	During Acute Phase	Treatment with Adrenal Steroids	Arteriosclerosis	Intimal proliferation of small arteries	Fibrinoid	Infarcts	Other pathol.* involvement	Comment
10	78	F	1	28 yrs.		230/110			NO	+	+			Oes., L.	Died from cerebral haemorrhage.
11	76	F	2	46 yrs.	200/100	220/120	45	—	NO	+	+			H.	Died from cerebral haemorrhage.

* H = heart, L = lung, Oes. = oesophagus

However his condition rapidly deteriorated: he developed a pericardial friction rub and oliguria, the blood urea concentration rose from its admission level of 105 mg. per hundred ml. to 230 mg. per one hundred mg., and his death occurred three weeks after his admission to hospital.

At necropsy, there was a fibrinous pericarditis, the heart was moderately enlarged, the myocardium pale, but histologically normal. The lungs were oedematous and hemorrhagic with a region of consolidation in the right lung and histological findings of marked fibrosis and thickening of the walls of small arteries. The kidneys were rather small with a rather narrow cortex and showed mottled appearance both on the surface and on section and on histological examination showed moderate arteriosclerosis, marked intimal thickening of small arteries and patchy fibrinoid necrosis.

Comment: A patient with Type 3 scleroderma under treatment with adrenal steroids who suddenly developed hypertension, fulminating renal failure and death within a few weeks. Necropsy showed the characteristic findings of scleroderma kidney.

CASE 2: A woman aged fifty-three years was seen in 1957, with a history that over the past eight years she had suffered from cyanosis of her hands produced by cold and emotional disturbance and over the past ten months she had developed painful dark areas at the tips of her fingers, which healed to leave small scars. She had also noticed that her skin had become tighter. She had suffered from four attacks of pneumonia over the past twelve years and after the last attack two years ago she had been subject to palpitations and was also nervous.

On examination, her face had a pinched expression and the skin of her forehead and cheeks was rather stiff. Her hands were cold and cyanosed, the skin was thick and immobile and there were ulcers at the tips of some fingers. Her feet were cold and the toes cyanosed but the skin was not appreciably thickened. Her blood pressure was 155/90 mm. Hg. Her heart, lungs and abdomen were clinically normal. Radiography of the chest, electrocardiography, microscopy of urine and renal function tests gave normal findings. Radiography of the hands showed trophic changes in the terminal phalanges and a barium swallow examination showed deficient peristalsis.

Relief of the ischaemic episodes in the hands was obtained with oral tolazoline, but the skin of the hands became tighter and the sclerodermatous changes of her forearm and neck became more marked. Treatment with prednisolone twenty mg. per day was commenced, but the drug was stopped for a period because of elevation of blood pressure to 210/100 mm. Hg. Prednisolone was later recommenced in a dose of fifteen mg per day.

The patient was admitted to hospital in 1961, with a history of feeling generally unwell over the past month, vomiting and poor appetite for twelve days and severe headaches for five days. On examination she was a sick, dehydrated woman with a blood pressure of 230/100 mm. Hg. There were marked skin changes of scleroderma as previously noted. Her heart was enlarged and there was a triple rhythm. Examination of ocular fundi showed hemorrhages and papilloedema. The blood urea concentration was 60 mg. per one hundred ml. The electrocardiogram showed a left ventricular strain pattern. Radiography of the chest showed effusions at both bases. There were haematological features of a hemolytic anemia with a hemoglobin concentration of eight gm. per one hundred ml., and a reticulocyte count of twenty percent, but the serum bilirubin and urinary and fecal urobilinogen were normal. The erythrocyte sedimention rate (Wintrobe method) was thirty mm. in one hour. An intravenous pyelogram showed the kidneys to be very small. A renal biopsy was attempted but an inadequate specimen was obtained. The blood pressure was reduced with the use of ganglion blocking drugs and the prednisolone was continued at a dose of fifteen mg. per day. Her general condition at first improved, but later her blood urea rose to eighty-five mg. percent and she deteriorated rapidly over the next few days and was not helped by an increase of her prednisolone dosage to sixty mg. per day. Her death occurred one month after admission to hospital.

At necropsy, the kidneys were small and the cortex slightly narowed and mottled. Histological examination revealed marked thickening of the intima of small arteries and fibrinoid changes in the vessels. Other significant autopsy findings were increase in the submucous fibrous tissue in the esophagus, patchy fibrosis and emphysema in the lungs and a severe cystitis.

Comment: This is a case of a middle-aged woman with Type 2 scleroderma. Her main problems at first concerned her peripheral circulation. She later developed mild symptoms of gastro-intestinal involvement, became hypertensive during treatment with adrenal steroids and suddenly developed fulminating renal failure. Necropsy showed the typical features of scleroderma kidney.

CASE 3: A woman aged forty-five years was seen in January, 1969 with the complaint that she had developed progressive stiffness of the skin of her feet, legs, hands and face over the past eighteen months and that also during the past fifteen months the tips of her fingers became white, blue and cold on exposure to cold. Otherwise she was in good health, apart from some mild dyspepsia present for several years.

On examination she was a thin, rather pigmented woman with small mouth and tight skin of her hands, arms, neck, face and lower part of her legs. Her blood pressure was 160/60 mm. Hg. Otherwise there were no significant findings on clinical examination.

She was admitted to hospital for various tests with the following results: barium swallow and meal showed a small sliding hiatus hernia but no other abnormality. Intravenous pyelogram showed normal renal function. The *L.E. cells* test was positive but there was no other hematological abnormality and the fluorescent antibody tests were negative. The fasting blood urea concentration was thirty-two mg. per one hundred ml. The liver function tests and concentrations of plasma proteins were normal. Although there were no urinary symptoms, urine culture grew β hemolytic streptococci and she received a course of nitrofurantoin. The electrocardiograph was normal. She was discharged from hospital without specific treatment.

She returned to the clinic in June 1969 with complaints of backache, anorexia and vomiting over the previous two months and frequency of mucturition for one day. On examination she was still thin, her blood pressure was 160/90 mm. Hg., her skin was generally softer, but there was marked pigmentation.

Microscopy of the urine showed more than one hundred polymorphs per c. mm., but no growth of organisms on culture. An intravenous pyelogram was normal. She was treated with sulphamethizole for her urinary infection.

She did not attend again until two months later when it was apparent that her health had greatly deteriorated. She had lost weight, her appetite had been very poor, she had been short of breath and had had a hemoptysis five days previously; she was very nervous and unable to sleep. On examination she was a thin, anxious, pale woman with a coated tongue, blood pressure 150/110 mm. Hg., pulse rate 120 per minute, raised jugular venous pressure, cardiac triple rhythm, crepitations at lung bases, hepatic enlargement, but no peripheral edema. She was admitted to hospital and the blood urea level was found to be 206 mg. per one hundred ml. An electrocardiogram showed widespread ST-T ischaemic changes. A radiograph of the chest showed cardiomegaly, pulmonary vascular congestion and edema. The hemogloblin concentration was nine gm. per one hundred ml. The erythrocyte sedimentation rate (Wintrobe method) was fifty mm. in one hour. The antinuclear factor was positive. She was treated with diuretics, digoxin, prednisolone, hypotensive agents and later the addition of cyclophosphamide twenty-five mg. daily but all these were of no avail—the uremia became more marked and she died twelve days after admission.

At necropsy, the kidneys were of normal size and there were scattered areas of petechial hemorrhages in the sub-capsular area. Histological examination showed concentric intimal fibrosis of small arteries and complete or partial infarction of several glomeruli and fibrinoid changes in some small arteries. Fibrosis and cystic changes were seen in the lungs, but the small arteries appeared normal.

Comment: This is a case of a patient with Type 2 scleroderma who, when first assessed, was found to have no evidence of visceral disturbance. She was treated with prednisolone. She suddenly developed fulminating renal failure and necropsy showed the characteristic features of scleroderma kidney.

CASE 4: A woman aged forty-four years was admitted to hospital in July 1961 for stabilization of diabetes mellitus, which had been diagnosed twelve months previously. Enquiry revealed that she had suffered from Raynaud's phenomenon of the hands for about four years and had noticed thickening of the skin of her hands, forearms, fingers and face for about one year. On examination there were marked sclerodermatous changes in the fingers, hands, forearms and face and Raynaud's phenomenon was readily demonstrated. Her blood pressure was 140/90 mm. Hg. The jugular venous pressure was two cm. above the sternal angle, but the heart was not clinically enlarged. There was a soft systolic murmur at the cardiac apex. The diabetes was stabilized but no specific treatment was given for the scleroderma. She was again admitted to hospital in March 1962 in coma, apparently due to prolonged hypoglycemia. Following the recovery, she was depressed and psychiatric testing indicated some organic brain damage. Stabilization of her diabetes now proved difficult but was eventually achieved and she was discharged.

She continued to have Raynaud's phenomenon and the sclerodermatous changes progressed. Corticosteroid treatment was given with a maintenance dose of prednisolone of twenty to thirty mg. per day. In May 1962 she was admitted to the hospital severely ill with a history of a five-day swelling of the eyes and blurring of vision and stated she had albumin in the urine on routine testing. She was found to be flushed with a pulse rate of 140 per minute, blood pressure was 226/125 mm. Hg., jugular venous pressure raised four cm., presystolic triple rhythm and systolic bruit over the cardiac apex. A few crepitations were heard at the lung bases and there was moderate edema of the ankles. An electrocardiogram showed sinus tachycardia and flat T waves in the left ventricular leads. The blood urea concentration was 125 mg. per one hundred ml. and sugar of 455 mg. per one hundred ml. She was digitalized and given diuretic treatment with marked diuresis and alleviation of the signs of congestive cardiac failure over the next three days. However five days after admission she began to complain of nausea and vomiting. Her urine contained much sugar. The digoxin was ceased but the vomiting continued and increased in severity and she also developed diarrhoea, became dehydrated and mentally confused. Intravenous therapy was instituted but her condition deteriorated and she died after a period of thirty-six hours of anuria.

At necropsy, the pericardium contained three hundred ml. of fluid. The heart showed some degree of left ventricular hypertrophy, some thickening of the mitral valve cusps, some patchy interstitial fibrosis of the myocardium, but no coronary artery atheroma. The lungs showed bronchopenumonia and patchy interstitial fibrosis. There was a hemorrhagic condition of the small bowel and digestion of the mucosa and a similar condition in the large bowel almost as far as the splenic flexure. The kidneys showed small areas of subcapsular infarction, marked intimal and medial thickening of small medium sized arteries, fibrinoid necrosis of the walls of small vessels, marked interstitial fibrosis and tubular loss. There was thrombosis of some radicles of the left renal vein associated with areas of infarction.

Comment: This patient had fairly rapidly progressive sclerodermatous changes and also diabetes mellitus. There was a rapid terminal illness with features of congestive cardiac failure and uremia and at necropsy, marked features of scleroderma kidney, also scleroderma heart disease and complicating hemorrhagic entereo-colitis.

Recently there has been exciting new work on the treatment of renal failure in scleroderma by hemodialysis followed by nephrectomy and kidney transplantation. Richardson (1973) has reported a case in which this treatment was successfully carried out. The grafted kidney showed no evidence of disease after eighteen months. Not only were the hypertension and renal failure relieved, but other manifestations of the disease (arthralgia and Raynaud's phenomenon) disappeared and the skin became less tightly bound to underlying structures.

CHRONIC RENAL CHANGES IN SCLERODERMA

In most of the patients referred to above who died in acute renal failure, there had been no clinical evidence of renal impairment until the final episode. Only rarely has previous chronic renal impairment (as in one case described by Levine and Boshell, 1960) been noted. In view of the chronic nature of the involvement of other viscera—alimentary tract, lungs, heart

—it seems strange that chronic involvement should not also occur in the kidneys and perhaps be the precursor of the acute renal failure. Although pathological changes are sometimes found in the kidneys of scleroderma patients in whom renal involvement has not been expected during life, these are usually not similar to those found in those with acute renal failure. Rottenberg *et al.* (1959), in a necropsy study of the kidneys of nine patients with diffuse scleroderma, found the typical pathological changes described above in three patients who died in uraemia, but that the kidneys of six patients without uremia were normal or showed minor changes only.

Urai *et al.* (1958) estimated the renal plasma flow by the clearance of para-amino hippuric acid and the glomerular filtration rate by the creatinine clearance in twenty-five patients with scleroderma. They found that 80 percent of the patients showed a reduced clearance of para-amino hippuric acid and a normal creatinine clearance with a resulting increased filtration fraction. They interpreted these findings as indicating structural narrowing in the preglomerular arteries accompanied by spasm of the efferent vessels. However, Barnett and Coventry (1969b) found a reduced creatinine clearance (less than seventy ml. per minute) in fourteen of twenty-eight patients without renal symptoms. It would seem that further study is required concerning renal function and pathology of patients with scleroderma without acute renal failure.

SUMMARY

Although there had previously been several references to pathological changes in the kidney in scleroderma, recognition of severe renal disease as one of the features of this disease has come rather late. Severe renal disease is rather uncommon and, when it occurs, it usually does so early Clinically there is onset of acute renal failure and hypertension in a patient without previous renal symptoms or elevated blood pressure. Until now, the illness has progressed inexorably to death in uremia within a few weeks. New hope for the sufferers of this grim condition has been afforded by a report of successful treatment by hemodialysis followed by nephrectomy and kidney transplantation. Pathologically the main feature is marked thickening of the intima of interlobular arteries by a mucoid connective tissue. Other common features are fibrinoid necrosis of small arteries and cortical infarcts. The changes are similar (and according to some, identical) with those of malignant hypertension.

The changes in the kidneys in scleroderma patients without renal failure have not been adequately studied. There are observations of disturbed renal function in some cases, but other workers have failed to find any significant pathological changes in the kidneys of patients with scleroderma but without renal failure.

Chapter XIII

OTHER SYSTEMIC DISTURBANCE

NEUROLOGICAL INVOLVEMENT

NEUROLOGICAL INVOLVEMENT in scleroderma is rare. A mild peripheral neuritis with paraesthesia and sensory defect is sometimes seen in the diffuse forms. The rarity and mildness of these symptoms is somewhat surprising in the light of the changes in the peripheral nerve network described by Pawlowski (1963) who studied horizontal sections of skin stained by methylene blue and found various stages of degeneration characterized by fragmentation and disintegration of the network.

Involvement of the larger nerves is rare. Richter (1954) described a patient with severe peripheral neuropathy, associated with cachexia, pigmentation, atrophy and tightness of the skin of the digits and who was found at necropsy to have a widespread increase in connective tissue throughout the body, particularly around the lymph glands and in the capsule of the kidney. There was incarceration of the spinal peripheral nerves in the generalized sclerosing process and extensive degeneration of nerve fibres. Although there were features of scleroderma in this case, it was a most unusual one as diffuse connective tissue overgrowth to this degree is not a feature of this disease.

A case of scleroderma with polyneuritis and swelling of lymph glands described by Ofstad (1960) can hardly be accepted as neuritis complicating scleroderma, as the neuritis occurred first and the case was complicated in various ways. Tightness of skin and subcutaneous tissue might be expected to compress nerves but this is rare. A case of carpal tunnel syndrome has been reported in a forty-five-year-old woman with scleroderma (Quinones *et al.*, 1966), but the carpal tunnel syndrome is common in women of this age without scleroderma.

Central nervous systemic disturbance due to scleroderma is also rare. The earliest report is attributed to Steven (1898), who described the post mortem findings in a case of scleroderma with hemiatrophy and found that the arteries throughout the spinal cord, medulla and pons, especially those in the grey matter, were surrounded by spaces containing homogeneous structureless material. Their coats seemed thicker than normal. Also nerve fibres from the cervical and lumbar plexuses showed well marked degeneration. There have been no similar reports and some other pathological process must be suspected. Also this type of scleroderma is not usually associated with systemic disturbance.

Lee and Haynes (1967) reported what they believed was the first case of carotid arteritis and cerebral infarction due to scleroderma. The patient, a man aged forty-three years with diffuse scleroderma, was admitted to hospital after developing a right-sided hemiparesis. Arteriography showed a long stenosis of his left carotid artery. At necropsy the affected part of the carotid artery showed fibrous proliferation of the intima, with thickening of the walls and patchy fibrinoid necrosis of the vasa vasorum. There was a large left-sided cerebral infarct and micro-infarcts in the right cerebral hemisphere associated with fibrosis of small vessels some of which were occluded by collagenous material. Kohle *et al.* (1970) have described a patient with scleroderma who suffered from a small stroke, dizziness and visual disturbance and in whom aortography showed occlusion of the left carotid arteries and stenosis of origins of vertebral arteries. A biopsy of the superficial temporal artery showed changes indicative of scleroderma.

The question of neurologic manifestations of scleroderma was the subject of special study by Gordon and Silverstein (1970) who reviewed the records of 130 patients with this disease admitted to the Mount Sinai Hospital. Although there were twenty-eight instances of problems involving the nervous system, only six, all myopathy, were related to the primary disease, the others being iatrogenic, secondary to disease elsewhere or coincidental. (Myopathy is not strictly a neurological disease and in this book has been dealt with when considering involvement of the skeletal system.) The authors accept only two cases from the literature: that of Lee and Haynes of internal carotid stenosis and that of Richter of peripheral neuropathy.

The escape of the central nervous system is remarkable. It may be related to the special type of supporting tissue (glia) with absence of fibroblasts. However the small arteries have a similar structure to those elsewhere, except that the wall thickness/lumen ratio is less.

OCULAR MANIFESTATIONS

Chronic ocular changes in scleroderma comprise tightness of lids, decreased secretion of tears and possibly cataract. Kirkham (1969) reported a case of a patient with scleroderma who presented with *gritty eyes*, was found to have inelastic skin of the eyelids and narrowed palpebral fissures, diminished tear secretion and moderately severe cortical lens opacities, and who eventually developed a corneal abscess resulting in loss of one eye. He summarized the ocular findings in ten women, aged forty-seven to seventy-six years, with scleroderma (including the one described above) and found narrowed palpebral fissures in four, presenile cataracts in three, and reduced lacrimal secretion in five (including one with Sjögren's syndrome).

Horan (1969) compared the ocular findings in twenty-three patients with scleroderma with those in twenty-three control subjects matched for age and sex. In the patients he found a significant increase of tightness of the lids—as indicated by a decrease in the size of the palpebral fissure in fifteen cases, shallow fornices in five, hyposecretion of tears in eleven, with none of these abnormalities in the control subjects. Seven patients had keratoconjunctivitis sicca and two had Sjögren's syndrome (keratoconjunctivitis sicca, enlarged salivary glands and arthritis). However there was no significant difference between the two groups in the incidence of lens opacities, which were found in eighteen patients but also in seventeen control subjects.

The retinopathy occurring in cases of acute renal failure in scleroderma has already been mentioned in the chapter on renal involvement. The changes are very similar to those in malignant hypertension and comprise arteriolar narrowing, cotton wool patches, exudates, hemorrhages and sometimes papilloedema. However the blood pressure is usually not as high as in cases of similar retinopathy due to hypertension.

The nature of the cotton wool patches has been the subject of considerable study. Pollack and Beckner (1962) described *cytoid bodies* in these patches. These occur in a variety of pathological states and are believed to represent degenerated nerve fibres. Klien (1965) found that the cotton wool patches contain scattered small necrotic foci within which there were a variety of vascular lesions (collapse, fibroid necrosis and thrombosis) and stated that these lesions were ischaemic infarcts due to vascular occlusion due to various causes. Ashton *et al.* (1968) reported that the clinical and pathological changes of the fundi in two patients with renal failure from scleroderma and blurred vision were similar to those in malignant hypertension, although they occurred with moderate elevation of blood pressure. Maclean and Guthrie (1969) reported the findings in two patients, one with uremia and characteristic retinopathy; and one dying from heart failure and with normal retinae one month before death. At necropsy the retina of the first patient showed cotton wool spots, thickening of the intima of arterioles and occlusion of small vessels; in the second case there was intimal thickening only. They suggest that the vascular lesions result from increased permeability (*dysoria*).

ENDOCRINAL INVOLVEMENT

Pathological Findings

Early pathologists describing the necropsy findings in scleroderma reported changes in the endocrine glands. Thus Hektoen (1897) found atrophy and fibrosis of the thyroid gland with endarteritis of the small vessels and increase in the number of chomophil cells in the pituitary gland. Matsui (1924) found atrophy of the suprarenal gland, a reduction of the chromophil cells and basophil cells and increase of the chromophobe cells of the pituitary gland, fibrosis and intimal thickening of the small arteries of the thyroid gland and reduction in number of follicles and sclerosis of small arteries in the ovaries. Kraus (1924) described fibrosis and infiltration by lymphocytes and plasma cells in the pancreas and parathyroid glands. Heine (1926) described fibrosis of pancreas, thyroid gland and anterior lobe of the pituitary gland with intimal thickening of the small arteries and infiltration with lymphocytes. Modern pathologists have paid less attention to endocrine gland involvement in scleroderma. D'Angelo *et al.* (1969) found the same incidence of fibrosis of the pancreas in the scleroderma patients as in the controls; atrophy of the adrenal glands was more common in the scleroderma patients than in the controls (but many had probably been treated with steroid drugs); fibrosis of the thyroid gland was much more common in the scleroderma patients (24 percent) than in the controls (7 percent). No figures are given for the pituitary and parathyroid glands which are not routinely examined.

Involvement of Particular Endocrine Glands

Thyroid Gland

Disorder of the endocrine glands was considered by some of the early writers to play a part in the symptomatology and possibly the pathogenesis of scleroderma and treatment was based on this idea. Thyroid dysfunction was particularly suspected and Osler (1898) used *thyroid* extract in treatment. The early literature was reviewed by Castle (1923) who considered the thyroid gland was involved. However O'Leary and Nomland (1930) failed to find a basal metabolic rate below normal in any of their cases of diffuse scleroderma; in seven cases there was evidence of hyperthyroidism and in one exophthalmic goitre.

Parathyroid Glands

The frequent occurrence of metastatic calcification in scleroderma has suggested parathyroid dysfunction and at one time parathyroidectomy was an accepted form of treatment (Bernheim and Garlock, 1935; Leriche *et al.*, 1937; Cornbleet and Struck, 1937). An interest in disturbance of the parathyroid glands in scleroderma has persisted until modern times and as recently as 1965, Samuelsson and Werner reported a case of scleroderma in which three of the four parathyroid glands showed hyperplasia. He listed forty-one reports in which a high serum calcium level had been found in cases of scleroderma and considered that mild hyperparathyroidism was probably not uncommon, although this was probably of the secondary type.

Pituitary Gland

The detailed description of pathological findings in the *pituitary* by Hektoen have already been mentioned. Subsequent writers (Foerster, 1916; Castle, 1923; Rake, 1931) considered that the pituitary was involved in the pathogenesis of scleroderma and posterior pituitary extract was used in treatment (Oliver and Lerman, 1936).

Adrenal Glands

The pigmentation and malnutrition in some cases of scleroderma obviously suggests dysfunction of the adrenal glands and it is therefore not surprising that substitution with adrenal gland extract was tried for this condition (Winfield, 1904; Millard, 1905). Other writers, convinced of endocrine factors in scleroderma, have included adrenal gland involvement among their suspects (Castle, 1923; Rake, 1931; O'Leary and Nomland, 1930).

Gil (1951), in a study of eight cases, stated that hypoadrenalism was indicated by an increased blood potassium concentration, a positive Kepler test, a low urinary excretion of ketosteroids, a lymphocytosis and evidence of disturbed metabolism in the form of a low serum cholesterol concentration and a flat glucose tolerance curve. Adrenal function in scleroderma does not seem to have been studied by modern techniques such as plasma cortisol estimations.

Pancreas

Dysfunction of the islet cells of the *pancreas* was also blamed and insulin therapy used (Wahl, 1930). More recently Fleischmajer and associates (Fleischmajer and Fogel, 1970; Fleischmajer and Piamphongsant, 1970; and Fleischmajer and Bansiddhi, 1970) have reported cases of scleroderma with various abnormalities in the glucose tolerance curve (chemical diabetes, flat curve, high two-hour blood-sugar level) and refer to a study of sixteen cases in whom eleven showed an abnormal glucose tolerance curve and all had an abnormal immuno-reactive insulin response (hyperinsulinism and/or delayed curve).

Other Endocrine Glands

Involvement of the *thymus gland* and *gonads* has also been suspected (Brooks, 1934). Recently, following the appreciation of the importance of the thymus in immunity, disturbance of this gland must be reconsidered.

Comment

In view of the great emphasis that has been placed by earlier workers on possible endocrine factors in the pathogenesis of scleroderma, it is rather surprising in the survey of 727 cases from the Mayo Clinic by Tuffanelli and Winkelmann (1961), that apart from the statement that in twenty-one of forty-six patients studied, the level of 17-ketosteroids in the urine was low, there is no reference to endocrine disturbance. Basal metabolic rate was normal or near normal in 177 patients, protein bound iodine was normal in twelve patients, serum calcium was normal in all but one of 173 patients and serum phosphorus was normal in all of eighty-seven patients studied.

The general view at present is that involvement of the endocrine glands may occur in scleroderma but clinical manifestations are uncommon. With the possible exception of the thymus, the involvement is part of the disease process and not of pathogenetic importance. The earlier writers were probably mistaken in ascribing a basic role to endocrine dysfunction in the pathogenesis of the disease.

METABOLIC DISTURBANCE

Metabolic disturbance in scleroderma may arise from involvement of a particular organ as part of the disease, for example, the malabsorption syndrome secondary to small bowel involvement and uremia in fulminating renal involvement. The metabolic changes are similar to those resulting from involvement of the particular organ from other causes and will not be discussed here.

Other metabolic changes have been described relating to the fundamental disturbance or to a supposed mechanism in production of the pathological changes. Scleroderma may be regarded as a disease of connective tissue metabolism and this aspect is so important that a chapter has been devoted to observations of the metabolism of connective tissue, mainly its two chief components: collagen and mucopolysaccharides (see Chapter IV). As indicated, recent observations have indicated a disturbance in collagen metabolism and the possibility of modifying it by drugs.

For completeness, it is necessary to discuss briefly some other aspects of metabolism which have been considered to be important in the pathogenesis of scleroderma.

Tryptophan Metabolism

Interest in tryptophan metabolism in scleroderma arises largely from the fact that it is the precursor of serotonin (5-hydroxytryptamine) which was at one time considered to be important in the pathogenesis of scleroderma (see Chapter V: Vascular Disturbance).

Tryptophan has two metabolic pathways: a major tryptophan-niacin pathway and a minor tryptophan-serotonin pathway as indicated schematically below (Fig. 13–1).

Price *et al.* (1957) studied tryptophan metabolism in three patients with acrosclerosis. They found that after an oral dose of two gm. of tryptophan there was an abnormally large excretion of certain metabolities (kynurenine, hydroxykynurenine and kynurenic acid). This defect was

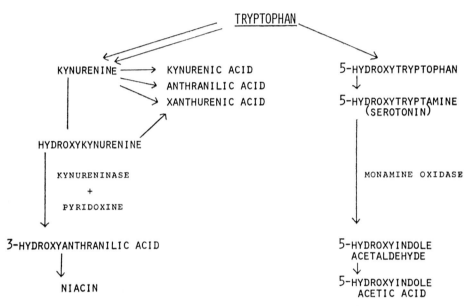

Figure 13–1. Tryptophan metabolism. Adapted from Birk, R. E. and Rupe, C. F., 1962, *Henry Ford Hosp Med Bull,* 10:523–553.

partly corrected by administration of disodium edetate (EDTA) and further improvement occurred after nicotinic acid. They suggested that EDTA acted by removing calcium and thereby *unlocking* magnesium which was required by the enzyme system necessary for the normal metabolism of tryptophan. Birk and Rupe (1962) claimed success from the treatment of fourteen patients with systemic sclerosis with disodium edatate and/or pyroxidine. They reviewed the literature concerning abnormal tryptophan metabolism, and evidence that pyridoxine activity as a co-factor for kynurenase depended on a normal heavy metal balance, restored by chelation. They suggested that increased diversion of tryptophan to the major niacin pathway following treatment with edetate might decrease the amount utilized in the minor serotonin pathway. Support for the observations of Price *et al.* has recently been given by Sonnischen *et al.* (1968). They found that after an oral dose of ten gm. of tryptophan there was an increased excretion of the metabolities kynurenine and xanthurenic acid in five of eleven subjects with scleroderma and that in two patients who were restudied after treatment with edetate there was a return towards normal.

The significance of these findings is obscure. If there were a block in one (niacin) metabolic pathway leading to increased utilization of the other (serotonin) pathway one would expect evidence of increased production of serotonin by increased urinary excretion of its metabolite 5-hydroxyindole acetic acid, which does not seem to have been demonstrated. It is also of note that the defect in tryptophan metabolism is only demonstrated after a loading dose. The observations are subject to various interpretations. Increased excretion of kynurenine, hydroxykynurenine and kynurenic acid results from the induction of tryptophan oxidase by corticosteroids and in stress conditions and is not specific to scleroderma. EDTA chelates other metals besides calcium and its effect might be explained by removal of a toxic metallic substance.

Phenylalanine and Tyrosine

Phenylalanine, an essential amino acid, is irreversibly converted to tyrosine which in addition to being a component of various proteins, is the precursor of the biologically active substances thyroxine, noradrenaline and adrenaline and also of the pigment melanin. Some of the biological pathways are shown in Figure 13–2.

Various disease are believed to be associated with particular blocks at the positions indicated [(1) phenylketonuria, (2) albinism, (3) tyrosinosis, (4) alkaptonuria]. Nishimura *et al.* (1958) reported the detection of 2,5-dihydroxyphenylpyruvic acid in the urine of patients with diffuse collagen disease including scleroderma, but not in other persons, including unaffected relatives and patients with other diseases. The administration of 1-tyrosine aggravated the clinical signs of the collagen disease. They postulated a fifth site of block in the position shown specific for collagen disease. As indicated in the diagram, melanin is derived from tyrosine and the possibility (not suggested by the above authors) arises that the pigmentation common in some cases of scleroderma might arise from a block of one metabolic pathway and diversion to another.

Kvyatkovskaya *et al.* (1963) measured the blood and urine levels of total amino-acids and of tyrosine in rheumatic conditions and collagen diseases. In scleroderma both the blood and urine levels of amino acids were raised; but although the blood level of tyrosine was raised, the urinary level was normal. The authors suggest that the increased level of tyrosine in the blood might be due to increased metabolism not only of collagen but of the protein moiety of protein-mucopolysaccharide complexes. Liver enzymes are concerned in the breakdown of tyrosine and they suggested that these enzymes were apparently inadequate to cope with the increased demand and that the deficiency of liver enzymes might

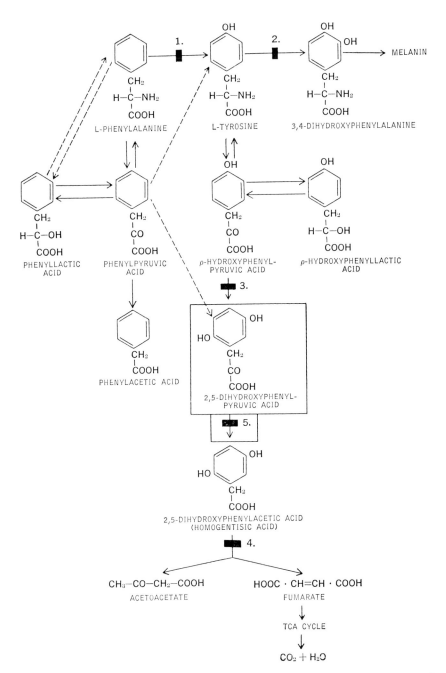

Figure 13–2. Phenylaline and tyrosine metabolism. Reproduced with permission from Nishimura *et. al.*, 1958, *Arch Derm and Syph*, 77:255–262.

be related to adrenal insufficiency. Although not mentioned by the authors, a metabolic block further down the pathway of tyrosine metabolism, as discussed above, has also to be considered.

Amino Acid Excretion

Winkelmann *et al.* (1971) reported on the urinary excretion of thirteen amino acids studied by microbiologic assay before and after treatment with the chelating agent disodium edetate (EDTA). In twelve women the levels were low or normal and increased after chelation treatment; in five men the levels were variable and decreased after chelation treatment. They concluded that the data indicated that scleroderma is not related to a specific amino aciduria and that disodium edetate has no specific effect on amino acids in scleroderma. These results might seem to conflict with some of the results described earlier concerning excretion of hydroxyproline and the findings described immediately above concerning possible abnormalities of tryptophan and tyrosine metabolism. However the latter results relate mainly to intermediate metabolites and refer usually to abnormalities detected in the urine after a loading dose of the amino acid. The urinary excretion of the individual amino acids is apparently normal.

Catecholamine Metabolism

The vascular disturbance in scleroderma suggests the possibility of some disturbance of metabolism of the catecholamines adrenaline (epinephrine) and noradrenaline (norepinephrine) in the form of either increased production or decreased breakdown.

The metabolic pathways for these substances are shown in Figure 13–3.

Brunjes *et al.* (1964) measured the urinary excretion of catecholamines and their metabolites in fourteen patients with scleroderma and twenty control subjects. They found that compared with the control subjects, the scleroderma patients showed decreased urinary excretion of free epinephrine, free norepinephrine and vanilylmandelic acid, but no significant difference in the excretion of free and conjugated metanephrine, and free and conjugated normetanephrine. It will be seen from inspection of the schema that monoamine oxidase (MAO) is not involved in the production of metanephrine (M) and normetanephrine (NM) but is involved at some stage in the production of all the vanilylmandelic acid (VMA). The authors calculated the ratio M + NM/VMA which they found to be significantly high, and which they interpreted as indicating decreased monoamine oxidase (MAO) activity in scleroderma. They considered the significance of this finding and suggested that decreased oxidative deamination of norepinephrine at its site of release could allow it to persist and produce hypertension, vasospasm and skin changes.

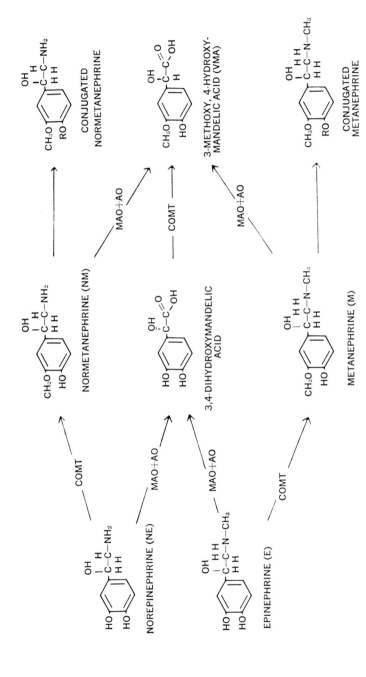

Figure 13–3. Catecholamine metabolism. Reproduced with permission from Brunjes, S. et al., 1964, *Arthritis and Rheum,* 7:138–152.

There are some strange findings in these results which are not explained. The excretion of free epinephrine, free norepinephrine and of the total amount of catecholamines and their metabolites is decreased. If the postulated mechanism operated one might have expected the excretion of substances not affected by MAO to be increased (unless for some reason the epinephrine and norepinephrine were immediately re-utilized by the nerve endings).

Sapiro *et al.* (1972) studied the resting venous cathecholamine concentrations and urinary excretion of catecholamines in patients with Raynaud's phenomenon associated with scleroderma and could not find evidence for excess of norepinephrine or epinephrine in this condition. They criticized the paper of Brunjes *et al.* on various methological grounds (no control of drug intake, no regulation of physical activity, no control of mental stress, urine collections too short).

It appears therefore that there is conflict between the findings of different groups, but no convincing evidence of abnormal catecholamine metabolism in scleroderma.

Porphyrin Metabolism

The occasional occurrence in patients of features both of scleroderma and of porphyria cutanea tarda led to a suspicion that there may be abnormal prophyrin metabolism in scleroderma. However the urinary and fecal porphyrin excretion in eight patients with *acrosclerotic scleroderma* was shown to be normal (Redeker and Bronow, 1962).

CLINICAL LABORATORY FINDINGS

Various abnormal laboratory findings which may occur in blood or urine in patients with scleroderma have been mentioned in various sections concerned with metabolism or immunology. These will now be briefly summarized.

Biochemistry

Blood Chemistry

ELECTROLYTES: These are generally normal. A raised blood calcium has been reported (Samuelsson and Werner, 1965). In a recent large series the levels of serum calcium and phosphorus were normal (Tuffanelli and Winkelmann, 1961).

GLUCOSE: A high incidence of abnormal glucose tolerance curves has been reported by one group (Fleischmajer *et al.*, 1970) but are not specific.

PLASMA PROTEINS: Abnormalities in the plasma globulin fractions include a frequent increase in the γ globulin concentration and a less frequent increase in the a_1 and a_2 globulin concentrations (Štáva, 1958; Gamp, 1961; Zlotnick and Rodnan, 1961; Corcos *et al.*, 1961; Barnett and Coventry, 1969b; Clark *et al.*, 1971). Fleischmajer (1964b) found a characteristic feature to be an increase in a_2 globulins and decrease in β globulins so that the β/a_2 ratio was decreased. Zlotnick and Rodnan (1961) compared the plasma proteins as studied by immuno-electrophoresis in fifteen patients with systemic sclerosis and fifteen healthy individuals. They found the main abnormalities to be increase in a_1 globulin (seven cases), in a_2 globulin (nine) and β_2M (six) and splitting of the anodic extremity of the a globulin. The findings by immuno-electrophoresis did not correlate with those of paper strip electrophoresis. The plasma albumin concentration may be low (Štáva, 1958) in association with raised plasma globulin levels.

The significance of these abnormalities is not clear. Stava stated that the increase in γ globulin concentration was more pronounced in the slowly progressing acrosclerosis than in the generalized diffuse scleroderma rapidly advancing to a fatal outcome. Gamp believed that the abnormal protein pattern was one of subacute or chronic inflammation and not diagnostic, although it might be useful in follow-up studies. He stated that, with long term observation, there was a tendency of the abnormality in the lowered albumin level and raised a globulin levels to return to normal, but there was varying behaviour of the γ fraction.

Spencer and Winkelmann (1971) studied the *immunoglobulins* in twenty-two patients. They found that there was no specific pattern of IgA or IgM levels, but the IgG level was elevated in two patients who died after a fulminating course.

MUCOPOLYSACCHARIDES: There have been several reports of raised serum concentrations of mucopolysaccharides or mucoproteins in scleroderma: *mucopolysaccharides* (Rodnan, 1963; Gamp, 1961; Balabanov and Samsonova, 1968), *seromucoid* (Gamp, 1961; Panja *et al.*, 1964), *bound hexose* (Winkelmann and McGuckin, 1965).

Urinary Findings

There are no specific urinary abnormalities in scleroderma. There is no specific amino aciduria (Winkelmann *et al.*, 1971). Although increased excretion of total hydroxyproline in the urine has been found by some workers (Smith *et al.*, 1965), others have found no change (Ziff *et al.*, 1956). The urinary 5-hydroxyindole acetic acid excretion is normal (Tufanelli, 1963); the vanilylmandelic acid excretion is not increased (Brunjes *et al.*, 1964).

Serology

ANTINUCLEAR FACTOR: A high percentage of sera from scleroderma patients is positive for antinuclear factor (See Chapter VI: Immunology).

LATEX RHEUMATOID FACTOR: This is positive in approximately 35 percent to 40 percent of cases irrespective of the presence of arthritic symptoms (Bartfield, 1960; Corcos *et al.*, 1961; McGiven *et al.*, 1968; Clark *et al.*, 1971).

OTHER SEROLOGICAL TESTS: A positive *L.E. test* without clinical systemic lupus erythematosus and false positive serological tests for syphilis are found in a small percentage of cases (Clark *et al.*, 1971).

Hematology

ANEMIA: Fifty of the 727 patients (approximately 7 percent) in Mayo Clinic series had an unexplained anemia (hemogloblin concentration less than twelve gm. per one hundred ml.,), usually mild and of the hypochromic microcytic type (Tuffanelli and Winkelmann, 1961). Occasional cases of auto-immune hemolytic anemia (A.I.H.A.) in association with scleroderma have been mentioned in the chapter on immunological aspects (Chapter VI).

ERYTHROCYTE SEDIMENTATION TEST: The sedimentation rate (E.S.R.) is elevated in 60 to 70 percent of patients and a markedly elevated E.S.R. is usually associated with rapidly progressive disease (Tuffanelli and Winkelmann, 1961; Clark *et al.*, 1971).

Chromosomal Abnormalities

Recently Emerit *et al.*, (1971) found a significantly increased number of chromosomal abnormalities in leucocytes of scleroderma patients compared with healthy persons or hospitalized patients with other diseases (Table XIX).

The abnormalities were more frequent in patients with Type 2 and 3 scleroderma than with Type 1 (of Barnett and Coventry).

The authors considered the various possible causes of these findings. The effect of diagnostic X-radiation is excluded as the patients did not have more radiation than Controls II. The effect of drugs is difficult to evaluate. Viral infection is considered a possibility as viruses are known to produce chromosomal damage. There may be some link with auto-immunity as chromosomal abnormalities may be responsible for the development of auto-immunity or auto-immunity may affect chromosomal stability (See Chapter VI).

TABLE XIX *

CHROMOSOMAL ABNORMALITIES IN PATIENTS WITH SCLERODERMA

Study Group	Number of subjects	Number of mitoses examined	Percent of mitoses with structural chromosomal abnormality	Percent of mitoses with more than one abnormality
Scleroderma patients	27	1867	32.67	8.78
Controls I	10	800	9.00	0.13
Controls II	12	650	12.31	1.54

Controls I :   Ten healthy males and females aged between twenty-five and thirty-five years.

Controls II: Six males and six females, aged forty-three to seventy-one years, hospitalized for various illnesses.

* From Emerit *et al.*: *Rev Europ Etud Clin Biol, 16*:684–694, 1971.

Similar but less frequent chromosomal abnormalities have been observed in patients in our series and who have not received drugs likely to cause these effects (Garson, 1971).

PSYCHOLOGICAL DISTURBANCE

Psychological disturbances, particularly anxiety and depression, are fairly frequent in patients with scleroderma, but it is difficult to determine whether this is an integral part of the disease or a nonspecific effect which might be expected in any chronic illness. Mufson (1953) described scleroderma patients with a specific personality defect with undue dependance on others. McMahon *et al.* (1953) gave a history of a case with obvious emotional factors both at the onset of the illness and coincidental with each flare-up of symptoms. They suggested that scleroderma might be a psychosomatic disorder. However a careful study involving assessment by a panel of three psychiatrists and a battery of psychological tests did not reveal any excess psychological disturbance in a group of twelve scleroderma patients in my series when compared with a group of matched patients from a general dermatological clinic.

Gulledge (1968) discussed the psychiatric aspects of progressive systemic sclerosis based on a study of the case notes of seventy-three cases. Psychiatric problems were recognized in twenty-six patients. These were mainly in those with serious emotional problems prior to the onset of the scleroderma, and comprised depression, anxiety and tension. Psychiatric symptoms occurring for the first time after the scleroderma symptoms were mainly of the anxiety type. Psychotic reactions were infrequent. It would seem that the disease was instrumental in bringing to light pre-existing emotional problems, as might be expected with any chronic distressing condition.

SUMMARY

This chapter has described various abnormalities found in patients with scleroderma and not included in the previous chapters concerned with the more major or frequent types of disturbance.

Although a mild peripheral neuritis is sometimes found and there is histological and physiological evidence of involvement of nerve terminals in the skin, major neurological involvement is very rare and in some of the reported cases the association of the neurological features with scleroderma is of doubtful significance. An exception is the occasional occurrence of central nervous systemic lesions secondary to involvement of cerebral arteries.

Chronic ocular changes comprise tightness of the lids, shallow fornices and hyposecretion of tears, which may occasionally be complicated by corneal ulcer. In patients developing renal failure there is commonly an acute retinopathy very similar to that in malignant hypertension.

Much prominence was given by early workers to endocrine gland disturbances. The modern view is that this is uncommon except for fibrosis of the thyroid gland. There have recently been reports of abnormality of the glucose tolerance curve and of the insulin response after glucose suggesting abnormality of the islet cell tissue of the pancreas.

There have been reports of abnormality in the metabolism of certain amino acids. In the case of tryptophan, there have been reports that after a loading dose of the amino acid there is increased excretion of certain intermediate metabolites on the tryptophan-niacin pathway, and improvement following treatment with disodium edatate (EDTA) and pyridoxine, suggesting deficiency of an enzyme system dependant on pyridoxine and heavy metal balance (? adequate megnesium). In the case of tyrosine, there has been a report of urinary excretion of a previously undetected intermediate metabolite along the pathway to aceto-acetic acid and fumaric acid, suggesting a metabolic block. The significance of these observations is not clear.

The urinary excretion of amino acids studied has shown no abnormality, suggesting therefore that scleroderma is not related to a specific amino-aciduria.

Although one group of investigators have claimed to have shown abnormality in the metabolism of catecholamines, consisting in deficiency of monoamine oxidase (MOA) others have failed to show evidence of excess of epinephrine or norepinephrine in scleroderma. The position is still not clear but it seems unlikely that there is abnormal catecholamine metabolism in scleroderma.

The various biochemical abnormalities in scleroderma have been described. There is a variable disturbance of plasma proteins consisting of elevation of the γ globulin and less frequently a, and a_2 fractions and decrease in the albumin level. It is probable that these changes are non-specific and are those of a chronic inflammatory process. The levels of serum mucopolysaccharides (or fractions detected by various ways) are elevated. The serum immunoglobulin levels are usually normal. There are no characteristic urinary findings.

Serological disturbances indicative of a disturbed immunological state are common and include positive test for antinuclear factor (A.N.F.), latex agglutinating test for rheumatoid arthritis and false positive tests for syphilis.

Unexplained anemia occurs in a small proportion of cases. The erythrocyte sedimentation test (E.S.R.) is frequently elevated.

Although psychological disturbance is fairly common in scleroderma patients, this seems to be non-specific and it appears that the chronic disease merely brings to light previous underlying emotional problems.

Chapter XIV

DIAGNOSIS AND DIFFERENTIAL DIAGNOSIS

DIFFICULTIES ARISING FROM CONFUSING TERMS

REFERENCE HAS BEEN MADE in Chapter I to the variety of terms used in connection with scleroderma and similar conditions. Although the meaning of the terms has since become better defined, confusion may still occur from the use of like-sounding words. Some writers group together systemic sclerosis and morphoea, which are both described as scleroderma, although most clinicians now regard them as distinct conditions.

The term *scleroderma* is used to indicate a condition in which the skin is hard, inelastic and tight, and is now commonly applied to pathological states in which this occurs. As discussed in detail in Chapter VII, most workers at present recognize two such conditions: progressive systemic sclerosis (with various subdivisions) and circumscribed (morphoea type) scleroderma (again with several subdivisions). The word *sclerodermatous* is also applied in certain situations in which the skin, either locally or generally resembles that found in these conditions, even though the underlying pathological condition is different.

The term *sclerema* was apparently used by some early writers in cases which would now be regarded as scleroderma. It is now restricted to *sclerema neonatorun*, a disease of newborn infants, and manifested by induration of the skin, usually of the trunk and proximal part of the limbs. The affected infants are usually extremely ill, often premature and many do not survive, but if they do, the lesions resolve during neonatal life. It is a disorder mainly of the subcutaneous connective tissue and has no relationship with scleroderma.

The term *scleroedema* is now used only for *scleroedema adultorum* of Bushke. This is usually a benign condition in which there occurs, usually after an acute infection, a progressive swelling and hardening of the skin usually commencing on the posterior and lateral aspects of the neck and spreading within a few days to involve the face and other parts, chiefly the upper part of the body (Curtis and Shulak, 1965). It is misnamed as the water content of the skin is not increased and it may affect children (Fleischmajer and Lara, 1965). It has no relation to scleroderma.

Scleromyxoedema (Gottron, 1954) is a somewhat allied condition in which there is a progressive thickening of the skin (pachyderma) involving most anatomic areas with the exception of the scalp, breasts, intermammary, mid-back and crural regions. A striking feature is the dense aggregation of lichenoid papules, particularly on the glabella, producing deep longitudinal furrows of the brow. In spite of the possible implication from the name, the patients are not hypothyroid and the disease has no relationship to scleroderma (Rudner *et al.*, 1966).

The term *scleroderma* sometimes appears in other names, such as *sclerodermatomyositis*, indicating that the presence of hard skin is a component of the disease (see later).

DIFFERENTIATION OF SCLERODERMA FROM OTHER DISEASES CAUSING STIFF OR HARD SKIN

The differentiation of scleroderma from scleroedema and scleromyxoedema should not be difficult. The nature and distribution of the skin involvement is different. In *scleroedema* the skin involvement begins in the nape of the neck and spreads to involve other areas. This is different from the case in scleroderma where, in the acrosclerotic form, changes are first in the hands and later in the forearms and face, or in the diffuse form, where changes may be prominent initially in the trunk and upper arms. The nature of the skin involvement (brawny thickening in scleroedema, tight and glossy in scleroderma) is different. Raynaud's phenomenon and systemic manifestations are not characteristic of scleroedema. The time course is different—usually rapid progression followed by resolution in scleroedema, steady progression in scleroderma.

Also in *scleromyxoedema*, the appearance of the skin (thickening plus lichenoid papules) is different from that in scleroderma. Also the clinical associations are different, with absence of Raynaud's phenomenon and the visceral changes characteristic of scleroderma.

The histological picture of the skin is different in the various conditions. In scleroderma, the characteristic picture is tightly packed, relatively hypocellular collagen. In scleroedema the dermis is usually thick and contains large swollen collagen bundles, separated by clear spaces in which mucopolysaccharides can be demonstrated by special stains (Cohn *et al.*, 1970). In scleromyxoedema histological changes are most marked in the upper third of the dermis, which contains large stellate and elongated fibroblasts in a dense mucinous stroma which stains positively for mucopolysaccharides (Rudner *et al.*, 1966).

Skin changes have been described in four of the six *mucopolysaccharidoses:* Hurler type (MPS I), Hunter syndrome (MPS II) Morquio syndrome (MPS IV) and Schier type (MPS V). The most common finding is a diffuse thickening of the skin of the hands and feet. Some patients have papular and nodular plaques with an orange-peel texture on the upper part of the back, chest and arms (Esterley and McKusick, 1971). Recently Esterley and McKusik have described another *stiff skin syndrome* characterized by localized, stony-hard skin, affecting the buttocks and thighs. It occurs in children and, although not present at birth, and has probably a genetic origin. In the conditions mentioned above, the appearance of the skin is not really like that of scleroderma and any similarity lies in the stiffness of the skin to touch.

In *Werner's syndrome* however (Werner, 1904), the skin develops a taut, shiny hyperkeratotic appearance similar to that in scleroderma. The typical features of this syndrome comprise premature senility with cataract, short stature with spindly extremities and sclerodermatous skin changes. Other findings include generalized deficiency of muscle mass and subcutaneous tissue, subcutaneous calcification, skin ulcers, peripheral arterial calcification and tendency to formation of malignant tumours (Rosen *et al.*, 1970). Histologically, the skin shows thinning of epidermis and loss of papillae, almost complete disappearance of the appendages and hyalinization of collagen. Atrophy is more marked than sclerosis, but it may be difficult to distinguish the skin of Werner's syndrome from the late stage of scleroderma (Degreef, 1971). However the diagnosis of Werner's syndrome should be readily made from the clinical picture if one is aware of the condition.

Severe scleroderma-like changes may be seen on the regions exposed to light (such as the hands, face and neck) in *porphyria cutanea tarda* (Holti, 1970), but the distribution and lack of other features should readily distinguish this condition from scleroderma. Also there is no abnormal excretion of porphyrins in scleroderma.

A certain degree of sclerosis may occur in the other connective tissue diseases, in malignancy and certain rare congenital syndromes (Winkelmann, 1963), but owing to the associated features, confusion with systemic sclerosis is unlikely.

THE TWO SCLERODERMAS: PROGRESSIVE SYSTEMIC SCLEROSIS AND MORPHOEA

As discussed in Chapter VII, a great step forward in the study of scleroderma was made when Sellei (1934) clearly distinguished between the acrosclerotic type of scleroderma with associated systemic disturbance and the non-systemic type (circumscribed or morphoea). Although some of the early accounts included both types, most modern writers have written on one type only, regarding them as two separate diseases.

As this book deals particularly with the progressive systemic sclerosis type of scleroderma, only brief mention will be made of the circumscribed (morphoea) type which occurs in various forms. Typical *morphoea* are patches of hard skin occurring over various parts of the body surrounded in the early stages by a violet ring. Sometimes the lesions are very widespread and may affect most of the body, the condition then being termed generalized morphoea (Vickers, 1960; Feiwel, 1964). In other instances, there are linear, scar-like lesions often involving subcutaneous tissues which, when occurring on the face are referred to as *en coup de sabre.* Similar linear lesions of the limb may be associated with atrophy, not only of the subcutaneous tissue under the scar-like lesion but of the whole limb. If both the upper and lower limb of one side are affected the condition is called *scleroderma with hemiatrophy.* Patients with patches of morphoea described above commonly also have small white patches a few millimeters in diameter, called *guttate morphoea,* which sometimes occur alone.

Another condition sometimes occurring in association with morphoea is *lichen sclerosus et atrophicus* consisting of small white macules or papules with brown follicular centres most often on the back of the neck, upper part of the trunk, elbow flexures, wrists and anogenital regions. (This may also occur without morphoea, when it is generally regarded as a separate condition).

Reference has already been made in earlier chapters to the histological and biochemical differences between the two types. The skin in morphoea is thicker (Black *et al.,* 1970), oedema and proliferation of connective tissue are prominent but vessel changes are inconspicuous (O'Leary *et al.,* 1957), hexoses and hexosamines are increased in the skin (Fleischmajer *et al.,* 1966). Curtis and Jansen (1958) studied the prognosis in 106 patients, 75 percent of whom had been observed for more than five years. They found that a large percentage improved spontaneously, but the linear types had a greater tendency to progress than the plaque or guttate forms. Although benefit has been claimed for some remedies, for example the administration of potassium paramino benzoate (Zarafonetis, 1962), assessment of response is difficult because of the tendency to spontaneous remission, and it is doubtful if any treatment is of benefit.

An interesting finding by Curtis and Jansen was that diffuse systemic sclerosis could follow the onset of any type of circumscribed scleroderma and occurred in six of their 106 patients, suggesting a connection between these two diseases. It has previously been observed that morphoea-like patches may occur in progressive systemic sclerosis. Jablonska *et al.* (1962) studied seventy-five cases with particular reference to the possible relationship of morphoea to the systemic type of scleroderma. Features in morphoea included absence of changes in internal organs, absence of Raynaud's phenomena, higher incidence in young people, relatively greater incidence in males and a more favourable prognosis. Similarities included appearance of the skin, histological features, myositis in both, altered sensory chronaxie * in both and a relation to nervous system in both (Raynaud's phenomenon attributed to neuro-vascular disturbance in systemic sclerosis, segmental distribution in linear scleroderma). They concluded that morphoea and diffuse scleroderma are varieties of basically the same morbid process. Some of the similarities seem rather tenuous. Many conditions can give a similar appearance of the skin, or even histological features (for example scar tissue) and the relation to the nervous system is not convincing. Two features of particular interest are the associated myositis and altered sensory chronaxie. In morphoea the myositis affects only the muscle underlying the skin lesions, while in progressive systemic sclerosis it is widespread. The altered sensory chronaxie is widespread in both types, occurring in both affected and apparently healthy skin. Although the relationship between morphoea and progressive systemic sclerosis is an intriguing one, the clinical pictures are so distinct that it is best to regard them as different diseases, but with certain interesting overlap features.

OVERLAP SYNDROMES

Reference has already been made in Chapter VI to the relationship between scleroderma and certain other diseases believed to have an auto-immune basis, and this has been regarded by some as evidence for an auto-immune basis of scleroderma. The diseases particularly concerned are the other so called collagen (or connective tissue) diseases—dermatomyosus, systemic lupus erythematosus, rheumatoid arthritis and Sjögrens syndrome. Although these diseases usually present as distinctive clinical entities, they have certain features in common including a fairly high incidence of auto-immune phenomena, particularly positive auto-antibody tests, arteritis and the occurrence of various types of systemic disturbance (Black, 1961). Scleroderma is mainly distinguished from the other members by the characteristic skin involvement, frequent peripheral vascular disturbance and the distinctive nature of the involvement of certain viscera, particularly the esophagus. The other diseases also have their characteristic features such as acute vasculitis and early nephritis in systemic lupus erythematosus, distinctive joint changes in rheumatoid arthritis, predominant muscle involvement and association with malignancy in dermatomyositis.

Tuffanelli and Winkelmann (1962) discussed the association of scleroderma with other collagenoses based on a study of 727 patients from the Mayo Clinic. Thirty-six of these had features of scleroderma plus dermatomyositis, five had positive *L.E. tests* (two with clinical features of

---

* Chronaxie is the time taken to excite a tissue when the current is twice the rheobase; the latter being the minimal current necessary for excitation if flowing for an unlimited time.

systemic lupus erythematosus), thirty-one had scleroderma plus rheumatoid arthritis, and seven had scleroderma plus Sjögrens disease.

The greatest overlap is between scleroderma and *dermatomyositis* which have as common features: cutaneous sclerosis, vasomotor disturbance, dysphagia, gastro-intestinal disturbance, oedema, muscle weakness, calcification of soft tissues and telangiectasia. The myopathy is the most striking feature in dermatomyositis, but muscle involvement may also occur in scleroderma. Cutaneous sclerosis is usually the most prominent feature in scleroderma but may also occur in dermatomyositis when the descriptive term *sclerodermatomyositis* is sometimes used (Corson, 1967).

Most large series of scleroderma patients contain a few with a positive *L.E. test,* but the clinical and pathological picture of systemic lupus erythematosus in addition to scleroderma is probably not common. The criteria for diagnosis of systemic lupus erythematosus vary in strictness but generally one would require, in addition to a positive *L.E. test,* some of the common clinical manifestations (acute arthritis, skin rash, hyperglobulinaemia) and histological evidence from biopsy of skin, muscle or kidney. Bianchi *et al.,* (1966) reported two cases of probable association of scleroderma and systemic lupus erythematosus, searched the literature of that time and concluded that "of fourteen cases stated to be a combination of scleroderma and S.L.E. in the literature, only five will stand scrutiny in the light of current knowledge."

Joint involvement in scleroderma is common and there are marked similarities to *rheumatoid arthritis* in the form of acute polyarthritis, flexion deformity (in the late stage), glossy skin and positive rheumatoid factor in a high proportion of cases. However the typical rheumatoid joints with spindle shaped swelling and ulnar deviation do not usually occur. However occasionally the two diseases co-exist.

There have been several reports of *Sjögren's syndrome* in association with scleroderma (See Chapter VI). There were seven such cases in the Mayo Clinic series.

Occasional cases are seen with features of several connective tissue diseases. One case from the Mayo Clinic series had features of scleroderma, dermatomyositis, systemic lupus erythematosis and rheumatoid arthritis.

Toth and Alpert (1971) reported a case of long-standing scleroderma with marked gastro-intestinal features who developed fulminating renal failure and who was found, at necropsy, to have, in addition to the vascular lesions characteristic of scleroderma, necrotizing lesions of small arteries with aneurysm formation, characteristic of *polyarteritis nodosa.* Fibrinoid necrosis of the small arteries and arterioles is the rule in patients with scleroderma dying with renal failure and in such cases fibrinoid necrosis is sometimes found in vessels in other regions and it is not surprising that the destructive process may sometimes affect larger arteries.

Recently Sharp *et al.* (1971, 1972) have described an apparently distinct rheumatic disease syndrome which they have termed *mixed connective tissue disease*. The clinical characteristics include a combination of features similar to those of systemic lupus erythematosus, scleroderma and polymositis, and a responsiveness to corticosteroid therapy. All the patients had hemagglutinating antibody to an extractable nuclear antigen (ENA) which consists mainly of protein and ribo-nucleic acid (RNA). Serum from patients with mixed connective tissue disease also contains high titres of *speckled* pattern anti-nuclear antibody. It is possible that some, but not all, of the overlap syndromes mentioned above were cases of mixed connective tissue disease.

Diagnosis in these overlap syndromes is largely a matter of terminology. When one disease predominates, diagnosis is usually made under its heading; if there are features of two diseases, it is probably best to make a double diagnosis, recognizing that such combinations occur; if several connective tissue diseases are intermingled, the possibility of *mixed connective tissue disease* must be considered.

DIAGNOSIS WITH MINIMAL SKIN CHANGES

Early Cases

In early cases presenting ischaemic episodes of the fingers, the diagnosis from other causes of Raynaud's phenomenon, particularly primary Raynaud's disease may be difficult, as skin changes may not yet be evident. However alertness to the possibility may lead to the recognition of slight skin changes of the fingers which would otherwise be missed. In cases of doubtfully significant skin signs, I have found the *neck sign* (tightness of the skin of the neck on extension of the head) is very helpful. In some early cases it is sometimes not possible to make a firm diagnosis. If the onset of Raynaud's phenomenon is in early life (under thirty years) and the patient is female, primary Raynaud's disease is the more likely diagnosis; if the onset is later (after forty years) or the patient is male, primary Raynaud's disease is excluded and the Raynaud's phenomenon is *secondary* to some other disease. Although other causes of secondary Raynaud's phenomenon, such as thromboangitis obliterans, vibration syndrome, cryoglobulinemia, cold agglutination, thoracic outlet syndrome and systemic lupus erythematosus, have to be considered, these can usually be excluded by history, examination of the pulses and appropriate special tests; if no such cause is found it is probable that the case will prove to be scleroderma. Tests are usually of little help at this stage.

A positive latex test, or antinuclear factor or impaired esophageal peristalsis would increase the probability of scleroderma, but their absence would by no means invalidate it. By the time of presentation, most patients have some skin changes which, even though minimal, are adequate for diagnosis. In the cases without adequate skin changes, the diagnosis is "secondary Raynaud's phenomenon, probably early scleroderma" and a firm diagnosis is usually possible within one or two years.

Visceral Involvement with Minimal or Absent Skin Changes

Reference has been made in the previous chapters to the occasional occurrence of severe visceral disturbance, particularly gastro-intestinal, of the nature found in systemic sclerosis, with minimal or even absent skin changes. In my cases, skin changes have been present on careful inspection, although not apparent to the patient. Cases with no skin changes are probably very rare. It is important that in disturbances of obscure origin, such as vague abdominal symptoms and bloating, malabsorption syndrome, cardiomyopathy and pulmonary fibrosis, scleroderma should be considered and a careful inspection should be made of the skin, particularly of the fingers, and an inquiry should be made concerning vascular disturbance.

The above discussion raises the question of the minimal criteria for the diagnosis of scleroderma. The criteria used by D'Angelo *et al.* (1969) of typical skin changes plus characteristic involvement of one internal organ, or characteristic involvement of at least two internal organs in the absence of characteristic skin changes, seems reasonable for selection of subjects for a pathological study. However, in the clinical situation, one wishes to make the diagnosis at an early stage, before evidence of visceral disturbance, in which case characteristic skin changes plus ischaemic episodes of the digits would be adequate.

DIAGNOSTIC AIDS

There are no specific diagnostic tests for scleroderma. A skin biopsy is usually taken and in obvious cases shows the characteristic changes, but is of no use in the early cases where changes are often more easily discernable by eye and touch. *Serological tests* (latex agglutination, rheumatoid factor, antinuclear factor) are useful when positive. Numerous *radiological* changes have been described in soft tissues, bones, lung fields, heart and gastro-intestinal tract. Harper and Jackson (1965) found that common abnormalities were absorption of phalanges (80 percent), esophageal changes (80 percent), subcutaneous calcification of hands (60 percent), and colonic changes (50 percent). However these figures are based on established cases, diagnosed clinically and radiology is not very helpful in early cases. However radiological demonstration of characteristic findings not only in the clinically affected organ, but elsewhere is helpful in cases with minimal skin involvement. Gough (1965) has drawn attention to the similarity between the radiological picture of the lung in scleroderma and asbestosis. In a study on the correlation between the lung asbestos count at necropsy and the radiological appearances before death, of ten patients with positive radiological appearances for asbestosis, the only case without a positive asbestos count at necropsy had scleroderma (McPherson and Davidson, 1969).

Claims have been made, based on only a few cases, that *thermography* gives a characteristic picture in scleroderma (Herma van Voss, 1968; Haberman *et al.*, 1968), but this method has not yet been evaluated. Also preliminary work has been done on *skin elasticity* (Pace and Potter, 1966) but there are no extensive studies. The claim that *skin chronaxie* is a valuable method in diagnosis (Jablónska *et al.*, 1962) does not seem to have been followed up. *Nail fold capillaroscopy* (Redisch *et al.*, 1970) has shown distinctive features in established cases, but it is not clear whether these are also present in the early cases where diagnosis presents difficulty. It is clear that there is scope for more work in refining methods for the early diagnosis of scleroderma.

SUMMARY

In the past, difficulties in diagnosis of scleroderma have arisen from confusing terms. The like-sounding terms scleroedema and sclerema are now confined to rare and well defined conditions distinct from scleroderma.

Scleroderma has to be differentiated from various other conditions causing stiff or hard skin. These comprise two main groups. In one (scleroedema and mucopolysaccharidoses) the skin feels stiff, but the appearance is different from scleroderma. In the other group (including Werner's syndrome and some cases of porphyria cutanea tarda) the appearance of the skin is similar to that in scleroderma. The various conditions can usually be distinguished by difference in distribution of the changes, frequent vascular disturbance in scleroderma but not in the other conditions and other characteristic features of the particular disease.

It is now recognized that the diagnosis *scleroderma* is used for two distinct conditions: the non-systemic type (morphoea) and the systemic type (progressive systemic sclerosis). Each of these has several subdivisions. Although there is some overlap between these two major conditions, it is best to regard them as separate diseases, with occasional overlap features.

Cases have been reported with overlap between the features of scleroderma with other connective tissue diseases or diseases with auto-immune phenomena. It is suggested that the diagnosis adopted be that of the condition with the predominant features. In cases with overlap of features of several diseases, a diagnosis of the recently described condition of *mixed connective tissue disease* should be considered.

Early diagnosis in a patient with Raynaud's phenomenon and as yet unconvincing skin signs may be difficult. The neck sign is very helpful. The probable diagnosis is suggested by the age and sex of the patient and the exclusion of other causes of Raynaud's phenomenon, but sometimes it is necessary to wait one to two years before making a firm diagnosis.

Difficulty arises in arriving at the correct diagnosis in patients with the visceral manifestations of systemic sclerosis but minimal or even absent skin changes. It is suggested that skin changes are rarely completely absent and it is important in patients with visceral disturbance of obscure origin to look carefully for the skin changes of scleroderma.

There is no specific test for scleroderma. Skin biopsy findings are confirmatory, but by the time the changes are definite, the diagnosis can be made on clinical grounds. Results of special tests (serological, radiological) may be confirmatory but not diagnostic. Other measures claimed by some workers to be diagnostic have not yet been adequately evaluated.

Chapter XV

TREATMENT

THE AETIOLOGY OF SCLERODERMA remains unknown and there is therefore no specific curative treatment. However numerous remedies have been used, based on some manifestation of the disease or some supposed pathogenetic process. In practically all cases benefit in a high proportion of cases has been claimed by the originators of the treatment and their immediate successors, although later workers have not been so successful and many of the treatments are no longer in use. Early workers relied largely on the patients' impressions or qualitative assessments such as healing of ulcers or softening of skin. Such methods are obviously fallible in a chronic condition with superadded psychological disturbance, with episodic disturbances such as ulceration and with dependence of symptoms on extraneous factors, particularly weather. The modern techniques of clinical trials using objective measurements, controls and *double-blind* assessment have still not been widely employed in this condition.

Although no specific treatment has been established as curative in scleroderma, there is much that practitioners can do in the management of this condition which may affect practically all systems and demands the skills of the physician, sometimes the help of his specialist colleagues. In the following pages, the various treatments used will be outlined, and then the problems of general management discussed.

PARTICULAR TREATMENT METHODS

In presenting the treatments, an attempt will be made to group them according to their pharmacological action or supposed action in scleroderma.

Drug Treatment

Hormones

There was a widespread belief among early workers that scleroderma was due to a disorder of the ductless glands (see Chapter XIII) and replacement therapy with gland extracts was used by various workers and successes claimed (Castle, 1923; Oliver and Lerman, 1936; Burch, 1939). As recently as 1962 Asboe-Hansen claimed benefit from treatment with d-thyroxine (the non-calorigenic isomer of the thyroid hormone, 1-thyroxine) in a dose of four to ten mg. per day over a period up to two years. However Winkelmann *et al.* (1965) using a double-blind trial found no significant difference in results between a group of seventeen patients who received the drug and a group of fifteen who received a placebo.

The theory of an endocrine basis for scleroderma has generally been discarded and hormones are not now used as replacement therapy. However hormones have again been used because of their pharmacological effects, such as anti-inflammatory action or anti-fibrotic effects and will be discussed later with other drugs believed to have these actions.

Vitamin D

Cornbleet and Struck (1937) reported studies in two scleroderma patients showing a positive calcium and phosphorus balance which became negative after treatment with 200,000 to 300,000 units of Vitamin D daily. These two patients and seven others improved clinically with this treatment. The mechanism of action of Vitamin D in these cases was obscure.

Ethylene-diamino-tetra-acetic Acid

Treatment with the chelating agent ethylene-diamino-tetra-acetic acid (EDTA) is discussed at this stage as its introduction by Klein and Harris (1955) was based on disturbed calcium metabolism shown by calcific deposits in the skin and subcutaneous tissues. It is given by intravenous infusion of the sodium salt (*disodium edetate*) three gm. in five hundred ml. of a 5% solution of dextrose in water over about three and a half hours with careful monitoring of the serum calcium level. Courses consist of daily infusion for about a week, with intervals of about a week between courses. Klein and Harris reported not only decrease in the calcific deposits, but regression of the sclerodermatous changes in the skin (confirmed by biopsy) and marked general improvement, particularly in respect to joint mobility.

Subsequent studies on skin histology have not been so favourable, reporting either no change or slight improvement (Rukavina *et al.*, 1957; Muller *et al.*, 1959), although Keech *et al.* (1966) found improvement in three of four cases. Reports on the early clinical effects have been encouraging (Winkelmann, 1959; Winder and Curtis, 1960; Birk and Rupe, 1962), but Neldner *et al.* (1962) found the late results (assessed two to four years after treatment) disappointing and considered that the immediate benefit could have been due to bed rest and concomitant physiotherapy. The clinical course of the disease was not altered and they did not think the routine use of the method warranted. Fuleihan *et al.* (1968) could not demonstrate any improvement of lung function following treatment with E.D.T.A., reserpine and pyridoxine. There was no benefit from the treatment in two patients with severe calcinosis in my series.

The mode of action of the treatment is conjectural. The amount of calcium removed in the treatment is not large compared with that present in the deposits. Rukavina *et al.* obtained clinical benefit in non-calcific cases. Price *et al.* (1957) found that E.D.T.A. could partially or completely correct a defect in tryptophan metabolism consisting of increased excretion of kynurine and other metabolites after a loading dose of tryptophan. They suggested that the removal of calcium *unlocked* magnesium needed for the operation of an enzyme system concerned in the metabolism of tryptophane. They suggested that in deficiency of this enzyme system the metabolic pathway of tryptophan is shifted to an alternative route with increased production of serotonin.

Adrenal steroids and A.C.T.H.

Soon after the demonstration of beneficial effect from adrenal steroids and A.C.T.H. in rheumatic and collagen disease, these drugs were used in the treatment of scleroderma. Most of the early workers reported benefit (Bayles *et al.*, 1949; Hines *et al.*, 1950; Sauer *et al.*, 1951; Taubenhaus and Lev, 1951; Frank and Levitt, 1952; Zion *et al.*, 1955), although others were not impressed (Thorn *et al.*, 1950; Briggs and Illingworth, 1952). Histological changes produced by these drugs include atrophy of hypertrophied collagen bundles and fibrils and reduction in hyalinization (Mancini *et al.*, 1960). In spite of improvement in the skin and subjective improvement, pulmonary function tests are unchanged (Salomon *et al.*, 1955). As mentioned in Chapter XII, some writers have blamed adrenal steroids for the precipitation of acute renal failure, but this is probably unjustified.

Although a relatively large dose (two hundred mg. of cortisone or forty mg. of prednisolone) is commonly used initially, this is usually reduced to a maintenance dose of about one hundred mg. of cortisone or twenty mg. of prednisolone after several weeks and treatment at this dose continued for months or years. Barnett and Coventry observed no benefit in Type 1 or 2 cases, but in several Type 3 cases there was definite improvement in the skin in which the changes regressed in a centrifugal direction. No improvement has been observed in the visceral manifestations and acute renal failure may occur while the patient is still receiving steroids.

Other anti-inflammatory drugs

Other anti-inflammatory drugs, which have been found of benefit in rheumatic diseases, have been used from time to time with variable results. An extensive series of patients with rheumatic disorders treated with indomethacin in a dose increasing from twenty-five to seventy-five mg. per day (Thompson and Percy, 1966) included one with scleroderma who was not helped.

COLCHICINE DERIVATIVE: Housset (1967) treated nine cases with acid trimethyl colchicine (a derivative of colchicine claimed to be better tolerated and with less side effects) in a dose of fifty to one hundred mg. per day for several months. Results were not impressive: failure in three, temporary softening of the skin in four, lasting softening of the skin in two, no effect on visceral manifestations, erythrocyte sedimentation rate or immunofluorescent tests.

SALAZOPYRIN: * Recently Dover (1971) has claimed marked benefit from salozopyrin in nineteen patients with scleroderma of various types, including eleven with systemic sclerosis. Beneficial effects claimed include subjective improvement, wider range of joint movements, softening of skin, growth of hair and decrease in pigmentation. The drug is used in an initial dose of one to seven gm. per day for two to three weeks, followed by a maintenance dose of 0.25 to one gm. per day and has been continued for up to thirty-five months. Unfortunately there have been frequent side effects (fever, rash, nausea, leukopenia, leucocytosis, thrombocytopenia) but these have disappeared following a reduction in dose.

Anti-fibrotic drugs

Since scleroderma has been considered to be a disorder of connective tissue which appears to be increased in amount and densely packed in various locations, attempts have been made to decrease or soften this tissue by anti-fibrotic drugs.

POTASSIUM PARA-AMINO BENZOIC ACID (POTABA): This drug was introduced in the treatment of scleroderma by Zarafonetis (1959, 1964) who claimed remarkable beneficial results (marked improvement in skin of fifty-eight of sixty patients after three months). The dose is twelve gm. per day over several weeks or months. Although success has been reported from one double blind trial (Bushnell *et al.*, 1966), others have shown no benefit (Barnett and Coventry, 1969a).

PENICILLAMINE: Harris and Sjöerdsma (1966b) reported what they claimed to be the first direct demonstration of an effect of a drug on human collagen. They found that in scleroderma patients there was a decrease in the percentage of collagen soluble in 0.5 N acetic acid, although the α-β ratio (ratio of single strand to double strand chains in collagen extract) was normal. Following treatment with penicillamine in two patients there was an increase in the percentage of collagen soluble in 0.5 N acetic acid and the α-β ratio also increased. However they were unable to demonstrate an increase in the urinary excretion of hydroxyproline. Böni *et al.* (1969) treated three cases with D-penicillamine in a dose of 1.8 gm. per day for

---

* Other names: sulfasalazine, salicylsulfapyridine, azulfidine.

four months. They found that the drug was well tolerated and reported benefit as judged from skin fold measurements. However Fulghum and Katz (1968) using a dose of one gm. per day increased to three to four gm. per day for periods of ten to 363 days (over one month in four patients) found no objective benefit in any of five patients but side effects in all. Bluestone *et al.* (1970) treated ten patients for two weeks to sixteen months with a dose commencing at 150 mg. per day and increased gradually over the first month to the maximum tolerated up to three gm. per day, with the addition of pyridoxine thirty mg. per day. Although there was improvement in skin elasticity measurements in six patients and the palm prints of three patients improved following cessation of treatment, there was no clinical improvement and eight patients suffered severe side effects (rash, fever, malaise, proteinuria, pruritus, dyspepsia, anorexia). Jaffe *et al.* (1968) reported development of nephropathy, confirmed by renal biopsy and electron-microscopy, in two patients treated with D-penicillamine, 0.5 gm. per day increased to two gm. per day, for four months in one case and six months in the other. Immunofluorescent staining of the kidney sections showed a positive reaction with antisera to IgG and complement. Both patients improved after the drug was discontinued.

Although the effects of D-penicillamine on the collagen in scleroderma are of great theoretical interest, the clinical effects are too small and the toxic effects are too severe for the drug to be recommended for clinical use.

Similar effects to those from D-penicillamine have been demonstrated with beta-aminopropionitrile (Keiser and Sjoerdsma, 1967), but the toxic effects have precluded further clinical trial.

RELAXIN: Casten and Boucek (1958) reported significant improvement in skin tightness, Raynaud's phenomenon and trophic ulceration in twenty three patients with scleroderma treated for six to thirty months with *relaxin,* the hormone responsible for softening of the ligament of the symphysis pubis during pregnancy. Evans (1959) reported favourable results in eleven patients treated with sympathectomy, plus diethylstilboestriol (one mg. per day) plus relaxin given either by intravenous injection (2.5 mg. to eighty mg. in 5 percent dextrose), intramuscular injection of a gel (thirty to fifty mg.) or by rectal suppositories (forty mg.). There was a fatal anaphylactic reaction following an intravenous injection in one patient previously treated by other routes.

PANCREATIC COLLAGENASE: Nellas *et al.* (1965) employed pancreatic collagenase in an attempt to break down the supposed excessive accumulation of collagen in scleroderma.

The preparation, obtained from porcine pancreas, was given daily by intramuscular injection of one hundred mg. per day, subsequently decreased to sixty mg. per day, for several months. There was, at first, clinical improvement, increase in the urinary hydroxyproline, and decrease in the skin content of hydroxyproline but later in the treatment program clinical improvement was not maintained and the laboratory results reverted to their pre-treatment levels.

DIMETHYL SULPHOXIDE (DMSO): This substance $\left(\begin{smallmatrix} CH_3 \\ CH_3 \end{smallmatrix} > S = O\right)$, a by-product of the paper industry, has the remarkable property of being extremely soluble in both water and oils and passes readily through the skin. It was found to have a softening effect on collagen and benefit was reported from its use in scleroderma and muscular skeletal disorders (Scherbel *et al.*, 1965; Rosenbaum *et al.*, 1965; Ehrlich *et al.*, 1965). It was usually applied locally in a dose of up to fifteen ml. of a 60% to 90% solution which was allowed to soak through the skin. In successful cases there was reduction in skin pigmentation, increased joint movement and healing of ulcers. However one worker (Tuffanelli, 1966) failed to find improvement in any of the parameters studied—cutaneous sclerosis, joint mobility, ulceration, biopsy appearance, anti-nuclear factor titres, protein electrophoretic patterns or esophageal mobility. There have been further reports of dramatic benefit (Scherbel *et al.*, 1967; Engel, 1967), although others have had only limited success (Kappert, 1968). The method of use has been extended to include application to the whole body of a 30% to 100% preparation, immersion of hands and wrists in a 50% solution in increasing periods of one to ten minutes twice daily and injection of five to ten ml. of a one percent to five percent solution in physiological saline on four days per week for two to four weeks (Scherbel *et al.*, 1967). The drug was found to cause lens opacities in animals (although these have not been reported in man) and its use has been restricted to investigational studies. Its place in therapy has not yet been established.

GESTAGENS: Recently Korting and Holzmann have claimed that progesterone and related substances (*gestagens*) have a beneficial effect on the collagen in scleroderma (Korting and Holzmann, 1967; Holzmann *et al.*, 1968b). They have found that in the skin in scleroderma there is an increase in collagen soluble in neutral salt solution corresponding to an increase in fine fibrils. They found that in eleven treated cases there was improved blood flow, decreased severity of Raynaud's phenomenon, softening of the skin and delayed wound healing (Holzmann *et al.*, 1968b).

Treatment in post-menopausal women consists of injections of hydroxy-progesterone in oil (Proluton depot, Schering A.G.) with a weekly dose of 125 to 250 mg. Alternatively norethisterone acetate may be given orally in a commencing dose of 5 mg. twice daily during the first month, 5 mg. three times daily in the second and third months, 10 mg. twice daily in the fourth month, 10 mg. three times daily in the fifth and six months, and 10 mg. twice daily in the succeeding months. In the pre-menopausal women, treatment with norethisterone acetate orally may be given in a dose of 5 mg. three times a day in conformity with the menstrual cycle. In men, injection treatment with hydroxyprogesterone acetate is preferred as this has a less marked action on the anterior pituitary gland. The recommended dose is less than for women, namely 10 to 50 mg. weekly.

HYALURODINASE: Petter and Bellmann (1971a,b) have suggested that the cause of the fibrotic changes in scleroderma may be accumulation in the tissues of acid mucopolysaccharides which are concerned both in the intracellular formation of collagen and the extracellular laying down into fibrils, and that this process may be modified by the use of hyaluronidase which decreases the concentration of mucopolysaccharides. They also postulate that acid mucopolysaccharides are concerned in the initiation of calcium deposition by binding calcium and influencing its deposition in calcium phosphate crystals or collagen fibrils. They have given hyaluronidase to two patients with scleroderma in a dose of 1,500 international units intravenously three times a week (one patient receiving 90,000 units over five month) with favourable results: softening of skin, healing of ulcers and disappearance of calcium deposits in the skin.

CARNITINE (KARNITIN): This is a betaine with the formula $L(-) - (CH_3)_3^+ NCH_2CHONCH_2 COO^-$ which is stated to have a very wide activity in influencing various types of intermediate metabolism and to exert a favourable effect on connective tissue diseases (Strack *et al.*, 1970; Nitzschmer and Liebsch, 1971). It may be obtained from meat extracts or synthesized and is administered in a dose of two gm. orally (in tea or fruit juices) per day. Remarkable softening of the skin has been reported, apparently in one case as soon as after five days of treatment, although there was no effect on muscle or joint pain. The mode of action of the drug is not clear.

Antibiotic Treatment

A supposition of a possible infective agent and participation of the nervous system in the etiology of scleroderma led Ottolenghi (1961) to try treatment with the diethylamino ethylester hydriodide salt of penicillin G, which has a high capacity for penetration into the cerebrospinal fluid. He treated eight cases of various types of scleroderma by the intramuscular injection of 500,000 units daily for periods up to one month and claimed that this produced softening of the skin, particularly in the more recent cases. Øhlenschlaeger and Tissot (1967) used the drug in the same dosage in courses of ten to twenty days in eight patients with *localized* and eight patients with *diffuse* scleroderma. In the latter group, improvement (judged from softening of skin, increased mobility of joints, reduction in Raynaud's phenomena, healing of ulcers) occurred in response to eleven of thirteen treatments.

Immunosuppressant Drugs

As outlined earlier, there is much evidence for an immunological disturbance in many cases of scleroderma and some writers believe that auto-immunity may play a fundamental role in its pathogenesis. It is therefore natural that immunosuppressive drugs should be tried in treatment. Demis *et al.* (1964) included two patients with scleroderma in a group of patients with auto-immune features treated with the immunosuppressive drug 6-thioguanine. The results were not impressive (some softening of the skin in one case and questionable softening in the other). Jansen *et al.*, 1968 treated eighteen patients with azothioprine (*Imuran*) using a starting dose of 150 mg. per day, increasing gradually to 250 mg. per day. Again the results were not impressive. Although eight improved symptomatically, there was no significant change in laboratory tests or in skin biopsy appearance. Side effects were frequent and serious (nausea and/or vomiting in three, granulocytopenia in four, anaemia in three, thrombocytopenia in two, serum sickness-like reaction in three) and necessitated cessation of the treatment in three cases.

Serotonin antagonists

Following the papers suggesting that serotonin was implicated in scleroderma, serotonin antagonists were used in treatment. Grin *et al.* (1964) used methergide (*Deseril*) given orally or by injection in eight patients and claimed good results with no side effects.

Epsilon amino-caproid acid (EACA)

Rotstein *et al.* (1963) reported remarkably good results in twenty-eight patients from the administration of epsilon amino-caproid acid. The drug was given intravenously in a dose totalling 210 gm. in seven days and then orally in a liquid in a dose of sixteen or thirty-two gm. per day for thirty months. They obtained fair to excellent improvement in twenty-two of twenty-eight patients, benefit being shown not only in the skin manifestations, but in joints, amelioration of Raynaud's phenomenon, and relief of pulmonary symptoms and dysphagia. Reque (1965) used the drug in a dose of one to four gm. daily for periods up to twenty-five months in nine patients and claimed subjective improvement and marked softening of the skin.

The rationale seems to have been based on the idea that the pathological changes in scleroderma are due to the products of lysis of clots and may be ameliorated by preventing this lysis. There is no evidence that the changes in scleroderma are due to clot lysis, but if blood clotting were important it would seem more reasonable to inhibit the clotting. Hall and Scott (1966) found no improvement in any of seven patients treated with EACA (forty-five gm. orally per day or intravenously up to three hundred gm. over six days).

Miscellaneous Measures of Doubtful Value

Parathyroidectomy

As discussed in Chapter XIII, there was, at one stage, a strong belief that parathyroid hyperplasia was involved in the pathogenesis of scleroderma. Leriche *et al.* (1937) reported on thirteen patients treated by parathyroidectomy with improvement in twelve. Several of the patients were also treated with concurrent sympathectomy and it is difficult to determine how much of the improvement was due to the latter procedure. This treatment is no longer used.

Scorbutic diet

A strange recent treatment was the use of a scorbutic diet. The idea was that since scleroderma is characterized by hyperplasia of collagen, it might be reversed by depletion of Vitamin C, a substance believed to be required for collagen biosynthesis. Lazarus *et al.* (1970) treated eleven patients with a scorbutogenic diet (one to three mg. Vitamin C per day) for two to twenty-four months. None of the signs or symptoms of scleroderma were alleviated in any patient. One patient developed clinical scurvy!

Vegetable extracts

A more attractive, even if not more scientific treatment is the administration of an extract of the total unsaponifiable oils of avocado and of soya bean (given as six capsules per day each containing fifty mg. of the *active principle*) a method which Lamberton (1970) attributes to Thiers (1961) and found beneficial in 50 percent of fifty cases.

Procedures for Treatment of Ischaemia

One of the prominent clinical features of scleroderma is ischaemia of the digits and one of the constant pathological features is thickening of the wall and corresponding decrease in the lumen of blood vessels. It is reasonable therefore that measures should be directed toward improving the blood flow or improving the nutrition of ischaemic tissue.

Sympathectomy

Sympathectomy (cervical or lumbar) for ischaemia of the digits has been practiced for many years. Early reports for its use in scleroderma were published by Adson *et al.* (1930) who treated sixteen cases with improvement, at least in the early follow-up period, and by Leriche *et al.* (1937) who obtained marked or moderate improvement in nine of thirteen cases. It has continued to be used in certain cases but the results are variable. Barnett and Coventry (1969a) considered that worthwhile benefit in respect to ischaemic symptoms was obtained in twelve of twenty cases.

Low molecular weight dextran

Solutions of low molecular weight dextran (*Dextran 40*, or *Rheomacrodex*), which are believed to increase capillary blood flow by decreasing viscosity and preventing sludging of blood cells, were used by Holti for the treatment of scleroderma in 1965. He gave a slow infusion of two litres of a 10% solution over forty-eight hours, repeated at intervals of five to eight weeks in winter and at longer intervals in summer, and reported a good or satisfactory response in ten of twelve patients.

Although some workers have reported improvement in small numbers of cases (Fountain and Stevens, 1966; Kantor, 1966; Tonkin, 1968) and it is still being used with success by its originator (Holti, 1971), others have reported no worthwhile improvement (Kirk and Dixon, 1969; Zackheim *et al.*, 1969; Lane, 1970). It is doubtful whether it constitutes a major advance in therapy.

Hyperbaric oxygen

Copeman and Ashfield (1967) used hyperbaric oxygen at two atmospheres absolute for two sessions each of two hours per day for ten to fourteen days for treatment of six patients with Raynaud's phenomenon. Not only were the Raynaud's phenomena alleviated, but in five patients the skin became softer and in the four patients with ulcers, these healed in one to three weeks.

Intra-arterial reserpine

Romeo *et al.* (1970) have described treatment of patients with Raynaud's disease and Raynaud's phenomenon by the intra-arterial injection of reserpine (one mg. in 2.5 ml. of saline injected over one minute). Their patients included eleven with scleroderma of whom eight obtained benefit in decreased frequency and more ready termination of ischaemic episodes. The period of clinical effectiveness after a single injection varied from one to thirteen months.

MANAGEMENT OF THE PATIENT

From the foregoing it is apparent that, although there have been many remedies for scleroderma, none of the older ones have stood the test of time and the newer ones need further evaluation. We are still left with the problem of the management of the patient, which may be required over a considerable period.

Treatment Related to Different Types

It must be appreciated that the prognosis of patients with scleroderma is very variable, although some indication of this may be obtained by the *type* which is established soon after presentation. Type 1 patients commonly live out a normal expectancy and die from causes not related to scleroderma. Their main problems are usually related to digital ischaemia. It would not be justifiable in such cases to use potent drugs such as adrenal steroids. Type 2 cases usually live for a considerable time, but eventually develop visceral disturbances—gastro-intestinal, pulmonary, cardiac, which require their own particular management. Type 3 cases have a poor prognosis and most do not survive five years and it is justifiable to use potent drugs in spite of the possible side effects if there is a possibility that they will diminish symptoms or prolong life. Unfortunately, to date no drug has been shown to prolong life or indeed prevent or diminish the visceral manifestations in these cases. I have used corticosteroids in several such patients (usually in the form of prednisone twenty mg. per day), and this treatment has been associated with softening of the skin in some cases and increased sense of well being although probably not by prolongation of life. Fatal renal failure has occurred in spite of treatment with corticosteroids and according to some, has been precipitated by it.

Treatment of Ischaemia

Raynaud's phenomenon is a common early manifestation of scleroderma. Treatment is usually medical, consisting of administration of an alpha-adrenergic blocking drug such as tolazoline twenty-five mg. three times per day or phenoxybenzamine ten mg. twice daily on cold days, the inunction of a vasodilator ointment (such as the currently available chilblain preventatives containing nicotinic acid esters) and wearing of warm gloves. If ischaemic ulcers occur, a trial may be made of the intra-arterial injection of reserpine (one mg. in 2.5 ml. saline into the brachial artery) or the infusion of low molecular weight dextran (two liters of a ten percent solution over forty-eight hours) as discussed above, although the results are disappointing. If ischaemic episodes and skin ulceration are very troublesome, particularly at any early stage of the disease, cervicodorsal sympathectomy may be recommended, although worthwhile benefit can be expected in only about half of the cases.

Treatment of ulceration and superficial gangrene is conservative as long as possible, by careful debridement and application of an antibiotic cream. If pain is severe, temporary relief while waiting for the ulcer to heal may be obtained by crushing the appropriate digital nerves in the palm. However if there is repeated ulceration and shortening of the finger, amputation of the digit becomes obligatory. The amputation site usually heals surprisingly well.

Treatment of Joint Disturbances and Calcification

In long-standing cases, the fingers commonly are stiff and bent, largely because of sclerosis of the periarticular structures. Attempts must be made from the early stage to minimize deformity and stiffness by heat treatment and exercises. One method of exercising the fingers is to squeeze a plasticine-like material (*play dough*). If joints are painful, anti-inflammatory drugs are indicated. Of these corticosteroids are the most effective and joint symptoms may often be controlled by a relatively small dose (for example, ten mg. of prednisone daily).

In chronic cases with severe deformity, plastic surgical procedures (arthrodeses of interphalangeal joints and capsulotomy with arthroplasty of metacarpophalangeal joints) have been performed with benefit (Lipscomb *et al.*, 1969).

Calcification of soft tissues may create annoying problems interfering with joint mobility causing tenderness and ulceration over pressure points and tender discharging nodules of the hands. Although some have claimed benefit from infusion of ethylene diamino tetra acetic acid (EDTA), others have found this disappointing. Large areas of calcification (as in the buttocks in one of my cases) may be excised surgically. Calcific nodules in the fingers can be removed without damage to the fibrous septa by breaking up with a dental burr and irrigating with saline (MacDowell, 1969).

Treatment of Visceral Disturbances

Gastro-intestinal

Some of the commonest visceral problems in scleroderma are due to disturbances of the esophagus and gastro-esophageal region, causing dysphagia and symptoms of gastro-esophageal reflux, retrosternal pain and acid regurgitation. Generally these symptoms can be managed by simple medical measures: avoiding chunky food, chewing well and eating slowly to allow time for the esophagus to empty by gravity, sleeping with a head-up position and using a long-acting antacid mixture (such as aluminum hydroxide gel) bewteen meals and before retiring. In cases where a stricture develops, dilatation will be necessary and the patient will need to be instructed in the regular use of mercury filled esophageal bougies (Hurst's tubes). Surgical treatment is best avoided.

Patients with scleroderma are commonly thin and there is probably some degree of malabsorption. These patients may be helped by the administration of a food supplement containing calories, proteins, minerals and vitamins in a readily absorbable form.

Rarely patients may develop a frank malabsorption syndrome with loss of weight, abdominal bloating, diarrhoea and characteristic radiological findings (see Chapter IX). It is now believed that these symptoms are due to stasis and bacterial proliferation and that they may respond to antibiotics although these have to be given on a long term basis and the type has to be varied—tetracycline, sulphasuxidine, neomycin, erythromycin (Cliff *et al.*, 1966). Sometimes when the affection of the bowel is localized, surgical excision of the affected area may be appropriate.

Acute surgical abdominal symptoms in scleroderma present a difficult problem. *Pseudo-obstruction* should be suspected and, if diagnosed, treated medically by intravenous infusion and aspiration. However it must be remembered that occasionally there may in fact be a truly surgical problem such as a perforated, impacted diverticulum requiring operation.

Cardiac, Pulmonary and Renal

Cardiac involvement in scleroderma may occur in the form of right heart failure secondary to pulmonary failure, cardiomyopathy or arrhythmia—ectopic beats or tachyarrythmia or (rarely) heart block. The treatment of these conditions is along orthodox lines for these conditions from other causes.

Respiratory involvement is manifested more frequently on radiographic examination of the chest and pulmonary function tests than by symptoms. Occasionally respiratory symptoms may predominate and lead to severe dyspnoea. Unfortunately there is no specific remedy for these cases, which may eventually require continuous oxygen administration. The possibility of spontaneous pneumothorax must be remembered in cases of dyspnoea of acute onset. This will respond to continuous negative pressure aspiration, followed, if the lung fails to remain inflated after a few days, by pleuradhesis produced by painting of the pleural surface with silver nitrate.

Until recently no treatment has been effective in preventing death in acute renal failure in scleroderma but there is now cause for hope following a report of successful management by hemodialysis followed by nephrectomy and kidney transplantation.

Specific Treatment

No specific treatment is available for scleroderma. However the position is not without hope. Recently drugs have been introduced which have been demonstrated to have an effect on collagen metabolism. Penicillamine is too toxic for general use, but gestagens and high dose hyaluronidase have been used in small numbers of patients with reported benefit and no serious side effects.

The relationship of auto-immunity to scleroderma still needs clarification, but, pending further investigation, it is probably justifiable to use immunosuppressive drugs in severe (Type 3) cases where nothing else seems to be available, although the results to date are not impressive.

It must be admitted that the outlook for the individual patient with severe disease is not bright and the drugs mentioned immediately above are still experimental. Reports of good results in a few patients must be accepted with caution as they are reminiscent of similar reports with many drugs in the past. It is to be hoped that centres with reasonably large numbers of patients will be able to organize well-conducted trials with objective assessment, and if the circumstances permit, a *double-blind* technique to enable accurate assessment to be made for the guidance of physicians and help to patients in the future.

Chapter XVI

CONCLUSION

SCLERODERMA IS PROBABLY NOT a modern disease: there are some descriptions suggesting that it may have occurred in ancient time and there are numerous accounts in the nineteenth century. However knowledge of the nature of the disorder developed slowly and the fact that the skin and vascular disturbances are but part of a condition affecting many organs was not fully appreciated until about the middle of the twentieth century.

It is an uncommon but not rare disease and is distributed widely both geographically and racially. Its apparent rarity in certain Asian and African countries may be due to lack of awareness of the condition or difference in the clinical features in warm countries. Although there are many theories, the aetiology is unknown. It is not familial and although infective agents have been postulated by some writers, the evidence is not convincing. One intriguing feature is the higher incidence in persons exposed to silica dust—demonstrated in three countries, although such a factor is not present in the great majority of patients. Its onset is mainly in middle-age, and women are affected more commonly than men.

The pathological changes in the skin, blood vessels and other affected organs have now been described in detail. It is a multi-system disease with, however, a predilection for particular organs. The main changes are in blood vessels, in which there is increase in wall thickness mainly through hypertrophy of the intima with corresponding reduction in lumen, and in connective tissue which shows apparent increase and altered appearance (homogenization in the dermis, accumulation of cellular connective tissue in the heart). Although most of the other pathological features are explicable on the basis of parenchymatous degeneration secondary to diminished blood flow or replacement by fibrous tissue, this does not afford a complete explanation in all cases.

Cardiac and skeletal muscle may show accumulations of inflammatory cells and degenerative changes in muscle cells indicative of myocarditis or myositis. The pathological findings in the kidneys in cases with acute renal failure are particularly striking and contrast with the more chronic type of findings in other organs. The main features here are firstly hypertrophy of the intima of the interlobular arteries by proliferation of a mucoid type of connective tissue resulting in gross diminution of their lumen and secondly fibrinoid changes in afferent arterioles, sometimes extending into

216

glomerular tufts. The changes are very similar to those in malignant hypertension but may occur without marked elevation of the blood pressure.

There has been discussion concerning the primary importance of the vascular and connective tissue changes. However pathological studies indicate that although these two features are often associated they do not run parallel in severity in various sites, and it would therefore seem that they are both the result of some more fundamental disturbance.

The nature of the basic fault in scleroderma remains to be discovered. Since the most obvious histological changes are in connective tissue, whose chief constituent is collagen, extensive study has been made of the content, nature and metabolism of collagen in scleroderma. Early studies were disappointing. The chemical constitution, physical properties and electron microscopic appearance of the collagen in the skin of patients with scleroderma was normal. Although some workers reported increased activity of the enzyme concerned in the transformation of protocollagen to collagen, others could not confirm increased collagen metabolism. Recently however there have been important new findings. Collagen in scleroderma has been found to contain an increased fraction soluble in dilute sodium chloride and electron-microscope studies have shown an increased proportion of thin fibrils, and also the presence of *beaded filaments* otherwise found only in fetal tissues.

The other main component of connective tissue, ground substance composed largely of protein-mucopolysaccharide complexes, has been studied less intensively. However there are some indications that this substance may be abnormal in scleroderma. These include a reported abnormal response of the electrical potential following injection of hyaluronidase, and the finding of increased levels of mucopolysaccharides or their derivatives in the serum. Mucopolysaccharides and collagen are closely associated in connective tissue and it has been suggested that disturbance of mucopolysaccharides may be of primary importance.

Exciting new work on the disturbance of connective tissue in scleroderma has recently been published and includes findings of increased production of collagen and mucopolysaccharides in tissue slices and increased production of soluble collagen and "glycoproteins" by fibroblasts in tissue culture. These observations await confirmation and assessment.

There have been some attempts to demonstrate other metabolic disturbances in scleroderma. Although one group of workers claimed to have demonstrated abnormal catecholamine metabolism, suggesting decreased monoamine oxidase activity, this has not been confirmed by others. Some writers postulated that the vascular disturbance and fibrosis might result from serotonin excess; it has been suggested that this may be due to an abnormality of tryptophan metabolism with a partial enzymatic block in the major niacin pathway resulting in a diversion to the minor serotonin pathway. However excess serotonin production has not been demonstrated in scleroderma and an abnormality of tryptophan metabolism remains highly conjectural.

One group of workers have claimed to have demonstrated in the urine of patients with scleroderma and other connective tissue diseases the presence of an intermediate metabolite of phenylalamine and tyrosine. Various metabolic blocks in phenylaline and tyrosine have already been demonstrated and are associated with particular diseases. It has been suggested that there is another block specific to connective tissue diseases and leading to the accumulation of a previously undetected metabolite which is excreted in the urine. It is not clear whether such a block is of primary importance and how it brings about the changes found in scleroderma.

In common with other connective tissue diseases, scleroderma shows a high incidence of auto-immune phenomena, particularly the presence of auto-antibodies. One of these, the *speckled* type of antinuclear factor, occurs predominantly in scleroderma. It has been suggested that scleroderma may be an auto-immune disease. However auto-antibodies cannot be demonstrated in a large proportion of cases, their presence or absence does not seem to be related to the severity of the clinical course, and it has not been shown that they are harmful. It seems therefore that we are not justified at present in classifying scleroderma as an auto-immune disease and the significance of the auto-immune features is not clear. They may be the result of tissue damage rather than its cause.

Similarly the significance of the recently demonstrated high incidence of chromosomal abnormalities in leucocytes in scleroderma is conjectural. They may be a result of other changes rather than their cause.

Due to the great diversity in the clinical picture, the classification of scleroderma has presented a problem. It is now generally accepted that the form with vascular and systemic mainfestations (called progressive systemic sclerosis) is distinct from the form with purely dermatological changes (morphoea form). Most workers regard the more acute diffuse form and the more chronic acrosclerotic form as variants of the one disease although not all would also accept as scleroderma cases with Raynaud's phenomenon, sclerosis of the fingers and no obvious visceral disturbance. Argument has been produced in this book that these three conditions comprise one disease and they have been classified as Type 1 (sclerosis limited to fingers), Type 2 (acrosclerotic form with sclerosis predominantly on extremities and face) and Type 3 (with diffuse sclerosis of skin). This classification is useful in respect to prognosis in that Type 1 cases usually live to their normal expectancy, Type 2 cases frequently die from the disease after many years and Type 3 cases usually succumb within five years. However these *types* are not rigid as there is overlapping of the clinical features and some Type 1 cases have severe, fatal systemic disease.

Cutaneous and subcutaneous features in addition to skin sclerosis include calcinosis and telangiectasia. These are particularly prominent in some patients (whom some writers have suggested should be regarded as belonging to a special syndrome *CRST*). However, most would regard them as cases of scleroderma in which there is an association of certain common features.

Since the recognition towards the middle of this century that scleroderma is a multi-system disease, there have been extensive reports on detailed studies of functional and pathological changes in particular organs and it is difficult to understand why this systemic involvement was not recognized by the early writers. Joint involvement is frequent in scleroderma. Although limitation of joint movement may occur from sclerosis of surrounding structures, there is also a direct involvement of synovial membrane and secondary osteo-arthritic changes may also occur. It has recently been recognized that myositis is frequent in scleroderma—more often recognized histologically than clinically.

The most frequently involved viscera are the alimentary canal, lungs, heart and kidneys. Esophageal involvement in the form of impaired peristalsis occurs in almost all cases in which the disease has been present for more than a few years. Symptoms in the form of dysphagia and gastro-esophageal reflux occur in only a proportion of cases. Intestinal involvement is less common and includes bloating, abdominal pain, pseudo-obstruction, severe stasis and malabsorption.

Pulmonary function studies indicate that lung involvement, shown by an impaired diffusion or a restrictive defect, is very common. Radiological and clinical involvement is less frequent. Occasionally the lung disease is the dominating feature and leads to the death of the patient.

The commonest type of cardiac involvement is right-sided cardiac enlargement and sometimes failure secondary to increased pulmonary vascular resistance. Scleroderma cardiomyopathy in which there is replacement of cardiac muscle cells by connective tissue is well documented but rare. Other cardiac abnormalities in scleroderma include pericarditis and various arrhythmias.

Although there may be some mild chronic impairment of renal function in scleroderma, this has not been extensively studied and is not clinically apparent. The striking renal disturbance in this disease is acute, unheralded renal failure, sometimes associated with hypertension and consistently fatal within a few weeks. There is a characteristic pathological picture in the kidneys, the main features of which are (a) gross narrowing of the lumen of interlobular arteries due to hyperplasia of the connective tissue of the intima and (b) frequent occurrence of fibrinoid in the afferent glomerular arterioles.

Changes have been described in most other organs. However central nervous system disturbance is very rare and probably only occurs secondary to involvement of blood vessels supplying the brain.

The diagnosis of scleroderma depends mainly on recognition of the clinical features. Confirmation may be obtained by histological examination of biopsy material, by the presence of antinuclear factor of the *speckled* variety or by demonstration of characteristic involvement of some organ, particularly the esophagus, studied by barium swallow technique. There is no specific test. In some early cases in which Raynaud's phenomenon is the only symptom it may be necessary to wait two years before making a definite diagnosis.

A disease such as scleroderma which may continue for many years and which may affect practically every organ in the body is very demanding of the patience and skills of the physician. Symptomatic treatment of the disturbances of various organs is along similar lines to those used in affections due to other diseases. Unfortunately, in the absence of knowledge of the cause and pathogenesis of the disease, there is no curative treatment. Treatment with adrenal steroids is associated with regression of the skin changes in early diffuse cases but has not been shown to have any beneficial effect on the visceral disturbances or to prolong life. Numerous other treatments introduced based on some hypothesis concerning the etiology or pathogenesis of the disease or on a supposed action of the particular remedy on collagen have been discontinued because of disappointing results. Recently there have been claims that certain drugs, particularly penicillamine (which is too toxic for general use) and progesterone-like drugs, can be shown, by biochemical studies of biopsy material and determinations of urinary hydroxyproline excretion, to favourably influence collagen metabolism in scleroderma. This gives the hope that we may be on the verge of more rational and effective treatment of this condition. Recently there has been a report of successful treatment of a patient with scleroderma and renal failure by hemodialysis followed by nephrectomy and kidney transplantation giving new hope in the management of this hitherto uniformly fatal manifestation. However true curative treatment will probably not be possible until cause and pathogenesis of the disease have been discovered.

BIBLIOGRAPHY

Abrams, H. L., Carnes, W. H., and Eaton, J.: Alimentary tract in disseminated scleroderma with emphasis on small bowel. *Arch Int Med,* 94:61, 1954.

Adhikari, P. K., Bianchi, F. A., Boushy, S. F., Sakamoto, A., and Lewis, B. M.: Pulmonary function in scleroderma: its relation to changes in the chest roentgenogram and in the skin of the thorax. *Amer Rev Resp Dis,* 86:823, 1962.

Adson, A. W., O'Leary, P. A., and Brown, G. E.: Surgical treatment of vasospastic types of scleroderma by resection of sympathetic ganglia and trunks. *Ann Intern Med,* 4:555, 1930.

Ala, A. P.: Personal communication; 1971.

Alexander, W. R. M., Brenner, J. M., and Duthie, J. J. R.: Incidence of anti-nuclear factor in human sera. *Ann Rheum Dis,* 19:338, 1960.

Allen, E. V., Barker, N. W., and Hines, E. A. Jr.: *Peripheral Vascular Disease,* 2nd ed. Philadelphia, Saunders, 1955.

Aprosina, Z. G., Guseva, N. G., Potekaev, M. A., and Gritsman, N. M.: Affection of the liver and bile ducts in systemic scleroderma. *Klin Med* (Mosk), 48:119, 1970.

Arcilla, R., Bandler, M., Farber, M., and Olivar, A.: Gastrointestinal scleroderma simulating chronic and acute intestinal obstruction. *Gastroenterology,* 31:764, 1956.

Asboe-Hansen, G.: Scleroderma in carcinoid syndrome. *Acta Derm-Venereol* (Stockh), 39:270, 199.

Asboe-Hansen, G.: Treatment of scleroderma with dextro-thyroxine. *Exerpta Med Int Congr Ser,* No. 55:1305, 1962.

Ashba, J. K., and Ghanem, M. H.: The lungs in systemic sclerosis. *Dis Chest,* 47:52, 1965.

Ashton, N., Coomes, E. N., Garner, A., and Oliver, D. O.: Retinopathy due to progressive systemic sclerosis. *J Pathol Bacteriol,* 96:259, 1968.

Atlas, E.: Intestinal scleroderma with malabsorption. *JAMA,* 205:939, 1968.

Auspitz, H.: Ein Beitrag zur Lehre von Haut-Sklerem der Erwachsenen. *Wien Med Wochenschr,* 13:739, 1893. Quoted by Rodnan, G. P., and Benedek, T. G., 1962 (*loc. cit.*).

Bachman, D. M.: Quantitating skin mobility in scleroderma. *Arch Dermatol,* 83:598, 1961.

Balabanov, K., and Samsonova, S.: Untersuchungen über die Mukopolysaccharide im Blutserum bei manchen Kollagenosen. *Dermatol Wochenschr,* 151:876, 1965.

Baldwin, E. de F., Cournand, A., and Richards, D. W.: Pulmonary insufficiency, II; A study of thirty-nine cases of pulmonary fibrosis. *Medicine,* 28:1, 1949.

Bardawil, W. A., Toy, B. L., Galins, N., and Bayles, T. B.: Disseminated lupus erythematosus, scleroderma and dermatomyositis as manifestations of sensitization to DNA-protein, I; An immunohistochemical approach. *Amer J Pathol,* 34:607, 1952.

Barnett, A. J.: Scleroderma and Raynaud's disease. *Alfred Hosp Clin Rep* (Melbourne), 9:33, 1959.

Barnett, A. J., and Coventry, D. A.: Scleroderma: 1; Clinical features, course of illness and response to treatment in sixty-one cases. *Med J Aust, 1*:992, 1969a.

Barnett, A. J., and Coventry, D. A.: Scleroderma: 2; Incidence of systemic disturbance and assessment of possible aetiological factors. *Med J Aust, 1*:1040, 1969b.

Barr, I. M., Abramov, A., Dreyfuss, F., Yahini, J. H., and Neufeld, H. N.: Progressive heart block in a case of scleroderma. *J Med Sci, 6*:373, 1970.

Barritt, D. W., and O'Brien, W.: Heart disease in scleroderma. *Br Heart J, 14*:421, 1952.

Bartfeld, H.: Incidence and significance of seropositive tests for rheumatoid factor in non-rheumatoid diseases. *Ann Intern Med, 52*:1059, 1960.

Bartholomew, L. G., Cain, J. C., Winkelmann, R. K., and Baggenstoss, A. H.: Chronic diseases of the liver associated with systemic scleroderma. *Am J Dig Dis, 9*:43, 1964.

Batsakis, J. G., and Johnson, H. A.: Generalized scleroderma involving lungs and liver with pulmonary adenocarcinoma. *Arch Path, 69*:633, 1960.

Bauer, G. E.: Scleroderma with heart failure. *Aust Ann Med, 4*:149, 1955.

Bäumer, A. von, and Brinkmann, A.: Ergebnisse der immunfloureszenztechnischen Analyse antinuklearer Faktoren bei Patienten mit Kollagenkrankheiten und einer Kontrollgruppe mit verschiedenen internistischen Erkrankungen. *Z Rheumaforsch, 29*:352, 1970.

Bayles, T. B., Stout, C. F., Stillman, J. S., and Lever, W.: The treatment of scleroderma with adrenocorticotrophic hormone; preliminary observations. In Mote, J. F. (Ed.) *Proceedings of the 1st Clinical ACTH Conference, Chicago, 1949*. London Churchill, 447, 1950.

Beck, J. S.: Variations in the morphological patterns of *autoimmune* nuclear fluoresence. *Lancet, 1*:1203, 1961.

Beck, J. S.: Partial identification of the *speckled* nuclear antigen. *Lancet, 1*:241, 1962.

Beck, J. S.: Antinuclear antibodies: methods of detection and significance. *Mayo Clinic Proc, 44*:600, 1969.

Beck, J. S., Anderson, J. R., Gray, K. G., and Rowell, N. R.: Antinuclear and precipitating autoantibodies in progressive systemic sclerosis. *Lancet, 2*:1188, 1963.

Beerman, H.: The visceral manifestations of scleroderma; a review of the recent literature. *Am J Med Sci, 216*:458, 1948.

Beigelman, P. M.; Goldner, F., and Bayles, T. B.: Progressive systemic sclerosis (scleroderma). *N Engl J Med, 249*:45, 1953.

Bendixen, G., Jarnum, S., Ottesen, O., Schmidt, H., and Thomsen, K.: Gastrointestinal involvement in systemic scleroderma. *Dermatologica (Basel), 137*:26, 1968.

Bennett, G. A., and Dällenbach, F. D.: Synovial membrane changes in disseminated lupus erythematosus, observations of two autopsied cases. *Milit Surg, 109*:531, 1951.

Bernheim, A. R., and Garlock, J. H.: Parathyroidectomy for Raynaud's disease and scleroderma. *Ann Surg, 101*:1012, 1935.

Berris, B., Rother, I., and Rosen, P. S.: Telangiectases simulating hereditary hemorrhagic telangiectasia in scleroderma: report of two cases. *Can Med Ass J, 96*:1528, 1967.

Bevans, M.: Pathology of scleroderma with special reference to changes in the gastrointestinal tract. *Am J Pathol, 21*:25, 1945.

Bianchi, F. A., Bistue, A. R., Wendt, V. E., Puro, H. E., and Keech, M. K.: Analysis of twenty-seven cases of progressive systemic sclerosis (including two with combined systemic lupus erythematosus) and a review of the literature. *J Chronic Dis, 19:953,* 1966.

Bicks, R. O., Goldgraber, M. B., and Kirsner, J. B.: Generalized scleroderma associated with chronic ulcerative colitis. *Am J Med, 24:447,* 1958.

Biggart, J. D., and Nevin, N. C.: Hyperplasia of the thymus in progressive systemic sclerosis. *J Pathol Bacteriol, 93:334,* 1967.

Binford, R. T., Jr.: CRST syndrome with gastrointestinal bleeding. *Arch Dermatol, 97:603,* 1968.

Birk, R. E.: Treatment of systemic sclerosis. *Modern Treatment, 3:1287,* 1966.

Birk, R. E., and Rupe, C. E.: Systemic sclerosis: fourteen cases treated with chelation (disodium EDTA) and/or pyridoxine; with comments on the possible role of altered tryptophan metabolism in pathogenesis. *Henry Ford Hosp Bull, 10:523,* 1962.

Bjersand, A. J.: New bone formation and carpal synostosis in scleroderma; a case report. *Am J Roentgenol Radium Ther Nucl Med, 103:616,* 1968.

Black, M. M., Bottoms, E., and Shuster, S. L.: Skin collagen content and thickness in systemic sclerosis. *Br J Dermatol, 83:552,* 1970.

Black, R. L.: The characterization of polyarteritis nodosa, dermatomyositis and progressive systemic sclerosis. *Med Clin North Am, 45:1295,* 1961.

Blanchard, R. E., and Speed, R. M.: Scleroderma: periodontal membrane manifestations in two brothers. *Periodontics, 3:77,* 1965.

Bloom, W., and Fawcett, D. W.: *A Textbook of Histology,* 9th ed. Philadelphia, Saunders, 1968.

Bluestone, R., Grahame, R., Holloway, V., and Holt, P. J. L.: Treatment of systemic sclerosis with D-penicillamine. *Ann Rheum Dis, 29:153,* 1970.

Boas, N. F., and Foley, J. B.: Effects of growth, fasting and trauma on the concentrations of connective tissue hexosamine and water. *Proc Soc Exp Biol Med, 86:690,* 1954.

Boccardelli, V., and Fabbri, G.: Il cuore nella sclerodermia; studio clinico di 12 casi. *Minerva Cardioangiol, 4:157,* 1956.

Böni, A., Pavelka, K., and Kludas, M.: Behandlung der progressiven Sklerodermie mit D-Penicillamin (Metalcaptase). *Munch Med Wochenschr, 111:1580,* 1969.

Bornstein, P.: Disorders of connective tissues. In Bondy, P. K. (Ed.) *Duncan's Diseases of Metabolism,* 6th ed. Philadelphia, Saunders, 1969, pp. 654–710.

Bourel, M.; Gouffault, J., and Guillou, M.: L'atteinte cardiaque au cours de la sclérodermie. *Arch Mal Coeur, 59:1368,* 1966.

Bramwell, B.: Diffuse sclerodermia; its frequency; its occurrence in stone masons; its treatment by fibrolysin—elevations of temperature due to fibrolysin injections. *Edinb Med J, 12:387,* 1914.

Braun-Falco, O., and Rupec, M.: Collagen fibrils of scleroderma in ultra-thin skin sections. *Nature, 202:708,* 1964.

Briggs, J. N., and Illingworth, R. S.: A case of scleroderma; failure to respond to recent drugs. *Lancet, 1:346,* 1952.

Brock, G. W.: Dermatomyositis and diffuse scleroderma; differential diagnosis and reports of cases. *Arch Dermatol Syph, 30:227,* 1934.

Brooks, W. D. W.: Calcinosis. *Q J Med, 3:293,* 1934.

Brown, G. E., and O'Leary, P. A.: Skin capillaries in scleroderma. *Arch Intern Med, 36:73,* 1925.

Brown, G. E.; O'Leary, P. A., and Adson, A. W.: Diagnostic and physiologic studies in certain forms of scleroderma. *Ann Intern Med, 4:531,* 1930.

Brunjes, S., Arterberry, J. D., Shankel, S., and Johns, V. J. Jr.: Decreased oxidative deamination of catecholamines associated with clinical scleroderma. *Arthritis Rheum,* 7:138, 1964.

Buchanan, I. S., and Humpston, D. J.: Nail-fold capillaries in connective-tissue disorders. *Lancet,* 1:845, 1968.

Bunim, J. J.: A broader spectrum of Sjögren's syndrome and its pathogenic implications. *Ann Rheum Dis,* 20:1, 1961.

Burch, G. E.: Scleroderma; a symposium; etiology and abnormal physiology. *New Orleans Med Surg J,* 92:12, 1939.

Burch, P. R. J., and Rowell, N. R.: Autoimmunity; aetiological aspects of chronic discoid and systemic lupus erythematosus, systemic sclerosis, and Hashimoto's thyroiditis; some immunological implications. *Lancet,* 2:507, 1963.

Burge, K. M.; Perry, H. O., and Stickler, C. B.: Familial scleroderma. *Arch Dermatol,* 99:681, 1969.

Burnet, M.: *Self and Not-Self.* Melbourne, University Press, 1969.

Burnham, T. K., Neblett, T. R., and Fine, G.: Immunofluorescent tumour imprint technic, III; the diagnostic and prognostic significance of the *speckle*-inducing antinuclear antibody. *Am J Clin Pathol,* 50:683, 1968.

Burnham, T. K., Neblett, T. R., Fine, G., and Bank, P.: The immunofluorescent tumour imprint technique, IV: the significance of *thready* nuclear immunofluorescence. *Arch Dermatol,* 99:611, 1969.

Bushnell, W. J., Galens, G. J., Bartholemew, L. E., Thompson, G., and Duff, I. F.: The treatment of progressive systemic sclerosis: a comparison of para-aminobenzoate and placebo in a double-blind study. *Arthritis Rheum,* 9:495, 1966.

Bywaters, E. G. L., and Scott, J. T.: Systemic diseases of connective tissue. In Dixon, A. St. J. (Ed.): *Progress in Clinical Rheumatology.* Boston, Little, 1965, pp. 114–166.

Calvert, R. J., Barling, B., Sopher, M., and Feiwel, M.: Systemic scleroderma with portal hypertension. *Br Med J,* 1:22, 1958.

Calvert, R. J., and Owen, T. K.: True scleroderma kidney. *Lancet,* 2:19, 1956.

Cantwell, A. R. Jr., Craggs, E., Wilson, J. W., and Swatek, F.: Acid-fast bacteria as a possible cause of scleroderma. *Dermatologica (Basel),* 136:141, 1968.

Cantwell, A. R. Jr., and Kelso, D. W.: Acid-fast bacteria in scleroderma and morphoea. *Arch Dermatol,* 104:21, 1971.

Cantwell, A. R. Jr., and Wilson, J. W.: Scleroderma with ulceration secondary to atypical mycobacteria. *Arch Dermatol,* 94:663, 1966.

Caplan, H.: Honeycomb lungs and malignant pulmonary adenomatosis in scleroderma. *Thorax,* 14:89, 1959.

Carr, R. B.; Heisel, E. B., and Stevenson, T. D.: CRST syndrome; a benign variant of scleroderma. *Arch Dermatol,* 92:519, 1965.

Casals, S. P.; Friou, G. J., and Teague, P. O.: Specific nuclear reaction pattern of antibody to DNA in lupus erythematosus sera. *J Lab Clin Med,* 62:625, 1963.

Casten, G. G., and Boucek, R. J.: Use of relaxin in the treatment of scleroderma. *JAMA,* 166:319, 1958.

Castle, W. F.: The endocrine causation of scleroderma including morphoea. *Br J Dermatol Syph,* 35:255, 1923.

Catterall, M., and Rowell, N. R.: Respiratory function in progressive systemic sclerosis. *Thorax,* 18:10, 1963.

Catterall, M., and Rowell, N. R.: Respiratory function studies in patients with certain connective tissue diseases. *Br J Dermatol Syph,* 77:221, 1965.

Chaves, F. C.; Rodrigo, F. G.; Franco, M. L., and Esteves, J.: Systemic sclerosis associated with auto-immune haemolytic anaemia. *Br J Dermatol Syph,* 82:298, 1970.

Chorzelski, T., and Jablońska, S.: Co-existence of lupus erythematosus and scleroderma in the light of immunopathological investigations. *Acta Derm-venereol (Stockh),* 50:81, 1970.

Church, R. E., and Ellis, A. R. P.: Cystic pulmonary fibrosis in generalised scleroderma. *Lancet, 1:*392, 1950.

Clark, J. A., Winkelmann, R. K., and Ward, L. E.: Serologic alterations in scleroderma and sclerodermatomyositis. *Mayo Clin Proc,* 46:104, 1971.

Clark, M., and Fountain, R. B.: Oesophageal motility in connective tissue disease. *Br J Dermatol,* 79:449, 1967.

Cliff, I. S., Herber, R., and Demis, D. J.: Control of malabsorption in scleroderma. *J Invest Dermatol,* 47:475, 1966.

Code, C. F., and Schlegel, J. F.: The pressure profile of the gastroesophageal sphincter in man: an improved method of detection. *Mayo Clinic Proc,* 33:406, 1958.

Coffmann, J. D.: Skin blood flow in scleroderma. *J Lab Clin Med.* 76:480, 1970.

Cohn, B. A., Wheeler, C. E., and Briggaman, R. A.: Scleredema adultorum of Buschke and diabetes mellitus. *Arch Dermatol,* 101:27, 1970.

Comptom, R.: Scleroderma with diverticulosis and colonic obstruction. *Am J Surg,* 118:602, 1969.

Copeman, P. W. M., and Ashfield, R. (for Dowling, G. B.): Raynaud's phenomenon in scleroderma treated with hyperbaric oxygen. *Proc Roy Soc Med,* 60:1268, 1967.

Corcos, J. M., Robbins, W. C., Rogoff, B., and Heimer R.: Some serum protein abnormalities in patients with progressive systemic sclerosis and their relatives. *Arthritis Rheum,* 4:107, 1961.

Cornbleet, T., and Struck, H. C.: Calcium metabolism in scleroderma. *Arch Dermatol Syph (Chic),* 35:188, 1937.

Corson, J. K.: Sclerodermatomyositis. *Arch Dermatol,* 96:596, 1967.

Creamer, B., Andersen, H. A., and Code, C. F.: Esophageal motility in patients with scleroderma and related diseases. *Gastroenterologia (Basel),* 86:763, 1956.

Crown, S.: Visceral scleroderma without skin involvement. *Br Med J,* 2:1541, 1961.

Cullinan, E. R.: Scleroderma (diffuse systemic sclerosis). *Proc Roy Soc Med,* 46:507, 1953.

Curtis, A. C., and Jansen, T. G.: The prognosis of localized scleroderma. *Arch Dermatol,* 78:749, 1958.

Curtis, A. C., and Shulak, B. M.: Scleredema adultorum: not always a benign self-limited disease. *Arch Dermatol,* 92:526, 1965.

Curzio, C.: Discussioni anatomico pratiche di un raro, e stravagante morbo cutaneo in una giovane donna felicemente curato in questo grande Ospedale degl' Incurabili. Napoli, Giovanni de Simone. (1753). Quoted by Rodnan, G. P. and Benedek, T. G. (1962) *loc. cit.*

D'Angelo, W. A., Fries, J. F., Masi, A. T., and Shulman, L. E.: Pathologic observations in systemic sclerosis (scleroderma). *Am J Med,* 46:428, 1969.

Dawson, J. J. Y.: Scleroderma with pulmonary involvement and chronic bronchitis. *Proc Roy Soc Med,* 48:152, 1955.

Day, W.: Case of scleroderma or sclerema with autopsy and remarks. *Am J Med Sci,* 59:350, 1870. Quoted by Weaver, A. L. *et. al.,* 1967 (*loc. cit.*).

Degreef, H.: The Werner syndrome. *Dermatologica (Basel),* 142:45, 1971.

Dellipiani, A. W., and George, M.: Syndrome of sclerodactyly, calcinosis, Raynaud's phenomenon and telangiectasia. *Br Med J, 2*:334, 1967.

Delmotte, N., and van der Meiren, L.: Recherches bactériologiques et histologiques concernant la sclérodermie. *Dermatologica (Basel), 107*:177, 1953.

DeLuca, V. A. Jr., Spiro, H. M., and Thayer, W. R.: Ulcerative colitis and scleroderma. *Gastroenterology, 49*:433, 1965.

Demis, D. J., Brown, C. S., and Crosby, W. H.: Thioguanine in the treatment of certain autoimmune, immunologic and related diseases. *Am J Med, 37*:195, 1964.

DeMuth, G. R., Furstenberg, N. A., Dabich, L., and Zarafonetis, C. J. D.: Pulmonary manifestations of progressive systemic sclerosis. *Am J Med Sci, 255*:94, 1968.

Denko, C. W.: Mechanical vibration and ³⁵S incorporation. *Environ Res, 2*:143, 1969.

Denko, C. W., and Stoughton, R. B.: Fixation of ³⁵S in the skin of patients with progressive systemic sclerosis. *Arthritis Rheum, 1*:77, 1958.

de Takats, G., and Fowler, E. F.: Raynaud's phenomenon. *JAMA, 179*:1, 1962.

Dilke, T. F. W., and Richardson, A. T.: Systemic sclerosis with myocardial and pericardial involvement. *Proc Roy Soc Med, 64*:57, 1971.

Dines, D. E., Clagett, O. T., and Good, C. A.: Nontuberculous pulmonary parenchymal conditions predisposing to spontaneous pneumothorax. *J Thorac Cardiovasc Surg, 53*:726, 1967.

Dinkler, M.: Zur Lehre von der Sklerodermie. *Deutsch Arch Klin Med, 48*:514, 1891. Quoted by Sackner, M. A. (1962), *loc. cit.* (lung involvement) and Medsger, T. A. (1968) *loc. cit.* (joint involvement).

Dover, N.: Salazopyrin (azulfidine) treatment in scleroderma. *Isr J Med Sci, 7*:1301, 1971.

Drake, A. M., Le Feber, E. J., and Patterson, M.: Collagen disease primarily affecting the gastrointestinal tract. *Am J Dig Dis, 9*:872, 1964.

Durham, R. A.: Scleroderma and calcinosis. *Arch Intern Med, 42*:467, 1928.

East, T., and Oram, S.: The heart in scleroderma. *Br Heart J, 9*:167, 1947.

Ehrlich, G. E., and Joseph, R.: Dimethyl sulfoxide in scleroderma. *Penn Med J, 68*:51, 1965.

Ehrlich, P., and Morgenroth, J.: Über Hämolysine Funte Millheilung. In Himmelweit, F. (Ed.) *Collected Papers of Paul Ehrlich.* London, Pergamon, 1957, p. 234.

Ehrman, S.: Über die Beziehung der Sklerodermie zu den Autotoxischen Erythemen. *Wien Med Wochenschr, 53*:1097–1156 (1903). Quoted by Cullinan, E. R., 1952 (*loc. cit.*).

El Zawahry, M.: Systemic sclerosis; general consideration and report of a case. *J Egypt Med Assoc, 49*:185, 1966.

Emerit, I., Housset, E., and Camus, J. P.: Chromosome studies in patients with diffuse scleroderma and other collagen diseases. *Excerpta Medica Int Congr,* ser. no. 233:63, 1971.

Emerit, I., Housset, E., De Grouchy, J., and Camus, J. P.: Chromosomal breakage in diffuse scleroderma: a study of twenty-seven patients. *Rev Europ Etud Clin Biol, 16*:684, 1971.

Engel, M. F.: Indications and contra-indications for the use of DMSO in clinical dermatology. *Ann NY Acad Sci, 141*:638, 1967.

Erasmus, L. D.: Scleroderma in gold-miners on the Witwatersrand with particular reference to pulmonary manifestations. *S Afr J Lab Clin Med, 3*:209, 1957.

Escudero, J., and McDevitt, E.: The electrocardiogram in scleroderma: analysis of sixty cases and review of the literature. *Am Heart J, 56*:846, 1958.

Esterly, N. B., and McKusick, V. A.: Stiff skin syndrome. *Pediatrics, 47*:360, 1971.

Evans, J. A.: Relaxin (releasin) therapy in diffuse progressive scleroderma; a preliminary report. *Arch Dermatol,* 79:150, 1959.

Fallon, R. H.: Pneumatosis cystoides intestinalis, associated with scleroderma and presenting with pneumoperitoneum. *Mo Med,* 64:117, 1967.

Farmer, R. G., Gifford, R. W. Jr., and Hines, E. A. Jr.: Prognostic significance of Raynaud's phenomenon and other clinical characteristics of systemic scleroderma; a study of 271 cases. *Circulation,* 21:1088, 1960.

Farmer, R. G., Gifford, R. W. Jr., and Hines, E. A. Jr.: Raynaud's disease with sclerodactylia: a follow-up study of seventy-one patients. *Circulation,* 23:13, 1961.

Feiwel, M.: Generalized morphoea. *Proc Roy Soc Med,* 57:517, 1964.

Fennell, R. H., Maclachlan, M. J., and Rodnan, G. P.: The occurrence of antinuclear factors in the sera of relatives of patients with systemic rheumatic disease. *Arthritis Rheum,* 5:296, 1962.

Fennell, R. H., Reddy, C. R. R. M., and Vaquez, J. J.: Progressive systemic sclerosis and malignant hypertension; immunohistochemical study of renal lesions. *Arch Pathol,* 72:209, 1961.

Finlay, D. W.: Clinical notes: scleroderma. *Br J Derm,* 1:339, 1889.

Finlay, D. W.: Abstracts of exceptional cases. *Middlesex Hos Rep London,* 1891, p. 29.

Fisher, E. R., and Rodnan, G. P.: Pathologic observations concerning kidneys in progressive systemic sclerosis. *Arch Pathol,* 65:29, 1958.

Fisher, E. R., and Rodman, G. P.: Pathologic observations concerning the cutaneous lesion of progressive systemic sclerosis: an electron microscopic, histochemical and immunohistochemical study. *Arthritis Rheum,* 3:536, 1960.

Fite, G. L.: Acid-fast bacteria in scleroderma. *Arch Dermatol,* 104:560, 1971.

Fleischmajer, R.: The collagen in scleroderma. *Arch Dermatol,* 89:437, 1964a.

Fleischmajer, R.: Serum proteins and glycoproteins in scleroderma. *Arch Dermatol,* 89:749, 1964b.

Fleischmajer, R., and Bansiddhi, P.: Localized scleroderma. *Arch Dermatol,* 101:697, 1970.

Fleischmajer, R., Damiano, V., and Nedwick, A.: Scleroderma and the subcutaneous tissue. *Science,* 171:1019, 1971.

Fleischmajer, R., and Fogel, M.: Systemic scleroderma. *Arch Dermatol,* 101:696, 1970.

Fleischmajer, R., and Hyman, A. B.: Clinical significance of derangements of tryptophan metabolism; a review of pellagra, carcinoid and H disease. *Arch Dermatol,* 84:563, 1961.

Fleischmajer, R., and Krol, S.: Chemical analysis of the dermis in scleroderma. *Proc Soc Exp Biol Med,* 126:252, 1967.

Fleischmajer, R., and Lara, J. V.: Scleredema; a histochemical and biochemical study. *Arch Dermatol,* 92:643, 1965.

Fleischmajer, R., Lara, J. V., and Krol, S.: Localized scleroderma; a histochemical and chemical study. *Arch Dermatol,* 94:531, 1966.

Fleischmajer, R., and Piamphongsant, T.: Systemic scleroderma. *Arch Dermatol,* 101:696, 1970.

Fletcher, E., and Morton, P.: Scleroderma heart disease. *Br Med J,* 4:657, 1967.

Foerster, O. H.: The relation of internal secretions to cutaneous disease. *J Cutan Dis,* 34:1, 1916.

Forget, C.-P.: Mémoire sur le chorionitis où la sclérosténose cutanée (maladie non décrite par les auteurs). *Gaz Méd Strasbourg,* 7:200, 1847. Quoted by Rodnan, G. P. and Benedek, T. G. 1962 *(loc. cit.).*

Fountain, R. B., and Stevens, A.: Scleroderma treated with low molecular weight dextran. *Br J Dermatol,* 78:605, 1966.

Frank, L., and Levitt, L. M.: Scleroderma with Raynaud's syndrome treated with cortisone. *NY State J Med,* 52:353, 1952.

Friou, G. J., Finch, S. C., and Detre, K. D.: Interaction of nuclei and globulin from lupus erythematosus serum demonstrated with fluorescent antibody. *J Immunol,* 80:324, 1958.

Fudenberg, H., and Wintrobe, M. M.: Scleroderma with symptomatic hemolytic anemia: a case report. *Ann Intern Med,* 43:201, 1955.

Fuleihan, F. J. D., Kurban, A. K., Abboud, R. T.: Beidas-Jubran, N., and Farah, F. S.: An objective evaluation of the treatment of systemic scleroderma with disodium EDTA, pyridoxine and reserpine. *Br J Dermatol,* 80:184, 1968.

Fulghum, D. D., and Katz, R.: Penicillamine for scleroderma. *Arch Dermatol,* 98:51, 1968.

Galen: Traité de therapeutique. Cited by Durham, R. H. 1928 *(loc. cit.).*

Gamp, A.: Bluteiweissbefunde bei progressiver Sklerodermie. *Med Klin (Munchen),* 56:1741, 1961.

Garrett, J. M., Winkelmann, R. K., Schlegel, J. F., and Code, C. F.: Esophageal deterioration in scleroderma. *Mayo Clinic Proc,* 46:92, 1971.

Garson, M.: Chromosomal studies in scleroderma. Unpublished observations, 1972.

Getzowa, S.: Cystic and compact pulmonary sclerosis in progressive scleroderma. *Arch Pathol,* 40:99, 1945.

Gil, J. R.: Clinical study of visceral lesions and endocrine disturbances in eight cases of diffuse scleroderma. *Ann Intern Med,* 34:862, 1951.

Gillette, quoted by Kaposi in Hebra, F.: *Diseases of the Skin Including the Exanthemata.* London, *New Sydenham Society,* 3:104, 1854, translated by W. Tay.

Gintrac, E.: Note sur la sclérodermie. *Rev Med Chir (Paris),* 2:263, 1847. Quoted by Rodnan, G. P., and Benedek, T. G., 1962 *(loc. cit).*

Gluck, E., and Humerfelt, S.: Les manifestations viscérales de la sclérodermie; étude clinique et anatomo-pathologique de trois cas vérifiés par l'autopsie. *Ann Anat Pathol (Paris),* 2:529, 1957.

Godfrey, S., Bluestone, R., and Higgs, B. E.: Lung function and the response to exercise in systemic sclerosis. *Thorax,* 24:427, 1969.

Goetz, R. H.: The pathology of pressive systemic sclerosis (generalized scleroderma) with special reference to changes in viscera. *Clin Proc,* 4:337, 1945.

Goetz, R. H.: The heart in generalized scleroderma; progressive systemic sclerosis. *Angiology,* 2:555; 1951.

Goetz, R. H., and Rous, M.: Note on a case showing Raynaud's phenomenon and additional manifestations. *Clin Proc,* 1:244, 1942.

Goldgraber, M. B., and Kirsner, J. B.: Scleroderma of the gastrointestinal tract; a review. *Arch Pathol,* 64:255, 1957.

Goldman, M. J.: *Principles of Clinical Electrocardiography.* 6th ed. Los Altos, Lange, 1967.

Gompels, B. M.: Pneumatosis cystoides intestinalis associated with progressive systemic sclerosis. *J Radiol,* 42:701, 1969.

Gordon, R. M., and Silverstein, A.: Neurologic manifestations in progressive systemic sclerosis. *Arch Neurol,* 22:126, 1970.

Gottron, H. A.: Skleromyxödem (Eine eigenartige Erscheinungsform von Myxothe-saurodermie). *Arch Dermatol Syph (Berlin)*, 199:71, 1954.

Gough, J.: Differential diagnosis in the pathology of asbestosis. *Ann NY Acad Sci*, 132:368, 1965.

Green, D.: Scleroderma and its oral manifestations; report of three cases of progressive systemic sclerosis (diffuse scleroderma). *Oral Surg*, 15:1312, 1962.

Greenberger, N. J., Dobbins, W. O., Ruppert, R. D., and Jesseph, J. E.: Intestinal atony in progressive systemic sclerosis (scleroderma). *Am J Med*, 45:301, 1968.

Grilliat, J.-P., Rauber, G., Laurent, J., and Drouin, P.: Sclérose hépatosplénique et syndrome de Thibièrge-Weissenbach. *Presse Med*, 75:2235; 1967.

Grin, E.; Sălamon, T., and Stern-Sarajevo, P.: Über die Behandlung einiger Erkrankungen aus dem Formenkreis der Sklerodermie und des Erythematodes chronicus mit einem Serotonin-Antagonisten. *Arch Klin Exp Derm*, 219:527, 1964.

Grisolle, M.: Cas rare de maladie de la peau. *Gaz Hôp Civ Milit (Paris)*, 9:209, 1847. Quoted by Rodnan, G. P. and Benedek, T. G. 1962 *(loc. cit.)*.

Gulledge, A. D.: Scleroderma: some psychiatric aspects of progressive systemic sclerosis. *J Kans Med Soc*, 69:593, 1968.

Günther, G., and Schuchardt, E.: Silikose und progressive Sklerodermie. Besteht ein ätiologischer Zusammenhang? *Deutsch Med Wochenschr*, 95:467, 1970.

Haas, J. E., and Yunis, E. J.: Tubular inclusions of systemic lupus erythematosus. Ultrastructural observations regarding their possible viral nature. *Exp Molec Pathol*, 12:257, 1970.

Haberman, J. D., Ehrlich, G. E., and Levenson, C.: Thermography in rheumatic diseases. *Arch Phys Med*, 49:187, 1968.

Hagberg, B., Leonhardt, T., and Skogh, M.: Familial occurrence of collagen diseases. *Acta Med Scand*, 169:727, 1961.

Hale, C. H., and Schatzki, R.: The roentgenological appearance of the gastro-intestinal tract in scleroderma. *Am J Roentgenol*, 51:407, 1944.

Hall, A. P., Bardawil, W. A., Bayles, T. B., Mednis, A. D., and Galins, N.: The relations between the antinuclear, rheumatoid and L.E.-cell factors in the systemic rheumatic diseases. *N Engl J Med*, 263:769, 1960.

Hall, A. P., and Scott, J. T.: Failure of ε-aminoeaproic acid in the treatment of scleroderma. *Ann Rheum Dis*, 25:175, 1966.

Hallen, A.: Fibrosis in the carcinoid syndrome. *Lancet*, 1:746, 1964.

Hannigan, C. A., Hannigan, M. H., and Scott, E. L.: Scleroderma of the kidneys. *Am J Med*, 20:793, 1956.

Hardy, K. H., Rosevear, J. W., Sams, W. M., and Winkelmann, R. K.: Scleroderma and urinary excretion of acidic glycosaminoglycans. *Mayo Clinic Proc*, 46:119, 1971.

Hargraves, M. M., Richmond, H., and Morton, R.: Presentation of two bone marrow elements: the *Tart* cell and the *L.E.* cell. *Mayo Clinic Proc*, 23:25, 1948.

Harley, J.: A case of slowly advancing scleroderma attended by cardiac and gastric disorders. *Br. Med J*, 1:107, 1877, quoted by Sackner, M. A. *Arthritis Rheum*, 5:184, 1962.

Harper, R. A. K.: The radiological manifestations of diffuse systemic sclerosis (scleroderma). *Proc Roy Soc Med*, 46:512, 1953.

Harper, R. A. K., and Jackson, D. C.: Progressive systemic sclerosis. *Br J Radiol*, 38:825, 1965.

Harris, E. D. Jr., Jaffe, I., and Sjoerdsma, A.: Effect of penicillamine on collagen in man. *Arthritis Rheum,* 9:509, 1966.

Harris, E. D. Jr., and Sjoerdsma, A.: Collagen profile in various clinical conditions. *Lancet,* 2:707, 1966a.

Harris, E. D. Jr., and Sjoerdsma, A.: Effect of penicillamine on human collagen and its possible application to treatment of scleroderma. *Lancet,* 2:996, 1966b.

Hausmanowa-Petrusewicz, I., and Koźmińska, A.: Electromyographic findings in scleroderma. *Arch Neurol,* 4:281, 1961.

Hausmanowa-Petrusewicz, I., and Koźmińska, A.: Further studies on electromyographic findings in generalized scleroderma. *Acta Neuroveg (Wien),* 29:220, 1966.

Hay, D. R.: Malignant carcinoid syndrome with scleroderma. *NZ Med J,* 63:90, 1964.

Hayes, R. L., and Rodnan, G. P.: The ultrastructure of skin in progressive systemic sclerosis (scleroderma). *Am J Path,* 63:433, 1971.

Heerma van Voss, S. F. C.: Experiences with thermography in peripheral vascular disease. *Acta Chir Belg,* 67:457, 1968.

Heine, J.: Über ein eigenartiges Krankheitsbild von diffuser Sklerosis der Haut und innerer Organe. *Virchows Arch Pathol Anat,* 262:351, 1926.

Heinz, E. R., Steinberg, A. J., and Sackner, M. A.: Roentgenographic and pathologic aspects of intestinal scleroderma. *Ann Intern Med,* 59:822, 1963.

Hektoen, L.: Diffuse scleroderma associated with chronic fibrous changes in the thyroid and great diminution in the amount of thyroidin; increase in the chromophile cells and of the colloid in the hypophysis. *JAMA,* 28:1240, 1897.

Helm, F.: Seltene Roentgenbilder des Oesophagus. *Med Klin (Munchen), Juli-Dez,* 665, 1918.

Herrington, J. L. Jr.: Scleroderma as a cause of small-bowel obstruction; successful treatment of a case by intestinal resection. *Arch Surg,* 78:17, 1959.

Hines, E. A., Wakim, K. G., Roth, G. M., and Kierland, R. R.: The effect of cortisone and adrenocorticotrophic hormone (ACTH) on the peripheral circulation and blood pressure in scleroderma. *J Lab Clin Med,* 36:834, 1950.

Hippocrates. Quoted by Durham, R. A.: 1928 (*loc. cit.*).

Holti, G.: The effect of intermittent low molecular dextran infusions upon the digital circulation in systemic sclerosis. *Br J Dermatol,* 77:560, 1965.

Holti, G.: Scleroderma. *Practitioner,* 204:644, 1970.

Holti, G.: Low molecular weight dextran in systemic sclerosis. *Br Med J,* 1:405, 1971.

Holzmann, H., Korting, G. W., and Morsches, B.: Zur Beeinflussung der Mucopolysaccharide in Serum und Urin von Sklerodermiekranken durch Gestagen-Behandlung. *Arch Klin Exp Dermatol,* 231:156, 1968a.

Holzmann, H., Korting, G. W., and Morsches, B.: Gestagen treatment of scleroderma. *Aust J Derm,* 9:237, 1968b.

Holzmann, H., Korting, G. W., Morsches, B., and Schlaudecker, A.: Zum Verhalten des *collagen-like protein* in Serum von Sklerodermiekranken von und nach Therapie mit Gestagenen. *Arch Klin Exp Dermatol,* 230:69, 1967.

Hoppe-Seyler, G.: Zwei Falle von Sklerodermie. *Dtsch Arch Klin Med,* 44:581, 1889. Quoted by Rodnan, G. P. and Benedek, T. G. 1962 (*loc. cit*).

Horan, E. C.: Ophthalmic manifestations of progressive systemic sclerosis. *Br J Ophthal,* 53:388, 1969.

Horswell, R. R., Hargrove, M. D. Jr., Peete, W. P., and Ruffin, J. M.: Scleroderma presenting as the malabsorption syndrome; a case report. *Gastroenterology,* 40:580, 1961.

Hoskins, L. C., Norris, H. T., Gottlieb, L. S., and Zamcheck, N.: Functional and morphologic alterations of the gastrointestinal tract in progressive systemic sclerosis (scleroderma). *Am J Med*, 33:459, 1962.

Housset, E.: Interêt de certains dérivés de la colchicine dans le traitement des syndromes sclérodermiques. *Ann Dermatol Syph (Paris)*, 94:31, 1967.

Housset, E., Emerit, I., Baulon, A., and de Grouchy, J.: Anomalies chromosomiques dans la sclérodermie generalisée. Une étude de dix malades. *CR Acad Sci (Paris)*, 269:413, 1969.

Huang, C. T., and Lyons, H. A.: Comparison of pulmonary function in patients with systemic lupus erythematosus, scleroderma and rheumatoid arthritis. *Am Rev Resp Dis*, 93:865, 1966.

Hughes, D. T. D., Gordon, K. C. D., Swann, J. C., and Bolt, G. L.: Pneumatosis cystoides intestinalis, *Gut*, 7:553, 1966.

Hughes, D. T. D., and Lee, F. I.: Lung function in patients with systemic sclerosis. *Thorax*, 18:16, 1963.

Hurly, J., Coe, J., and Weber, L.: Scleroderma heart disease. *Am Heart J*, 42:758, 1951.

Hutchinson, J.: Congenital defects and inherited proclivities. *Arch Surg*, 4:305, 1893.

Hutchinson, J.: On morphoea and allied conditions. *Arch Surg*, 6:350, 1895.

Israel, M. S., and Harley, B. J. S.: Spontaneous pneumothorax in scleroderma. *Thorax*, 2:113, 1956.

Jabłońska, S., Bubnow, B., and Lukasiak, B.: Acrosclerosis: a disease *sui generis* or a variety of diffuse scleroderma? *Br J Dermatol*, 71:123, 1959.

Jabłońska, S., Bubnow, B., Lukasiak, B., and Kisiel, J.: Hautfunktionsprüfungen bei den Gefässkrankheiten und ihre Bedeutung fur die Diagnostik und Prognose. *Arch Klin Exp Dermatol*, 206:209, 1957.

Jabłońska, S., Bubnow, B., and Szczepanski, A.: Morphoea: is it a separate entity or a variety of scleroderma? *Dermatologica (Basel)*, 125:140, 1962.

Jackman, J.: Roentgen features of scleroderma and acrosclerosis. *Radiology*, 40:163, 1943.

Jaffe, I. A., Treser, G., Suzuki, Y., and Ehrenreich, T.: Nephropathy induced by D-penicillamine. *Ann Intern Med*, 60:549, 1968.

Jakubowska, K., Rondio, H., and Syzmańska-Jagiello, W.: The radiological appearance of osteoarticular changes in progressive systemic sclerosis in children. *Reumatologia (Warsz)*, 8:11, 1970.

Jansen, G. T., Barraza, D. F., Ballard, J. L., Honeycutt, W. M., and Dillaha, C. J.: Generalized scleroderma; treatment with an immunosuppressive agent. *Arch Dermatol* 97:690, 1968.

Jones, E. W.: Valvular disease of the heart in systemic scleroderma. *Br J Dermatol*, 74:183, 1962.

Jordan, R. E., Deheer, D., Schroeter, A., and Winkelmann, R. K.: Antinuclear antibodies: their significance in scleroderma. *Mayo Clinic Proc*, 46:111, 1971.

Kahn, I. J., Jeffries, G. H., and Sleisenger, M. H.: Malabsorption in intestinal scleroderma; correction by antibiotics. *N Engl J Med*, 274:1339, 1966.

Kantor, I.: Scleroderma treated with dextran 40 (rheomacrodex). *Arch Dermatol*, 94:675, 1966.

Kappert, A.: Über einige Wirkungen von Dimethylsulfoxyd (DMSO) bei percutaner Anwendung. *Schweiz Med Wochenschr*, 98:1829, 1968.

Karten, I.: CRST syndrome and *neuropathic* arthropathy. *Arthritis Rheum*, 12:636, 1969.

Kaufmann, H. J., Braverman, I. M., and Spiro, H. M.: Esophageal manometry in scleroderma. *Scan J Gastroenterol, 3*:246, 1968.

Keech, M. K., McCann, D. S., Boyle, A. J., and Pinkus, H.: Effect of ethylenediamine-tetraacetic acid (EDTA) and tetrahydroxyquinone on sclerodermatous skin; histologic and chemical studies. *J Invest Dermatol, 47*:235, 1966.

Keiser, H., LeRoy, E. C., Udenfriend, S., and Sjoerdsma, A.: Collagen-like protein in human plasma. *Science, 142*:1678, 1963.

Keiser, H. R., and Sjoerdsma, A.: Studies on beta-aminopropionitrile in patients with scleroderma. *Clin Pharmacol Ther, 8*:593, 1967.

Keiser, H. R., and Sjoerdsma, A.: Direct measurement of the rate of collagen synthesis in skin. *Clin Chim Acta, 23*:341, 1969.

Keiser, H. R., Stein, D., and Sjoerdsma, A.: Increased protocollagen proline hydroxylase activity in sclerodermatous skin. *Arch Dermatol, 104*:57, 1971.

Kelley, M. L. Jr.: The clinical application of esophageal motility tests. *Ann Intern Med, 59*:338, 1963.

Kirk, J. A., and Dixon, A. St. J.: Failure of low molecular weight dextran infusions in scleroderma. *Ann Rheum Dis, 28*:49, 1969.

Kirkham, T. H.: Scleroderma and Sjögren's syndrome. *Br J Ophthalmol, 53*:131, 1969.

Klein, R., and Harris, S. B.: Treatment of scleroderma, sclerodactylia and calcinosis by chelation (EDTA). *Am J Med, 19*:798, 1955.

Klemperer, P., Pollack, A. D., and Baehr, G.: Diffuse collagen disease; acute disseminated lupus erythematosus and diffuse scleroderma. *JAMA, 119*:331, 1942.

Klien, B. A.: Comments on the cotton-wool lesions of the retina. *Am J Ophthalmol, 59*:17, 1965.

Klingman, W. O.: Dermatoneuromyositis resulting in scleroderma. *Arch Neurol, 24*:1187, 1970.

Kohle, G. A., Roos, W., and Fischer, H.: Zur Beteiligung des Nervensystems an der progressiven Sklerodermie. *Med Welt, 10*:386, 1970.

Korting, G. W., and Holzmann, H.: Gestagen-Behandlung der Sklerodermie. *Aesthet Med (Berlin), 16*:291, 1967.

Korting, G. W., Holzmann, H., and Kühn, K.: Biochemische Bindegeweb-analysen bei progressiver Sklerodermie. *Klin Wochenschr, 42*:248, 1964.

Koźmińska, A.: The effect of direct and reflected heat upon peripheral blood vessels in scleroderma. *Arch Klin Exp Dermatol, 233*:146, 1968.

Kraus, E. J.: Zur pathogenese der diffusen Sklerodermie. Zugleich ein Beitrag zur Pathologie der Epithelkörperchen. *Virchows Archiv Pathol Anat, 253*:710, 1924.

Kunkel, H. G.: Immunological aspects of connective tissue disorders. *Fed Proc, 23*:623, 1964.

Kurland, L. T., Hauser, W. A., Ferguson, R. H., and Holley, K. E.: Epidemiologic features of diffuse connective tissue disorders in Rochester, 1951 through 1967 with special reference to systemic lupus erythematosus. *Mayo Clinic Proc, 44*:649, 1969.

Kvyatkovskaya, A. N., Kainova, A. S., and Mikhailova, I. N.: Blood and urinary tyrosine in patients with collagenosis and its clinical significance. *Fed Proc, 22*:T247, 1963.

Laitinen, O., Uitto, J., Hannuksela, M., and Mustakallio, K. K.: Increased soluble collagen content of affected and normal-looking skin in dermatomyositis, lupus erythematosus and scleroderma. *Ann Med Exp Biol Fenn, 44*:507, 1966.

Laitinen, O., Uitto, J., Hannuksela, M., and Mustakallio, K. K.: Solubility and turnover of collagen in collagen diseases. *Ann Clin Res, 1*:64, 1969.

Lamberton, J.-N.: Une therapeutique *anti-sclérose* de la sclérodermie; l'insaponifiable des huiles d'avocat et de soja: cinquante applications cliniques du traitement de H. Thiers. *Presse Med,* 78:1235, 1970.

Lane, P.: Low molecular weight dextran infusions in systemic sclerosis with Raynaud's phenomenon: a report of nine cases. *Br Med J,* 4:657, 1970.

Laskin, D., Engel, M. B., Joseph, N. R., and Pollack, V. E.: A test of connective tissue state and reactivity in collagen diseases. *J Clin Invest,* 40:2153, 1961.

Lazarus, R. J., Kaplan, D. A., Diamond, H. S., and Emmanuel, G.: Treatment of scleroderma patients with a scorbutic diet, *JAMA, 213:*2261, 1970.

Lee, J. E., and Haynes, J. M.: Carotid arteritis and cerebral infarction due to scleroderma. *Neurology, 17:*18, 1967.

Leinwand, I., Duryee, A. W., and Richter, M. N.: Scleroderma (based on a study of over 150 cases). *Ann Intern Med, 41:*1003, 1954.

Leneman, F., Fierst, S., Gabriel, J. B., and Ingegno, A. P.: Progressive systemic sclerosis of the intestine presenting as malabsorption syndrome. *Gastroenterology,* 42:175, 1962.

Leonhardt, T.: Familial occurrence of collagen diseases, II. Progressive systemic sclerosis and dermatomyositis. *Acta Med Scand, 169:*735, 1961.

Leontjewa, L. A.: Über Veranderungen der Knochen und Gelenke bei Sklerodermie. *Arch f Klin Chir, 128:*293, 1924.

Leriche, R., Jung, A., and DeBakey, M.: The surgical treatment of scleroderma; rationale of sympathectomy and parathyroidectomy (based on experimental investigations and a clinical study of twenty-six personal cases). *Surgery,* 1:6, 1937.

LeRoy, E. C.: Connective tissue synthesis by scleroderma skin fibroblasts in cell culture. *J. Exper. Med, 135:*1351, 1971.

LeRoy, E. C., Downey, J. A., and Cannon, P. J.: Skin capillary blood flow in scleroderma. *J Clin Invest, 50:*930, 1971.

Lev, M., Landowne, M., Matchar, J. C., and Wagner, J. A.: Systemic scleroderma with complete heart block; report of a case with comprehensive study of the conduction system. *Am Heart J,* 72:13, 1966.

Levine, R. J., and Boshell, B. R.: Renal involvement in progressive systemic sclerosis (scleroderma). *Ann Intern Med, 52:*517, 1960.

Lewen, G., and Heller, J.: Die Sklerodermie. Berlin, 1895, quoted by Durham, R. H.: *Arch Intern Med, 42:*467, 1928.

Lewis, T.: The pathological changes in the arteries supplying the fingers in warm-handed people and in cases of so-called Raynaud's disease. *Clin Sci, 3:*287, 1937/8.

Lewis, T., and Landis, E. M.: Further observations upon a variety of Raynaud's disease; with special reference to arteriolar defects and to scleroderma. *Heart, 15:*329, 1931.

Lindsay, J. R., Templeton, F. E., and Rothman, S.: Lesions of the esophagus in generalized progressive scleroderma, *JAMA, 123:*745, 1943.

Linenthal, H., and Talkov, R.: Pulmonary fibrosis in Raynaud's disease. *N Engl J Med,* 221:682, 1941.

Lipscomb, P. R., Simons, G. W., and Winkelmann, R. K.: Surgery for sclerodactylia of the hand. *J Bone Joint Surg, 51-A:*1112, 1969.

Lloyd, W. E., and Tonkin, R. D.: Pulmonary fibrosis in generalized scleroderma: review of the literature and report of four further cases. *Thorax, 3:*241, 1948.

Lockhart-Mummery, H. E., and Jones, F. A.: Diffuse systemic sclerosis presenting as infarction of colon. *Proc Roy Soc Med, 53:*877, 1960.

Lorber, S. H., and Zarafonetis, C. J. D.: Esophageal transport studies in scleroderma. *Am J Med Sci, 245:*654, 1963.

Lunseth, J. H., Baker, L. A., and Shifrin, A.: Chronic scleroderma with acute exacerbation during corticotropin therapy; report of a case with autopsy observations. *Arch Intern Med, 88:*783, 1951.

Lushbaugh, C. C., Rubin, L., and Rothman, S.: Scleroderma of the intestinal tract: first report of a fatal case. *Gastroenterology, 11:*382, 1948.

McAndrew, G. M., and Barnes, E. G.: Familiar scleroderma. *Ann Phys Med, 8:*128, 1965.

McBrien, D. J., and Mummery, H. E. L.: Steatorrhoea in progressive systemic sclerosis (scleroderma). *Br Med J, 2:*1653, 1962.

MacDonald, R. A., Robbins, S. L., and Mallory, G. K.: Dermal fibrosis following subcutaneous injections of serotonin creatinine sulphate. *Proc Soc Exp Biol Med, 97:*334, 1958.

MacDowell, F. Jr.: Digital involvement of extremities in scleroderma; method of treatment. *NY St J Med, 69:*935, 1969.

McGiven, A. R., De Boer, W. G. R. M., and Barnett, A. J.: Renal immune deposits in scleroderma. *Pathology, 3:*145, 1971.

McGiven, A. R., De Boer, W. G. R. M., Barnett, A. J., and Coventry, D. A.: Autoantibodies in scleroderma. *Med J Aust, 2:*533, 1968.

Mackay, I. M., and Burnet, F. M.: *Auto-immune Diseases: Pathogenesis, Chemistry and Therapy.* Springfield, Thomas, 1963.

MacLean, H., and Guthrie, W.: Retinopathy in scleroderma. *Trans Ophthalmol Soc UK, 89:*209, 1969.

McMahon, H. E.: Systemic scleroderma and massive infarction of intestine and liver. *Surg Gynecol Obstet, 134:*10, 1972.

McMahon, J. M., Monroe, R. R., and Craighead, C. C.: Emotional factors in scleroderma: case history. *Ann Intern Med, 39:*1295, 1953.

MacPherson, P., and Davidson, J. K.: Correlation between lung asbestos count at necropsy and radiological appearances. *Br Med J, 1:*355, 1969.

Mancini, R. E., Stringa, S. G., and Canepa, L.: The action of ACTH, cortisone and prednisone on the connective tissue of normal and sclerodermic human skin. *J Invest Dermatol, 34:*393, 1960.

Marshall, I.: Collagen disease of the small bowel. *N Engl J Med, 255:*978, 1956.

Masi, A. T., and D'Angelo, W. A.: Epidemiology of fatal systemic sclerosis (diffuse scleroderma); a fifteen year survey in Baltimore. *Ann Intern Med, 66:*870, 1967.

Masugi, M., and Yä-Shu: Die diffuse Sklerodermie und ihre Gefassveranderung. *Virchows Arch Pathol Anat, 302:*39, 1938.

Mathisen, A. K., and Palmer, J. D.: Diffuse scleroderma with involvement of the heart; report of a case. *Am Heart J, 33:*366, 1947.

Matsui, S.: Über die Pathologie und Pathogenese von Sclerodermia universalis. *Mitt a d Med Fakult d k Univ z Tokyo, 31:*55, 1924.

Medsger, T. A. Jr., and Masi, A. T.: Epidemiology of systemic sclerosis (scleroderma). *Ann Intern Med, 74:*714, 1971.

Medsger, T. A., Jr., Masi, A. T., Rodnan, G. P., and Benedek, T. G.: Survival with systemic sclerosis (scleroderma); a life-table analysis of clinical and demographic factors in 309 patients. *Ann Intern Med, 75:*369, 1971.

Medsger, T. A. Jr., Rodnan, G. P., Moosy, J., and Vester, J. W.: Skeletal muscle involvement in progressive systemic sclerosis (scleroderma). *Arthritis Rheum, 11:*554, 1968.

Meihoff, W. E., Hirschfield, J. S., and Kern, F. Jr.: Small intestinal scleroderma with malabsorption and pneumatosis cystoides intestinalis. *JAMA, 204*:854, 1968.

Meltzer, J. I.: Pericardial effusion in generalized scleroderma. *Am J Med, 20*:638, 1956.

Méry, H.: *Anatomie pathologique et nature de la sclérodermie.* Paris. G. Steinheil, 1889, quoted by Medsger, T. A. Jr. *et al.*: 1968 (*loc. cit.*).

Meszaros, W. T.: The regional manifestations of scleroderma. *Radiology, 70*:313, 1958.

Meszaros, W. T.: The colon in systemic sclerosis (scleroderma). *Am J Roentgenol, 82*:1000, 1959.

Meyer, P.: *Gaz Med Strasbourg, 46*:126, 135, 1887 and *47:1*, 1888. Quoted by Sackner, M. A. *Arthritis Rheum, 5*:184, 1962.

Michalowski, R., and Kudejko, J.: Electron microscopic observations on skeletal muscle in diffuse scleroderma. *Br J Dermatol, 78*:24, 1966.

Miercort, R. D., and Merrill, F. G.: Pneumatosis and pseudo-obstruction in scleroderma. *Radiology, 92*:359, 1969.

Miguères, J., Layssol, M., Moreau, G., Jover, A., and Tricoire, J.: Sclérodermie pulmonaire et silicose du spath flour associée; rapports entre sclérodermie et silicose. *J Fr Med Chir Thorac, 20*:603, 1966.

Mikkelsen, W. M., Duff, I. F., Castor, C. W., Zevely, H. A., and French, A. J.: The diagnostic value of punch biopsy of the knee synovium. *Arch Intern Med, 102*:977, 1958.

Milbradt, W.: Atypische diffuse Sklerodermie mit Oslerschem Syndrom und Leberstörung. *Dermatol Wochenschr, 99*:973, 1934.

Millard, M.: Sclérodermie améliorée par l'arrhenal. *Bull Et Mem Soc Med d Hôp d Paris, 22*:163, 1905.

Miller, R. D., Fowler, W. S., and Helmholz, F. H. Jr.: Scleroderma of the lungs. *Mayo Clinic Proc, 34*:66, 1959.

Monroe, L. S., and Knauer, C. M.: Gastro-intestinal manifestations of systemic sclerosis (scleroderma): a review. *Am Practit, 13*:636, 1962.

Moore, H. C., and Sheehan, H. L.: The kidney of scleroderma. *Lancet, 1*:68, 1952.

Mufson, I.: An etilogy of scleroderma. *Ann Intern Med, 39*:1219, 1953.

Muller, S. A., Brunsting, L. A., and Winkelmann, R. K.: The treatment of scleroderma with the new chelating agent, edathamil. *Arch Dermatol, 80*:187, 1959.

Murphy, J. R., Krainin, P., and Gerson, M. J.: Scleroderma with pulmonary fibrosis. *JAMA, 116*:499, 1941.

Murray-Lyon, I. M., Thompson, R. P. H., Ansell, I. D., and Williams, R.: Scleroderma and primary biliary cirrhosis. *Br Med J, 1*:258, 1970.

Mustakallio, K. K., and Sarajas, H. S. S.: Some aspects of scleroderma heart disease. *Am Heart J, 47*:437, 1954.

Nakashima, T., Tajiri, T., and Tashiro, T.: An autopsy case of visceral scleroderma with lethel ileus. *Kurume Med J, 13*:129, 1966.

Nash, A. G., and Fountain, R.: Surgical presentation of systemic sclerosis of the small intestine. *Br J Surg, 55*:667, 1968.

Nasser, W. K., Mishkin, M. E., Rosenbaum, D., and Genovese, P.D.: Pericardial and myocardial disease in progressive systemic sclerosis. *Am J Cardiol, 22*:538, 1968.

Neal, J. E.: Scleroderma and the structural basis of skin compliance. *Arch. Dermatol, 107*:699, 1973.

Neldner, K. H., Jones, J. D., and Winkelmann, R. K.: Scleroderma; dermal amino acid composition with particular reference to hydroxyproline. *Proc Soc Exp Biol Med, 122*:39, 1966.

Neldner, K. H., Winkelmann, R. K., and Perry, H. O.: Scleroderma; an evaluation of treatment with disodium edetate. *Arch Dermatol, 86*:305, 1962.

Nellas, C. L., Crawford, N., and Scherbel, A. L.: Pancreatic collagenase therapy for severe progressive systemic sclerosis; effect on skin and hydroxyproline content in urine. *Clin Pharmacol Ther, 6*:367, 1965.

Nice, C. M. Jr.: *Clinical Roentgenology of Collagen Diseases.* Springfield, Thomas, 1966, p. 64.

Nishimura, N., Yasui, M., Okamoto, H., Kanazawa, M., Kotake, Y., and Shibata, Y.: Intermediary metabolism of phenylalanine and tyrosine in diffuse collagen diseases, I. The presence of 2,5-dihydroxyphenylpyruvic acid in the urine of patients with collagen disease. *Arch Dermatol, 77*:255, 1958.

Nitzschner, H., and Liebsch, F.: Anwendung von Karnitin bei bindegewebigen Erkrankungen. *Dermatol Wochenschr, 157*:538, 1971.

Nong Ting: Personal communication (1971).

Norton, W. L.: Endothelial inclusions in active lesions of systemic lupus erythematosus. *J Lab Clin Med, 74*:369, 1969.

Norton, W. L., Hurd, E. R., Lewis, D. C., and Ziff, M.: Evidence of microvascular injury in scleroderma and systemic lupus erythematosus: quantitative study of the microvascular bed. *J Lab Clin Med, 71*:919, 1968.

Norton, W. L., Hurd, E. R., and Ziff, M.: A capillary abnormality in scleroderma. *Arthritis Rheum, 9*:870, 1966.

Norton, W. L., and Nardo, J. M.: Vascular disease in progressive systemic sclerosis (scleroderma). *Ann Intern Med, 73*:317, 1970.

Notthafft, A. Von: Neure Arbeiten und Ansichten uber Sklerodermie. *Zentralbl f Pathol, 9*:870, 1898. Quoted by Sackner, M. A. *Arthritis Rheum, 5*:184, 1962.

Oaks, W. W., and O'Malley, J. F.: Systemic involvement in the CRST syndrome. *Postgrad Med, 45* (3):94, 1969.

O'Brien, S. T., Eddy, W. M., and Krawitt, E. I.: Primary biliary cirrhosis associated with scleroderma. *Gastroenterology, 62*:118, 1972.

Öbrink, B.: The influence of glycosamino-glycans on the formation of fibers from monomeric tropocollagen in vitro. *Fur. J. Biochem, 31*:129, 1973.

Ochsner, A., and DeBakey, M.: Scleroderma. Surgical considerations. *New Orleans Med Surg J, 92*:24, 1939.

Ofstad, E.: Scleroderma (progressive systemic sclerosis); a case involving polyneuritis and swelling of the lymph nodes. *Acta Rheum Scand, 6*:65, 1960.

Øhlenschaeger, K., and Friman, C.: A normal urinary excretion of acid mucopolysaccharides in generalized scleroderma. *Scand J Clinic Lab Invest, 21*:364, 1968.

Øhlenschlaeger, K., and Tissot, J.: Scleroderma treatment with the diethylaminoethylester hydriodide salt of penicillin G. *Dermatologica (Basel), 134*:129, 1967.

O'Leary, P. A., Montgomery, H., and Ragsdale, W. E.: Dermatohistopathology of various types of scleroderma. *Arch Dermatol, 75*:78, 1957.

O'Leary, P. A., and Nomland, R.: A clinical study of one hundred and three cases of scleroderma. *Am J Med Sci, 180*:95, 1930.

O'Leary, P. A., and Waisman, M.: Acrosclerosis. *Arch Dermatol Syph, 47*:382, 1943.

Oliver, E. L., and Lerman, J.: Scleroderma treated with injections of posterior pituitary extract. *Arch Dermatol Syph, 34*:469, 1936.

Olsen, A. M., O'Leary, P. A., and Kirklin, B. R.: Esophageal lesions associated with acrosclerosis and scleroderma. *Arch Intern Med, 76*:189, 1945.

Opie, L. H.: The pulmonary manifestations of generalized scleroderma (progressive systemic sclerosis). *Dis Chest, 28*:665, 1955.

Orabona, M. L., and Albano, O.: Progressive systemic sclerosis (or visceral scleroderma); review of literature and report of cases. *Acta Med Scand, 160*, Suppl 333, 1958.

Oram, S., and Stokes, W.: The heart in scleroderma, *Br Heart J, 23*:243, 1961.

Osler, W.: *The Principles and Practice of Medicine.* New York, Appleton, 1892, p. 994.

Osler, W.: On diffuse scleroderma with special reference to diagnosis and to the use of thyroid-gland extract. *J Cutan Genito-Urinary Dis, 16*:49, 127; 1898.

Ottolenghi, F.: An antibiotic with antisclerodermic activity: the diethylaminoethylester hydriodide salt of penicillin G. *Dermatologica (Basel), 123*:331, 1961.

Pace, N. A., and Potter, J. L. New method for evaluating and following cutaneous involvement in scleroderma. *Arthritis Rheum, 9*:870, 1966.

Page, I. H.: Serotonin (5-hydroxytryptamine); the last four years. *Physiol Rev, 38*:277, 1958.

Page, I. H., and McCubbin, J. W.: Renal vascular and systemic arterial pressure responses to nervous and chemical stimulation of the kidney. *Am J Physiol, 173*:411, 1953.

Panja, R. K., Sengupta, K. P., and Aikat, B. K.: Seromucoid in lupus erythematosus and scleroderma. *J Clin Pathol, 17*:658, 1964.

Pawlowski, A.: The nerve network of the skin in diffuse scleroderma and clinically similar conditions. *Arch Dermatol, 88*:868, 1963.

Peachey, R. D. G., Creamer, B., and Pierce, J. W.: Sclerodermatous involvement of the stomach and the small and large bowel. *Gut, 10*:285, 1969.

Petter, O., and Bellmann, H.: Die Behandlung der progressiven Sklerodermie mit intravenös hochdosierter Hyaluronidase. *Hautartz, 22*:32, 1971a.

Petter, O., and Bellmann, H.: Theoretische Aspekte zu neuen Anwendungsmöglichkeiten der Hyaluronidase. *Z Gesamte Inn Med, 26*:171, 1971b.

Pimentel, J. C.: Tridimensional photographic reconstruction in a study of the pathogenesis of honeycomb lung. *Thorax, 22*:444, 1967.

Piper, W. N., and Helwig, E. B.: Progressive systemic sclerosis; visceral manifestations in generalized scleroderma. *Arch Dermatol, 72*:535, 1955.

Platt, R., and Davson, J.: A clinical and pathological study of renal disease, part II. Diseases other than nephritis. *Quart J Med, 19*:33, 1950.

Pollack, I. P., and Becker, B.: Cytoid bodies of the retina in a patient with scleroderma. *Am J Ophthalmol, 54*:655, 1962.

Price, J. M., Brown, R. R., Rukavina, J. G., Mendelson, C., and Johnson, S. A. M.: Scleroderma (acrosclerosis) II. Tryptophan metabolism before and during treatment by chelation (EDTA). *J Invest Dermatol, 29*:289, 1957.

Prinzmetal, M.: Studies of the mechanism of circulatory insufficiency in Raynaud's disease and in association with sclerodactylia. *Arch Intern Med, 58*:309, 1936.

Privat, Y., Rousselot, M., Faye, I., and Bellossi, A.: Sclérodermie généralisée chez un Africain. *Bull Soc Med Afr Noire Lang Fr, 13*:405, 1968.

Prowse, C. B.: Generalized scleroderma with intestinal involvement. *Lancet, 1*:989, 1951.

Quinones, C. A., Perry, H. O., and Rushton, J. G.: Carpal tunnel syndrome in dermatomyositis and scleroderma. *Arch Dermatol, 94*:20, 1966.

Rake, G.: On the pathology and pathogenesis of scleroderma. *Johns Hopk Hosp Bull, 48*:212, 1931.

Ramsey, A. S.: Acrosclerosis. *Br Med J.,* 2:877, 1951.

Raskin, J.: Fluorescent antibody studies of certain dermatoses. *Arch Dermatol,* 89:569, 1964.

Rasmussen, D. M., Wakim, K. G., and Winkelmann, R. K.: Isotonic and isometric thermal contraction of human dermis, III. Scleroderma and cicatrizing lesions. *J Invest Dermatol,* 43:349, 1964.

Rattan Singh. Personal communication, 1972.

Raynaud, M.: On local asphyzia and symmetrical gangrene of the extremities, 1862. Translated by Barlow, T. London. The New Sydenham Society, 1888.

Raynaud, R., Benatre, A., Brochier, M., Morand, P., and Raynaud, P.: Coeur scléro-dermique et bloc auriculo-ventriculaire complet. *Arch Mal Coeur,* 60:1865, 1870.

Redeker, A. G., and Bronow, R. S.: Porphyrin excretion in scleroderma (acrosclerosis); a study. *Arch Dermatol,* 85:705, 1962.

Redisch, W., Messina, E. J.; Hughes, G., and McEwen, C.: Capillaroscopic observations in rheumatic diseases. *Ann Rheum Dis,* 20:244, 1970.

Rees, R. B., and Bennett, J.: Localized scleroderma in father and daughter. *Arch Dermatol,* 68:360, 1953.

Reinhardt, J. F., and Barry, W. F.: Scleroderma of the small bowel. *Am J Roentgenol,* 88:687, 1962.

Reque, P. G.: The treatment of systemic sclerosis with special reference to epsilon aminocaproic acid. *Sth Med J,* 58:319, 1965.

Reynolds, T. B., Denison, E. K., Frankel, H. D., Lieberman, F. L., and Peters, R. L.: Primary biliary cirrhosis with scleroderma, Raynaud's phenomenon and telangiectasia; new syndrome. *Am J Med,* 50:302, 1971.

Rich, A. R.: Hypersensitivity in disease with special reference to periarteritis nodosa, rheumatic fever, disseminated lupus erythematosus and rheumatoid arthritis. *Harvey Lect,* 42:106, 1946/47.

Richardson, J. A.: Hemodialysis and kidney transplantation for renal failure from scleroderma. *Arthritis Rheum,* 15:265, 1973.

Richter, R. B.: Peripheral neuropathy and connective tissue disease. *J Neuropath Exp Neurol,* 13:168, 1954.

Ritchie, B.: Pulmonary function in scleroderma. *Thorax,* 19:28, 1964.

Ritchie, R. F.: The clinical significance of titered antinuclear antibodies. *Arthritis Rheum,* 10:544, 1967.

Ritchie, R. F. Two new antinuclear antibodies: their relationship to the homogeneous immunofluorescent pattern. *Arthritis Rheum,* 11:37, 1968.

Ritchie, R. F.: Antinucleolar antibodies; their frequency and diagnostic association. *N Engl J Med,* 282:1174, 1970.

Rodnan, G. P.: The nature of joint involvement in progressive systemic sclerosis (diffuse scleroderma): clinical study and pathologic examination of synovium in twenty-nine patients. *Ann Intern Med,* 56:422, 1962.

Rodnan, G. P.: A review of recent observations and current theories on the etiology and pathogenesis of progressive systemic sclerosis (diffuse scleroderma). *J Chronic Dis,* 16:929, 1963.

Rodnan, G. P.: Progressive systemic sclerosis (diffuse scleroderma). In Hill, A. G. S. (Ed.): *Modern Trends in Rheumatology.* London, Butterworths, 1966, pp. 303–316.

Rodnan, G. P., and Benedek, T. G.: An historical account of the study of progressive systemic sclerosis (diffuse scleroderma). *Ann Intern Med,* 57:305, 1962.

Rodnan, G. P., Benedek, T. G., Medsger, T. A. Jr., and Cammarata, R. J.: The association of progressive systemic sclerosis (scleroderma) with coal miners' pneumoconiosis and other forms of silicosis. *Ann Intern Med, 66*:323, 1967.

Rodnan, G. P., and Cammarata, R. J.: Urinary excretion of hydroxyproline in progressive systemic sclerosis (diffuse scleroderma). *Clin Res. 11*:179, 1963.

Rodnan, G. P., and Fennell, R. H.: Progressive systemic sclerosis *sine* scleroderma. *JAMA, 180*:665, 1962.

Rodnan, G. P., and Medsger, T. A.: Musculo-skeletal involvement in progressive systemic sclerosis (scleroderma). *Bull Rheum Dis, 17*:419, 1966.

Rodnan, G. P., Schreiner, G. E., and Black, R. L.: Renal involvement in progressive systemic sclerosis (generalized scleroderma). *Am J Med, 23*:445, 1957.

Romeo, S. G., Whalen, R. E., and Tindall, J. P.: Intra-arterial administration of reserpine; its use in patients with Raynaud's disease or Raynaud's phenomenon. *Arch Intern Med, 125*:825, 1970.

Rosen, R. S., Cimini, R., and Coblentz, D.: Werner's syndrome. *Br J Radiol, 43*:193, 1970.

Rosenbaum, E. E., Herschler, R. J., and Jacob, S. W.: Dimethyl sulfoxide in musculo-skeletal disorders. *JAMA, 192*:309, 1965.

Rosenthal, F. D.: Small intestinal lesions with steatorrhea in diffuse systemic sclerosis (scleroderma). *Gastroenterology, 32*:332, 1957.

Ross, J. B.: Nailfold capillaroscopy—a useful aid in the diagnosis of collagen vascular diseases. *J Invest Dermatol, 47*:282, 1966.

Rossier, P. H., and Hegglin-Volkmann, M.: Die Sklerodermie als internmedizinisches Problem. *Schweiz Med Wochenschr, 84*:1161, 1954.

Rosson, R. S., and Yesner, R.: Peroral duodenal biopsy in progressive systemic sclerosis. *N Engl J Med, 72*:391, 1965.

Roth, L. M., and Kissane, J. M.: Panaortitis and aortic valvulitis in progressive systemic sclerosis (scleroderma); report of a case with perforation of an aortic cusp. *Am J Clin Path, 41*:287, 1964.

Rothbard, S., and Watson, R. F.: Renal glomerular lesions induced by rabbit anti-rat collagen serum in rats prepared with adjuvants. *J Exp Med, 109*:633, 1959.

Rothfield, N. F., and Rodnan, G. P.: Serum antinuclear antibodies in progressive systemic sclerosis (scleroderma). *Arthritis Rheum, 11*:607, 1968.

Rotstein, J., Gilbert, M., and Estrin, I.: Antifibrinolytic drug in treatment of progressive systemic sclerosis. *JAMA, 184*:518, 1963.

Rottenberg, E. N., Slocumb, C. H., and Edwards, J. E.: Cardiac and renal manifestations in progressive systemic sclerosis. *Mayo Clinic Proc, 34*:77, 1959.

Rowell, N. R.: Lupus erythematosus cells in systemic sclerosis. *Ann Rheum Dis, 21*:70, 1962.

Rowell, N. R.: Systemic sclerosis. *Br Med J, 1*:514, 1968.

Rowell, N. R., and Beck, J. S.: The diagnostic value of an antinuclear antibody test in clinical dermatology. *Arch Dermatol, 96*:290, 1967.

Rudner, E. J., Mehregan, A., and Pinkus, H.: Scleromyxedema; a variant of lichen myxedematosis. *Arch Dermatol, 93*:3, 1966.

Rukavina, J. G., Mendelson, C., Price, J. M., Brown, R. R., and Johnson, S. A. M.: Scleroderma (acrosclerosis), I. Treatment of three cases of the non-calcific variety by chelation (EDTA). *J Invest Dermatol, 29*:273, 1957.

Sabour, M. S., and el Mahallawy, M. N.: Mitral and aortic valve disease in a patient with scleroderma. *Br J Dermatol, 78*:15, 1966.

Sackner, M. A.: *Scleroderma.* New York, Greene and Stratton, 1967.

Sackner, M. A., Akgun, N. Kimbel, P., and Lewis, D. H.: The pathophysiology of scleroderma involving the heart and respiratory system. *Ann Intern Med, 60*:611, 1964.

Sackner, M. A., Heinz, E. R., and Steinberg, A. J.: The heart in scleroderma. *Am J Cardiol, 17*:542, 1966.

Saladin, T. A., French, A. B., Zarafonetis, C. J. D., Pollard, H. M.: Esophageal motor abnormalities in scleroderma and related diseases. *Am J Dig Dis, 11*:522, 1966.

Salen, G., Goldstein, F., and Wirts, C. W.: Malabsorption in intestinal scleroderma; relation to bacterial flora and treatment with antibiotics. *Ann Intern Med, 64*:834, 1966.

Salomon, A., Appel, B., Dougherty, E. F., Herschfus, J. A., and Segal, M. S.: Scleroderma; pulmonary and skin studies before and after treatment with cortisone. *Arch Intern Med, 95*:103, 1955.

Samuelsson, S.-M., and Werner, I.: Systemic scleroderma, calcinosis cutis and parathyroid hyperplasia. *Acta Med Scand, 177*:673, 1965.

Sapiro, J. D., Rodnan, G. P., Schieb, E. T., Klaniecki, T., and Rizk, M.: Studies of endogenous catecholamines in patients with Raynaud's phenomenon secondary to progressive systemic sclerosis (scleroderma). *Am J Med, 52*:330, 1972.

Sardavar: Personal communication. 1971.

Sauer, G. C., Herrmann, F., Milberg, I. L., Prose, P. H., Baer, R. L., and Sulzberger, M. B.: Effects of ACTH on certain diseases and physiologic functions of the skin. In Mote, J. R.: *Proceedings of the Second Clinical ACTH Conference,* Vol. 2. London, Churchill, 1951, p. 529 ff.

Scharer, L., and Smith, D. W.: Resorption of the terminal phalanges in scleroderma. *Arthritis Rheum, 12*:51, 1969.

Scherbel, A. L.: The possible role of serotonin in rheumatoid arthritis and other collagen diseases. In Mills, L. C. and Moyer, J. H. (Eds.): *Inflammation and Diseases of Connective Tissue.* Philadelphia, Saunders, 1961, p. 153.

Scherbel, A. L., McCormack, L. J., and Layle, J. K.: Further observations on the effect of dimethyl sulfoxide in patients with generalized scleroderma (progressive systemic sclerosis). *Ann NY Acad Sci, 141*:613, 1967.

Scherbel, A. L., McCormack, L. J., and Poppo, M. J.: Alteration of collagen in generalized scleroderma (progressive systemic sclerosis) after treatment with dimethyl sulfoxide. *Cleveland Clin Quart, 32*:47, 1965.

Schimke, R. N., Kirkpatrick, C. H., and Delp, M. H.: Calcinosis, Raynaud's phenomenon, sclerodactyly and telangiectasia; the CRST syndrome. *Arch Intern Med, 119*:365, 1967.

Schmidt, R.: Wissenschlaftliche Gesellschaft deutscher Aertze in Boehmen: Sklerodermie mit Dysphagie. *Wien Klin Wochenschr, 29*:932, 1916.

Schmitt, F. O., Levine, L., Drake, M. P., Rubin, A. L., Pfahl, D., and Davison, P. F.: The antigenicity of tropocollagen. *Proc Natl Acad Sci, 51*:493, 1964.

Schober, R., and Klüken, N.: Angiographische Befunde bei Sklerodermia progressiva. *Fortschr Rontgenstr, 105*:239, 1966.

Scudamore, H. H., Green, P. A., Hoffman, H. N. 2nd., Rosevear, J. W., and Tauxe, W. N.: Scleroderma (progressive systemic sclerosis) of the small intestine with malabsorption; evaluation of intestinal absorption and pancreatic function. *Am J Gastroent, 49*:193, 1968.

Sellei, J.: Die Akrosklerosis (Sklerodaktylie) und deren Symptomenkomplex nebst neueren Untersuchungen bei Sklerodermie. *Arch Dermatol Syph (Berlin). 163*:343, 1931.

Sellei, J.: The diagnosis and treatment of scleroderma and acrosclerosis and some of their kindred diseases. *Br J Dermatol Syph, 46:*523, 1934.

Sharnoff, J. G., Carideo, H. L., and Stein, I. D.: Cortisone-treated scleroderma: report of a case with autopsy findings. *JAMA, 145:*1230, 1951.

Sharp, G. C., Irvin, W. S., LaRoque, R. L., Velez, C., Daly, V., Kaiser, A. D., and Holman, H. R.: Association of autoantibodies to different nuclear antigens with clinical patterns of rheumatic diseases and responsiveness to therapy. *J Clin Invest, 50:*350, 1971.

Sharp, G. S., Irvin, W. S., Tan, E. M., Gould, R. G., and Holman, H. F.: Mixed connective tissue disease—an apparently distinct rheumatic disease syndrome associated with a specific antibody to an extractable nuclear antigen (ENA). *Am J Med, 52:*148; 1972.

Shearn, M. A.: Sjögren's syndrome in association with scleroderma. *Ann Intern Med, 52:*1352, 1960.

Shulman, L. E., Kurban, A. K., and Harvey, A. McG.: Tendon friction rubs in progressive systemic sclerosis (scleroderma). *Arthritis Rheum, 4:*438, 1961.

Shuster, S., Raffle, E. J., and Bottoms, E.: Quantitative changes in skin collagen in morphoea. *Br J Dermatol, 79:*456, 1967.

Silberberg, F. G.: Personal communication, 1972.

Singh, R.: Information in letter from Dr. S. Padmavati. Personal communication, 1971.

Sjoerdsma, A., Udenfriend, G., Keiser, H., and LeRoy, H. C.: Hydroxyproline and collagen metabolism: clinical implications. *Ann Intern Med, 63:*672, 1965.

Skouby, A. P., and Teilum, G.: Progressive systemic sclerosis with dominating gastrointestinal disturbances. *Acta Med Scand, 137:*111, 1950.

Smith, D. B.: Scleroderma: its oral manifestations. *Oral Surg, 11:*865, 1958.

Smith, Q. T., Rukavina, J. G., and Haaland, E. M.: Urinary hydroxyproline in various diseases. *Acta Derm-venereol (Stockh), 45:*44, 1965.

Sokoloff, L.: Some aspects of the pathology of collagen diseases. *Bull NY Acad Med, 32:*760, 1956.

Sokoloff, L.: Biopsy in rheumatic diseases. *Med Clin N Amer, 45:*1171, 1961.

Sommerville, R. L., Bargen, J. A., and Pugh, D. G.: Scleroderma of the small intestine. *Postgrad Med, 26:*356, 1959.

Sonneveldt, H. A., Leeuwen, P. von, and Blom, P. S.: Malabsorption in acrosclerosis; disseminated scleroderma. *Acta Med Scand, 171:*391, 1962.

Sönnischsen, N., Feuerstein, M., and Kolzsch, J.: Untersuchungen über die Ausscheidung von Tryptophan-Metaboliten bei Kranken mit zirkumskripter und progressiver Sklerodermie. *Dermatol Wochenschr, 154:*601, 1968.

Spain, D. M., and Thomas, A. G.: The pulmonary manifestations of scleroderma: an anatomic-physiological correlation. *Ann Intern Med, 32:*152, 1950.

Spencer, S. K., and Winkelmann, R. K.: Immunoglobulins in systemic scleroderma. *Mayo Clinic Proc, 46:*108, 1971.

Spiro, R. G.: Glycoproteins. *Ann Rev Biochem, 39:*599, 1970.

Stafne, E. C., and Austin, L. T.: A characteristic dental finding in acrosclerosis and diffuse scleroderma. *Amer J Othod (Oral Surg Section), 30:*25, 1944.

Starr, H. G. Jr., and Clifford, N. J.: Absorption of pesticides in a chronic skin disease. *Arch Environ Health, 22:*397, 1971.

Stastny, P., Stembridge, V. A., and Ziff, M.: Homologous disease in the adult rat, a model for autoimmune disease, I. General features and cutaneous lesions. *J Exp Med, 118:*635, 1963.

Štáva, Z.: Serum proteins in scleroderma. *Dermatologica (Basel), 117:*147, 1958.

Stein, H. D., Keiser, H. R., and Sjoerdsma, A.: Proline-hydroxylase activity in human blood. *Lancet*, 1:106, 1970.

Steinberg, I., and Rothbard, S.: Pericardial effusion and cor pulmonale in progressive systemic sclerosis (scleroderma): Role of angiocardiography in diagnosis in two cases. *Am J Cardiol*, 9:953, 1962.

Steinberg, I., and Rothbard, S.: Roentgen features of sclerodermal pericarditis with effusion. *Radiology*, 83:292, 1964.

Steiner, H., Haeger-Aronsen, B., Nilsson, G., and Waldenström, J.: Porphyria cutanea tarda, Sklerodermie, Leukopenie und hämolytische Anämie; klinische, biochemische und pathologisch-anatomische Analyse eines ungewöhnlichen Syndroms. *Schweiz Med Wochenschr*, 97:538, 1967.

Steven, J. L.: Case of scleroderma with pronounced hemiatrophy of the face, body and extremities—death from ovarian tumour—account of the post mortem examination: a sequel. *Glasg Med J*, 50:401; 1898.

Stevens, M. B., Hookman, P., Siegel, C. I., Esterly, J. R., Shulman, L. E., and Hendrix, T. R.: Aperistalsis of the esophagus in patients with connective-tissue disorders and Raynaud's phenomenon. *N Engl J Med*, 270:1218, 1964.

Stoughton, R., and Wells, G.: A histochemical study of polysaccharides in normal and diseased skin. *J Invest Dermatol*, 14:37, 1950.

Strack, E., Nitschner, H., and Liebsch, F.: Carnitin und bindegewebige Erkrankungen. *Dtsch Gesundheitsw*, 25:1233, 1970.

Swischuk, L. E., and Welsh, J. D.: Roentgenographic mucosal patterns in the *malabsorption syndrome;* a schema for diagnosis. *Am J Dig Dis*, 13:59, 1968.

Szymańska-Jagiello, W., and Rondio, H.: Clinical picture of articular changes in progressive systemic sclerosis in children in the light of own observations. *Reumatologia*, 8:1, 1970.

Talbott, J. H., Gall, E. A., Consolazio, W. V., and Coombs, F. S.: Dermatomyositis with scleroderma, calcinosis and renal endarteritis associated with focal cortical necrosis; report of a case in which the condition simulated Addison's disease, with comment on metabolic and pathologic studies. *Arch Intern Med*, 63:476, 1939.

Tange, J. D.: Renal lesions in scleroderma: clinical and pathological features. *Australas Ann Med*, 8:27, 1959.

Taubenhaus, M., and Lev, M.: Clinical and histological observations on a case of scleroderma treated with cortisone. *Arch Intern Med*, 87:583, 1951.

Tay, C. H., and Khoo, O. T.: Progressive systemic sclerosis (scleroderma). *Australas Ann Med*, 19:145, 1970.

Thibierge, G., and Weissenbach, A. J.: Concrétions calcaries sous-cutanées et sclérodermie. *Ann Dermatol Syphiligr (Paris)*, 2:129, 1911.

Thieme, von E.: Silikose und viszerale Sklerodermie. *Med Klin*, 62:907, 1967.

Thiers, H.: 1961. Quoted by Lamberton, J. N., 1970 (*loc. cit.*).

Thirial, H.: Du sclérème chez les adultes. *J Med Paris*, 3:137,161, 1945.
  Quoted by Rodnan, G. P., and Benedek, T. G., 1962 (*loc. cit.*).

Thompson, G. R., and Castor, C. W.: The excretion of nondialyzable urinary mucopolysaccharide in rheumatic and other systemic disease states. *J Lab Clin Med*, 68:617, 1966.

Thompson, J. M., Bluestone, R., Bywaters, E. G. L., Darling, J., and Johnstone, M.: Skeletal muscle involvement in systemic sclerosis. *Ann Rheum Dis*, 28:281, 1969.

Thompson, M., and Percy, J. S.: Further experience with indomethacin in the treatment of rheumatic disorders. *Br Med J*, 1:80, 1966.

Thorn, G. W., Forsham, P. H., Frawley, T. F., Hill, S. R. Jr., Roche, M., Staehelin, D., and Wilson, D. L.: The clinical usefulness of ACTH and cortisone. *N Engl J Med,* 242:865, 1950.

Tonkin, J. R.: Rheomacrodex in the treatment of scleroderma. *Aust J Derm,* 9:241, 1968.

Toth, A., and Alpert, L. I.: Progressive systemic sclerosis terminating as periarteritis nodosa. *Arch Pathol,* 92:31, 1971.

Touraine, A., Golé, L., and Soulignac, R.: La cellulite sclérodermiforme extensive bénigne (scléroedème de Buschke, sclérodermie oedémateuse, sclérème oedémateux du nouveau-né, dermatomyosite). *Ann Dermatol Syphiligr (Paris),* 8:761, 841, 921; 1937.

Townes, A. S.: Topics in clinical medicine. Complement levels in Disease. *Johns Hopkins Med J,* 120:337, 1967.

Treacy, W. L., Baggenstoss, A. H., Slocumb, C. H., and Code, C. F.: Scleroderma of esophagus; a correlation of histologic and physiologic findings. *Ann Intern Med,* 59:351, 1963.

Treacy, W. L., Bunting, W. L., Gamble, E. E., and Code, C. F.: Scleroderma presenting as obstruction of the small bowel. *Mayo Clinic Proc,* 37:607, 1962.

Truelove, S. C., and Whyte, H. M.: Acrosclerosis. *Br Med J,* 2:873; 1951.

Tuffanelli, D. L.: Urinary 5-hydroxyindoleacetic acid excretion in scleroderma. *J Invest Dermatol,* 41:139, 1963.

Tuffanelli, D. L.: Cutaneous hypersensitivity to leukocytes in scleroderma. *J Invest Dermatol,* 42:179, 1964.

Tuffanelli, D. L.: A clinical trial with dimethyl sulfoxide in scleroderma. *Arch Dermatol,* 93:724, 1966.

Tuffanelli, D. L., and Winkelmann, R. K.: Systemic scleroderma: a clinical study of 727 cases. *Arch Dermatol,* 84:359, 1961.

Tuffanelli, D. L., and Winkelmann, R. K.: Scleroderma and its relationship to the *collagenoses:* dermatomyositis, lupus erythematosus, rheumatoid arthritis and Sjögren's syndrome. *Am J Med Sci,* 243:133, 1962a.

Tuffanelli, D. L., and Winkelmann, R. K.: Diffuse systemic scleroderma; a comparison with acrosclerosis. *Ann Intern Med,* 57:198, 1962b.

Uitto, J., Halme, J., Hannuksela, M., Peltokallio, P., and Kivirikko, K. T.: Protocollagen proline hydroylase activity in the skin of normal human subjects and of patients with scleroderma. *Scand J Clin Lab Invest,* 23:241, 1969.

Uitto, J., Hannuksela, M., and Rasmussen, O. G.: Protocollagen proline hydroxylase activity in scleroderma and other connective tissue disorders. *Ann Clin Res,* 2:235, 1970.

Uitto, J., Helin, P., Rasmussen, O. G., and Lorenzen, I.: Skin collagen in patients with scleroderma: biosynthesis and maturation in vitro and the effect of D-penicillamine. *Ann Clin Res,* 2:228, 1970.

Uitto, J., Laitinen, O., Hannuksela, M., and Mustakallio, K. K.: The collagen in dermatomyositis, lupus erythematosus and scleroderma. *Scand J Clin Lab Invest.* 19, Suppl. 95:41, 1967.

Uitto, J., Øhlenschläger, K., and Lorenzen, I. B.: Solubility of skin collagen in normal human subjects and in patients with generalized scleroderma. *Clin Chim Acta,* 31:13, 1971.

Urai, L., Munkácsi, I., and Szinay, G.: New data on the pathology of *true scleroderma kidney. Br Med J,* 1:713, 1961.

Urai, L., Nagy, Z., Szinay, G., and Wiltner, W.: Renal function in scleroderma. *Br Med J,* 2:1264, 1958.

Verel, D.: Telangiectasia in Raynaud's disease. *Lancet,* 2:914, 1956.

Vickers, H. R.: Localized scleroderma and generalized sclerosis (five cases). *Proc Roy Soc Med,* 53:973, 1960.

Vogler, E., and Gollmann, G.: Über angiographisch nachweisbare Gefässveränderungen bei Sklerodermia diffusa. *Fortschr Röntgenstr,* 78:329, 1953.

Wahl, E. F.: Scleroderma; insulin therapy; case report. *J. Med Assoc Ga,* 19:285, 1930.

Walder, B.: Solvents and scleroderma. *Lancet,* 2:436, 1965.

Watson, R. (1754), quoted by Willan, Robert: *On Cutaneous Diseases,* London, J. Johnson, 1808, p.1. Cited by Brown, G. E., O'Leary, P. A., and Adson, A. W., 1930 (*loc. cit.*).

Weaver, A. L., Divertie, M. B., and Titus, J. L.: The lung in scleroderma. *Mayo Clinic Proc,* 42:754, 1967.

Weaver, A. L., Divertie, M. B., and Titus, J. L.: Pulmonary scleroderma. *Dis Chest,* 54:490, 1968.

Weber, H.: *Cor-Bl f schwerz Aertze,* 1878, p. 622. Quoted by Durham, R. A., 1928 (*loc. cit.*).

Weeks, R. E., Bernatz, P. E., and Titus, J. L.: A patient with steatorrhea and Raynaud's phenomenon. *Mayo Clinic Proc,* 40:714, 1965.

Weiss, S., Stead, E. A. Jr., Warren, J. V., and Bailey, O.T.: Scleroderma heart disease; with a consideration of certain other visceral manifestations of scleroderma. *Arch Intern Med,* 71:749, 1943.

Werner, C. W. O.: Uber Katarak in Verbindung mit Sklerodermie. Inaug Diss Kiel (1904).

Westerman, M. P., Martinez, R. C., Medsger, T. A., Totten, R. S., and Rodnan, G. P.: Anemia and scleroderma; frequency, causes and marrow findings. *Arch Intern Med,* 122:90, 1968.

Wessler, E.: Determination of acidic glycosaminoglycans (mucopolysaccharides) in the urine by an ion exchange method. Application to *collagenoses,* gargoylism, the nail-patella syndrome and *Farber's disease. Clin Chim Acta,* 16:235, 1967.

Westphal, C. F. O.: Zwei Fälle von Sklerodermie. *Charité-Annalen (Berlin),* 3:341, 360; 1876. Quoted by Rodnan, G. P., and Benedek, T. G., 1962 (*loc. cit.*).

White, W. D., Treece, T. R., and Juniper, K. Jr.: Pneumatosis in scleroderma of the small bowel. *JAMA,* 212:1068, 1970.

Wilde, A. H., Mankin, H. J., and Rodnan, G. P.: Avascular necrosis of the femoral head in scleroderma. *Arthritis Rheum,* 13:445, 1970.

Wilson, R. J., Rodnan, G. P., and Robin, E. D.: An early pulmonary physiologic abnormality in progressive systemic sclerosis (diffuse scleroderma). *Am J Med,* 36:361, 1964.

Winder, P. R., and Curtis, A. C.: Edathamil in the treatment of scleroderma and calcinosis cutis. *Arch Dermatol,* 82:732, 1960.

Windesheim, J. H., and Parkin, T. W.: Electrocardiograms of ninety patients with acrosclerosis and progressive diffuse sclerosis (scleroderma). *Circulation,* 17:874, 1958.

Winfield, J. M.: A case of scleroderma with symptoms simulating Addison's and Raynaud's diseases: marked improvement from the administration of extract of suprarenal gland. *J. Cutan Dis,* 22:586, 1904.

Winkelmann, R. K.: Treatment of systemic scleroderma. *Mayo Clinic Proc,* 34:55, 1959.

Winkelmann, R. K.: The cutaneous diagnosis of dermatomyositis, lupus erythematosus and scleroderma. *NY St J Med, 63:*3080, 1963.

Winkelmann, R. K.: Classification and pathogenesis of scleroderma. *Mayo Clinic Proc, 46:*83, 1971.

Winkelmann, R. K., Jones, J. D., and Ulrich, J. A.: Urinary amino acid excretion in patients with scleroderma. *Mayo Clinic Proc, 46:*114, 1971.

Winkelmann, R. K., Kierland, R. R., Perry, H. O., and Muller, S. A.: Treatment of scleroderma with sodium dextrothyroxine. *Arch Dermatol, 91:*66, 1965.

Winkelmann, R. K., and McGuckin, W. F.: Bound hexose of the serum in scleroderma. *Acta Derm-venereol (Stockh), 45:*212, 1965.

Winterbauer, R. H.: Multiple telangiectasia, Raynaud's phenomenon, sclerodactyly and subcutaneous calcinosis: a syndrome mimicking hereditary hemorrhagic telangiectasia. *Johns Hopkins Hosp Bull, 114:*361, 1964.

Wren, F., and Govindaraj, M.: Scleroderma heart disease. *Br Med J, 1:*578, 1968.

Wuerthele-Caspe, V., Brodkin, E., and Mermod, C.: Etiology of scleroderma; a preliminary clinical report. *J Med Soc NJ, 44:*256, 1947.

Zackheim, H. S., Farber, E. M., and Aschheim, E.: Effect of low molecular weight dextran on acrocyanosis and scleroderma. *Dermatologica (Basel), 139:*145, 1969.

Zacutus. Quoted by Jadassohn, J.: *Handbuch der Haut- und Geschlechtskrankheiten.* Berlin, Springer, v.8. Quoted by Zion, M. M., Goldberg, B., and Suzman, M. M., 1955 (*loc. cit.*).

Zarafonetis, C. J. D.: Treatment of scleroderma. *Ann Intern Med, 50:*343, 1959.

Zarafonetis, C. J. D.: Treatment of localized forms of scleroderma. *Am J Med Sci, 243:*147, 1962.

Zarafonetis, C. J. D.: Antifibrotic therapy with potaba. *Am J Med Sci, 248:*550, 1964.

Zarafonetis, C. J. D., Lorber, S. H., and Hanson, S. M.: Association of functioning carcinoid syndrome and scleroderma, I; case report. *Am J Med Sci, 236:*1, 1958.

Ziff, M., Kibrick, A., Dresner, E., and Gribetz, H. J.: Excretion of hydroxyproline in patients with rheumatic and non-rheumatic diseases. *J. Clin Invest, 35:*579, 1956.

Zion, M. M., Goldberg, B., and Suzman, M. M.: Corticotrophin and cortisone in the treatment of scleroderma. *Quart J Med, 24:*215, 1955.

Zlotnick, A., and Rodnan, G. P.: Immunoelectrophoresis of serum in progressive systemic sclerosis (diffuse scleroderma). *Proc Soc Exp Biol Med, 107:*112, 1961.

INDEX*

* Only workers publishing before 1950 are included in the index.

247